A

D

CU01090752

"It is overdue, but Cameron's carefully nuanced biography of C. Everett Koop is worth the wait. We are all in his debt."

—GEORGE D. LUNDBERG, MD, former editor in chief at *JAMA* and editor at large at Medscape

"Cameron has written a lively biography of one of my heroes, a man who seized the moment and became a legend in the history of the AIDS epidemic. It captures the complexity of a doctor who followed his conscience throughout his career and emerged on the right side of history. An inspiring read for the public health community and young physicians with leadership aspirations."

—MICHAEL GOTTLIEB, who is known for his 1981 identification of AIDS as a new disease, and for his HIV/AIDS research, activism, and philanthropic efforts associated with treatment

"Cameron's in-depth look at one of the most interesting and complex figures in American public health provides unvarnished context for Koop's critically important leadership at the start of the AIDS epidemic and on other critical public health issues."

—JEFFREY LEVI, former executive director of the National Gay and Lesbian Task Force

"At a time when political and cultural divides seem unbridgeable, we need only look to the recent past to find a model of a principled leader who reached across the chasm to care for our neediest citizens."

—PHILIP YANCEY, author of *What's So Amazing About Grace*

"In this lively and comprehensive biography, Nigel M. de S. Cameron traces the life and work of one of the late twentieth century's most riveting figures. The portrait of C. Everett Koop that emerges in these pages is that of a deeply religious man and principled contrarian whose prodigious accomplishments—as a pediatric surgeon, public health official, prolife and anti-tobacco crusader, advocate for the victims of AIDS, and health reformer—were matched (and likely driven) by his monumental ego. This thoroughly researched and textured account will be the definitive biography for decades to come."

—RANDALL BALMER, author of *Redeemer: The Life of Jimmy Carter*

"It was a privilege to have Dr. Koop as my mentor for over thirty years. I witnessed personally his successes, trials, and tribulations, which are brilliantly illustrated in this outstanding biography. This book will establish his legacy."

—ALLEN I. GOLDBERG, MD, MBA, Master FCCP, and Past-President of the American College of CHEST Physicians

"At the heart of Nigel Cameron's comprehensive biography lies the blow-by-blow account of how 'Dr. Kook,' as some of his critics were calling him, became a hero to me—and to many millions of Americans—and the public health leader of his generation, as he turned his ferocious energies to battling the tobacco companies, championed the needs of handicapped children and victims of domestic abuse, and led the fight-back against AIDS. We've waited a long time for this story to be told, and as Washington gets yet more deeply divided there could be no better time to be reminded of a man who was driven not by politics but by principle and moral courage."

—HENRY WAXMAN, former Member of Congress

"No one did more for American public health than C. Everett Koop. And that came after no one did more for pediatric surgery than C. Everett Koop. Cameron's *Dr. Koop* tells this story with brilliance and luster."

—GREGG EASTERBROOK, author of *Surgeon Koop* and *It's Better Than It Looks*

"Chick Koop was the role model for the modern surgeon general. His positive impact on the public's health was profound by any measure and this biography is an opportunity for us all to better understand the life of such a remarkable individual. *Dr. Koop: The Many Lives of the Surgeon General* is a well-researched biography of the man who redefined the role of our nation's top doc."

—GEORGES C. BENJAMIN, MD, executive director, American Public Health Association

"Cameron's biography of Dr. C. Everett Koop is incisive, entertaining, and a comprehensive tour de force!"

—N. SCOTT ADZICK, MD, Surgeon-in-Chief of the Children's Hospital of Philadelphia

"Had Dr. Koop never been Surgeon General, his development of the field of pediatric surgery still would rank him as a foundational figure of 20th-century American medicine. His tenure as Surgeon General at the dawn of the AIDS pandemic, his work on tobacco control, his nuanced statements on abortion, elevated him to near-mythic status. Cameron's meticulous and balanced biography does justice to the extraordinary life of this complicated man."

—STEVEN BERNSTEIN, director of the C. Everett Koop Institute at Dartmouth

"Cameron masterfully and compassionately delivers on his title. Readers familiar with just one of these intriguing lives—innovative pediatric surgeon, outspoken Surgeon General, Reagan appointee—may be surprised to learn the fuller story of this multifaceted, often maddening (to liberals and conservatives alike), influential personality. For this treatment, we owe Cameron our thanks."

—ERIC M. MESLIN, former executive director, US National Bioethics Advisory Commission

"A must-read for those interested in a nuanced history of the intersection of medicine and the anti-abortion movement. In *Dr. Koop*, Cameron gives us a compelling portrait of the famed Surgeon General and his incredible role in shaping the current American approach to pediatric disability, smoking, and AIDS."

—ALYSSA BURGART, clinical associate professor, anesthesiology and pediatrics, Stanford University

"This is a beautifully written and meticulously documented account that goes behind the many landmark accomplishments of Dr. Koop. It is a study in leadership and greatness that will be appreciated by and inspiring to people from all walks of life."
—JACK HENNINGFIELD, Johns Hopkins School of Medicine

"Thanks to Cameron we have a rich, compelling, and authoritative biography of the most influential Surgeon General in US history. Hailed as a 'rock star,' Chick Koop was surgeon, prophet, and public health educator. American medicine and public health are better off because of C. Everett Koop, MD, and we are the better for having this biography."
—C. BEN MITCHELL, former Director of Biomedical and Life Issues, Southern Baptist Convention's Ethics and Religious Liberty Commission

"Cameron breaks past the reductive caricatures of Koop to give readers a balanced picture of this free thinker and controversial man who revolutionized the field of medicine, the office of the surgeon general, and the evangelical church. Cameron deserves applause for his striking biography of Koop."
—ANTHONY EAMES, author of *A Voice in Their Own Destiny: Reagan, Thatcher, and Public Diplomacy in the Nuclear 1980s*

"Chick Koop was a friend, a fellow surgeon, a mentor, and an icon whose selfless leadership and public persona redefined the role of the United States Surgeon General."
—RICHARD CARMONA, 17th US Surgeon General

"Dr. C. Everett Koop was a compelling, sometimes controversial, nationally influential figure at the nexus of medicine, politics, and evangelicalism before, during, and after his famous work as Surgeon General in the Reagan Administration. This book covers the full scope of Dr. Koop's vast network of personal connections and impressive list of important roles in public and private life. Through interesting anecdotes and intimate encounters with 'America's Doctor,' Cameron's research enables us to take the measure of a man who always seemed much larger than life, with exceptional talents, remarkable accomplishments, and inevitable flaws."
—PHILIP RYKEN, president of Wheaton College, Illinois

Dr. Koop

Dr. Koop

THE MANY LIVES OF
THE SURGEON GENERAL

NIGEL M. DE S. CAMERON

University of Massachusetts Press

Amherst and Boston

ISBN 978-1-62534-853-1 (paper); 854-8 (hardcover)

Designed by Sally Nichols
Set in Minion Pro
Printed and bound by Books International, Inc.

Cover design by adam b. bohannon

Cover photo by John Gilbert Fox, *C. Everett Koop in his office in the Hubert H. Humphrey building in Washington, DC, 1988.* Used with permission.

Library of Congress Cataloging-in-Publication Data

Names: Cameron, Nigel M. de S., author.
Title: Dr. Koop : the many lives of the Surgeon General / Nigel M. de S. Cameron.
Other titles: Many lives of the Surgeon General
Description: Amherst ; Boston : University of Massachusetts Press, [2025] | Includes bibliographical references and index. |
Identifiers: LCCN 2024043187 (print) | LCCN 2024043188 (ebook) | ISBN 9781625348531 (paperback) | ISBN 9781625348548 (hardcover) | ISBN 9781685751289 (ebook) | ISBN 9781685751296 (epub)
Subjects: LCSH: Koop, C. Everett (Charles Everett), 1916-2013. | Koop, C. Everett (Charles Everett), 1916-2013—Family. | Health officers—United States—Biography. | Public health—United States—History—20th century. | Pediatric surgeons—United States—Biography. | United States. Public Health Service. Office of the Surgeon General—Biography.
Classification: LCC R154.K45 C36 2025 (print) | LCC R154.K45 (ebook) | DDC 610/.92 [B—dc23/eng/20250124
LC record available at https://lccn.loc.gov/2024043187
LC ebook record available at https://lccn.loc.gov/2024043188

British Library Cataloguing-in-Publication Data
A catalog record for this book is available from the British Library.

The authorized representative in the EU for product safety and compliance is Mare-Nostrum Group.
Email: gpsr@mare-nostrum.co.uk
Physical address: Mare-Nostrum Group B.V., Mauritskade 21D, 1091 GC Amsterdam, The Netherlands

In loving memory of my parents,
Valerie Evelyn Mure (McKerrell) Cameron,
August 12, 1921, to May 12, 1985,
and Albert John Bailey Cameron,
May 16, 1916, to July 3, 1995.

And of my disabled little brother Bruce,
born and died March 19, 1958.

As he elevated the once-obscure post of Surgeon General, Koop was able to achieve far more than even the most powerful Cabinet secretary.

DAVID KESSLER, Commissioner, Food and Drug Administration, *Proceedings of the National Academy of Sciences*

By his willingness to rise to the moment, to respond from his faith in God and his powerful belief in his calling as a doctor, as his fellow humans called out from their fear and suffering, C. Everett Koop changed the course of history.

JOHN-MANUEL ANDRIOTE, *Atlantic* obituary

And that's the thing that I admire the most about him. It's also the reason that he's not gone into the pantheon of Washington figures. He's not referenced all that much, because people in Washington have no idea what to make of someone whose motivations are moral. What do you mean you're moral, who cares about that?

GREGG EASTERBROOK, author of *Surgeon Koop*, interview

The most utterly consistent public servant I have ever seen.

MICHAEL SPECTER, *New Yorker*

CONTENTS

Part VI
PERSPECTIVE 305

ILLUSTRATIONS

PREFACE

Charles Everett Koop is important for many reasons beyond his astonishing resume, and ripe for presentation to a new generation. Back in the 1940s and 1950s, as he rose to prominence as a pediatric surgeon, we find him fighting racism and what we now call ableism, standing up for Jewish colleagues, boosting women in surgery, and week by week spending long hours with the down-and-outs on Philadelphia's skid row. Appointed Surgeon General by Ronald Reagan, he proved a model of integrity under political pressure—of which Washington is now much lacking, and a byword for honesty in public health. A man of intensely strong moral and religious convictions, with a manner that many found gruff, in his quest for health and life he reached out across traditional divides. After Senator Edward Kennedy refused to vote for him, Koop refused to shake his hand. Congressman Henry Waxman led the opposition to his appointment, calling him "a man of tremendous intolerance." Ted and Henry would soon be friends as well as allies as Koop took on the tobacco companies and led the fight-back against AIDS.

It is remarkable that, more than forty years after he took office, there is still no full-length Koop biography. Potential writers have perhaps been put off by the sheer multiplicity of his endeavors, and the complexity of his convictions. The innovative pediatric surgeon, lauded as the father of the specialty. The deeply religious campaigner for the value of human life, before as well as after birth. The outsider nominee for Surgeon General, who by force of personality turned a backroom job into a steamroller shaping the federal approach to public health. Then came his third career, as he parlayed his fame as "America's family doctor" into a series of initiatives focused on health communication. As the twentieth century drew to a close the octogenarian Koop helmed the world's leading healthcare website.

Before embarking on this project I checked in with Anthony Fauci, who first met Koop as a young MD at NIH, tasked back in 1981 with giving this new government employee a physical. They were soon colleagues fighting AIDS and became close. No, Tony told me; he didn't know of anyone writing about Koop, and he was glad that I was. Next I sought out the counsel of old friends, whose conversations have stayed with me these past four years of research and writing. First off John Wyatt, Emeritus Professor of Neonatal Paediatrics at University College, London; and Mark Noll, formerly Francis A. McAnaney Professor of History at Notre Dame, and leading historian of twentieth-century American religion. From Washington, two more friends encouraged and helped shape my thinking in early conversations—Henry Olsen, political analyst and *Washington Post* columnist and Tevi Troy, former deputy secretary at the Department of Health and Human Services—each of whom happens to have written books about the presidency. Two other writers stand out for their generosity, each the author of a fine Koop essay. Gregg Easterbrook kindly invited me to make use of material from his, which includes some telling interviews, so I have. My friend Philip Yancey went an extra mile by sharing with me his Koop interview files.

Among physicians, spectacular thanks go to Moritz (Mory) Ziegler, one of Koop's final trainees at the Children's Hospital of Philadelphia, who graciously introduced me to a slew of others and has been a generous teacher during my exploration of the history of pediatric surgery. Scott Adzick, Koop's current successor as surgeon-in-chief at the Children's Hospital of Philadelphia, generously shared memories and documents, and invited me to tour the hospital. The current director of Dartmouth's C. Everett Koop Institute, Steven Bernstein, has been enthusiastically supportive and welcoming.

I was so glad early in the project to discover sagacity and fellow-ship in the New York City-based Biographers International Organization. Closer to my current home, the congenial lounge of the Brussels Press Club has hosted many creative sessions when coffee and the buzz of conversation have appealed more than the stillness of my files. My deep gratitude to Matt Becker and the University of Massachusetts Press for stepping up and proving consistently encouraging.

And very special thanks are due to my wife Anna, whose support has been unflagging during four pandemic-stained years.

A Personal Note

Back in 1985, midway through Koop's time as Surgeon General, I was directing a research project in the UK, and somewhat cheekily wrote to the famous man to invite him to come over and deliver a lecture. I was taken aback to get an enthusiastic phone call in reply. I can still hear his voice! "This government owes me vacation time, and there are things I can say more easily overseas." The following year we spent an engaging week together, traveling around the UK to medical schools and conferences. He was tickled that I had been able to arrange a dinner in his honor in the House of Lords. He dined also with our family in Edinburgh, and had fun presenting "Smoke-free Society 2,000" pins with mock formality to eldest daughters Anastasia and Lydia, then little girls of seven and five years of age. "Ladies," he boomed, "You are the only recipients in the UK outside the United States Embassy!" Two decades later, I was privileged to join the celebration of his ninetieth birthday in Washington's Cosmos Club. And to find an excuse, a couple years later, to fly up to Dartmouth and meet for a leisurely lunch in the Hanover Inn. Needless to say, he was sporting a new bow tie.

—*Nigel M. de S. Cameron*, March 2024

Dr. Koop

Introduction

On any accounting, Charles Everett Koop was one of the most interesting and influential Americans of the late twentieth century. A celebrated surgeon, but political novice, he was picked in 1981 to be Surgeon General in the insurgent Reagan administration. It was a shrewd sop to growing anti-abortion sentiment, particularly among evangelical Christians, since the seeming grandeur of the office was belied by its extremely limited functions.

As America progressed through the 1980s, Koop's image underwent a remarkable metamorphosis—from pro-life stooge, excoriated by the press, to the sheer celebrity of a folk hero. By dint of an extraordinary work ethic, a flamboyant media presence, and a series of astute political plays, he had redefined both his job and himself.

Koop was a household name well before all one hundred seven million US households were mailed his briefing on AIDS. There were Koop editorial cartoons by the hundred. There were Koop super-hero dolls. *The Simpsons* scripted him, for all the latest "medical poop."[1] Elizabeth Taylor blew him air kisses on-air.[2] He was the butt of jokes in Johnny Carson monologues.[3] He played himself in *Exorcist III*.[4] And Frank Zappa wrote a song about him.[5] By the late 1980s, chief of staff Admiral Edward D. Martin mused, "He was on everything. He was everywhere. Here was a guy with five people on his staff, who was getting more PR than the Secretary . . . more than the President!"[6]

Right from the start, as Food and Drug Administration Commissioner David Kessler put it, Koop "elevated" the post of Surgeon

General, despite concerted efforts in the Department of Health and Human Services (HHS) hierarchy to keep him in his place.[7] He came into office with what one scholar has termed a "self-dramatizing theatricality."[8] It was allied with a force of personality and deep-seated self-confidence, which brought gravitas to his every move. We shall see how he rapidly turned around his relations with the press by going after the tobacco companies—becoming an instant hero to their critics. And how he became adept at exploiting the anachronisms built into his much-diminished role.

Until the 1960s, the entire Public Health Service (PHS) had reported to the Surgeon General—including the Centers for Disease Control (CDC), the National Institutes of Health (NIH), and the Food and Drug Administration (FDA). Then, suddenly, the office was reduced to an advisory role. Yet the heads of these agencies, and other top players at the Department of Health and Human Services, still bore the honorific "Assistant Surgeon General"—including, bizarrely, the assistant secretary for health, who had inherited the PHS empire, and was the Surgeon General's boss! These officials were still "flag officers," with high ranks in the "Commissioned Corps" of the PHS, over which the Surgeon General, as a vice admiral and its top officer, retained symbolic command. Koop promptly convened regular meetings of flag officers and Assistant Surgeons General in the Stone House that sits at the heart of the NIH campus.

When, a few months after his confirmation, budget cuts elsewhere in HHS added to his portfolio the leadership of the Office of International Health, he grandly established an "Advisory Committee on International Health to the Surgeon General," with the agency heads, all of higher government rank than himself, as members, and with two weeks' notice to its first meeting.[9] In their confessedly "scathing and irreverent" Koop assessment, *Public Health Profiteering*, Washington professors James T. Bennett and Thomas J. DiLorenzo write, if with mild exaggeration, that "Koop treated this brummagem[i] job as a cross between Pope, Secretary of State, and Exalted Ruler of the

---

i Brummagem: "showy, but inferior and worthless"—*Random House Dictionary*.

Universe."[10] The rise and rise of the Surgeon General's office under Koop's flamboyant leadership during the 1980s has few parallels in the history of government.

In the chapters that follow, after first reviewing Koop's family life, his faith, and his career as a pediatric surgeon, we follow the nearly nine years in public office during which he "elevated" his much-diminished post, as he transformed himself from "Dr. Kook" the anti-abortion activist, as he had been portrayed in the press, into a household name across America—and the public health giant of his generation.

Once out of office, Koop was determined to remain, as he put it, the nation's health conscience. There were campaigns and business ventures, a prominent role in the doomed Clinton healthcare reform effort, and a fresh institutional base back at his beloved Dartmouth College from which he sought to project a new vision for the future of medicine. Ever confident and theatrical, Koop had grown into and with the office of Surgeon General. Some would say that, as he became a celebrity, it went to his head. It certainly redoubled his self-assurance, and helped set him up for some unfortunate choices in his later years that damaged his reputation and caused him distress.

Koop's diverse set of commitments rendered him subject to caricature at every turn. Was he the unsophisticated pro-life kook the press suggested? Did he get a serious case of what in Washington is known as "Potomac fever"—an unhealthy taste of power—that undercut his conservative values and led him to go liberal? On retirement, did he exploit his reputation in the crass pursuit of riches? These and other sketches are easy to draw. Like every caricature, they pick out an element of the truth, and then twist it out of proportion so it is true no longer. Koop was an extraordinarily complex individual, as we shall see, as we seek to unravel his history, his character, his motivations, and to make sense of his life.

A Life of Faith

While the Christian religion is still widely practiced within mainstream western culture, especially in the United States, its long decline

—especially among elites—has made it increasingly challenging for nonreligious writers to grasp what it actually means for believers. There is no simpler example than the tendency of so many journalists to write just one thing about Koop's faith: that it was "fundamentalist," which it was not. In his essay *Surgeon Koop*, Gregg Easterbrook suggests that churchgoing among Washington's press corps is likely as common as square-dancing. Serious writers and readers need to take the religion of their subject seriously. Koop was a conservative presbyterian, who spent much of his adult life as a member of the mainstream—that is, theologically diverse—presbyterian denomination. Actual "fundamentalists" lock themselves into like-minded faith communities, while they repudiate culture, the life of the mind, and participation in public affairs. They have also not been known to drink double martinis.

The frequent "fundamentalist" dismissal of his religion has helped fuel fundamental misunderstanding of how he understood the significance of his faith for his work as Surgeon General. It's a complete mistake to think that Koop somehow set it aside. Midway through his second term, he gave a remarkably personal speech on a visit to Scotland, which started out by facing head-on the fact that he had strong convictions. "Well, what happens when a person with strong, controversial, and publicly advertised ideas enters government? Must you deposit your religious beliefs in a blind trust? Should you donate your moral values to charity? Before you move to Washington, should you hide your ethics in an attic trunk? I say, No. . . . None of the above."[11]

A fine assessment of the Surgeon General appeared in an unlikely place—the magazine *Mademoiselle*. "Dr. Koop keeps surprising us—and, apparently, himself." The writer challenges John B. Judis, of *The New Republic*, for writing of Koop's "separation of professional responsibility from personal views of morality." Even Koop himself could sometimes parrot this way of speaking, separating "ideology, religion and other things from my sworn duty as a health officer in this country," so she challenges Koop too! "I think both Judis and Koop are selling the Surgeon General short," says *Mademoiselle*. "It seems to me that Koop, by exercising an agonized compassion for the poor, the wounded and the disenfranchised, has successfully and spectacularly *integrated* his religious and professional life."[12]

The Sanctity of Life

For many readers, Koop's opposition to abortion shapes their assessment of him. Yet as his conduct in office revealed, to the astonishment of friends and foes alike, he proved no cookie-cutter pro-life activist. "I came into the pro-life movement through my work with handicapped children," he later wrote.[13] He feared that acceptance of abortion would lead to the acceptance of infanticide. And after that? The euthanasia of the elderly. "I believe that life issues are like falling dominoes."[14] That was the theme of the documentary movie series that made him a pro-life hero.[15]

On his appointment as Surgeon General he surprised everyone by deciding to step aside from the abortion debate. There was much else to do in public health, he maintained, that would save lives. "I would espouse the cause of the disenfranchised. Mothers and babies, handicapped children, people who needed transplantation of organs and couldn't find them, women and children who were being battered and abused. . . ."[16] Koop's vision was unabashedly "pro-life," both before and after birth. In office, his focus was after. Despite his dramatic campaigns of the 1970s, abortion was not (for him) as it is for some, the kind of overwhelming priority that seems to suck the oxygen out of every other moral question. Reflecting on his time in office, he could write that, "in spite of my feeling that the fetus was an extraordinarily important being, I felt as a public health officer that the number of deaths each year from smoking made it the number one public health problem." And he was cognizant that "abortion had become so politicized that one's stand on the issue could render any other work unproductive."[17] Meanwhile, though he had written and spoken against abortion in vivid terms, he became increasingly disenchanted with the stridency of the attitudes and actions of many pro-lifers. In a striking speech at Wheaton College soon after he stood down, he went further and criticized their focus on "legal and constitutional issues" on what was at heart a moral question.[18] He remained a principled abortion opponent, but his position was all along nuanced, and it plainly evolved.[19]

Writing about Koop

Koop's retirement from the office of Surgeon General was followed by his memoir, *Koop: The Memoirs of America's Family Doctor*, which appeared promptly in 1991.[20] Also published in 1991 was Gregg Easterbrook's elegant essay *Surgeon Koop*; a year later, Anne Bianchi's *C. Everett Koop: The Health of the Nation*, a slim volume in a series for young adults.[21] Nearly a decade after, a fourth volume appeared, Bennett and DiLorenzo's *Public Health Profiteering*.[22] They go after Koop in knockabout language, portraying him as a decent surgeon who turned into a public health nag and then spent years profiteering off his reputation.[23] In addition, two important essays appeared after Koop stepped down. James S. Bowman writes fulsomely of him in a volume on *Exemplary Public Administrators*.[24] "The Embattled Career of Dr. Koop," by Philip Yancey, is anchored in Koop's religious faith.[25] A planned popular biography by two health reporters never got off the ground. They met with Koop in May of 1988 and had hopes of a book in print by the time he left office. His enthusiasm seems muted. Perhaps he was terminally put off by their planned first chapter: "Condom King of America."[26]

There's no question that Koop expected to be written about. He disliked the Easterbrook essay, which he said was too complimentary.[27] In later retirement, as he prepared to pass a substantial quantity of archives to the National Library of Medicine (NLM)—and the public domain—he wrote individual commentaries, some several pages in length, on nearly three hundred separate files he considered especially significant.

There are particular challenges in writing about a near-contemporary. Many of Koop's friends and colleagues are still around, and it has been my privilege to interview more than one hundred of them, some on multiple occasions; some on the record, others on background.[ii] Families tend to be queasy about biographies.[28] I am grateful to several members of the Koop family for gracious responses to my inquiries.

I'm expecting others to write about Koop. There is so much to discover and discuss in his long and extraordinarily productive years. I've presented one picture of his life, distilled from thousands of documents, hundreds of interviews, and nearly three decades of personal acquaintance. I'm hoping to spark interest in others in exploring more of the pioneering pediatric surgeon, the influential religious layman, the public health leader, the new media pioneer, and the visionary for healthcare reform and a fresh approach to medical education.

Like the rest of us, of course, Koop had feet of clay. As a devout evangelical Christian, who believed that "all have sinned and fallen short of the glory of God," he knew that well.[29] Like others who have lived great, public lives and achieved far more than the rest of us, he had the opportunity to reveal his failings on a grander scale, sometimes, embarrassingly, in the eye of the press. At the close of the narrative, we return to his personality and character, and reflect on the life that he lived.

Robert Caro, celebrated for his biographies of Robert Moses and Lyndon Johnson, wrote that he "never had the slightest interest in writing the life of a great man. From the very start I thought of writing biographies as a means of illuminating the times of the men I was writing about and the great forces that molded those times— particularly the force that is political power."[30] Koop's life continually sheds often startling light on his times, as he emerged as a major figure in both medicine and religion from midcentury; in the 1970s played his part in the rise of social conservatism within the GOP, though finally resisting its machinations; and as he was caught up in the dot-com boom and bust of the late 1990s.

His eclectic set of convictions led him to move freely between communities generally seen, not least by themselves, as exclusive of each other. In an age hallmarked by growing social and political conformity and division, Koop plowed his own furrow. That's what

---

ii   See the Acknowledgments appendix.

makes him so interesting as a subject, and as an example: his principled, contrarian inclinations; his bucking of trends; his deep lack of interest in fulfilling the expectations of others; and how that set of characteristics led to remarkable achievement across professions and communities and decades. At the wedding of young friends just two years before his passing he was introduced as someone who had saved millions of lives. Never unduly modest, he muttered with a wry smile: "You're probably right."[31]

A Party in Washington

I remember so many things that this wonderful man did. He became one of the most popular people ever in the history of government. And we all love him to this very day.

—SENATOR ARLEN SPECTER, at the party

September 13, 2006

As Koop's ninetieth birthday approached, a galaxy of medical and political leaders gathered in Washington's elite Cosmos Club to honor the grand old man of public health. The gold braid glittered, as scores of officers of the Commissioned Corps of the PHS, including his successors as Surgeon General, filled the saloons and stairwells.

The genesis of the evening lay in discussions between Koop and two longtime friends in the struggle for tobacco control, Michael Fiore and Jack Henningfield; and in his desire to make what might be a final statement on "the next great task for our century—obtaining health care for all Americans," as *Dartmouth Medicine* reported.[1] His speech, on "Health and Health Care for the 21st Century: For All the People," was published soon after in the *American Journal of Public Health*.[2]

The evening was hosted, in person, by Senators Hillary Clinton (D) and Orrin Hatch (R), with a sponsoring committee that included three former presidents—George H. W. Bush, Jimmy Carter, and Bill Clinton (who sent a video greeting).

Long after the crowds had dispersed, a little group remained with Koop—a reminder of the near-ninety-year-old's "phenomenal energy," as Fiore recalled. "We all sat around having some drinks till probably 1:00 or 2:00 a.m. And it really was a wonderful cap to what I know was an extraordinarily special night for him."[3]

Part I
FAMILY AND FAITH

Emerson wrote, "There is properly no history, only biography."
I agree with him.

—CEK

The year 1947, in which Koop came to newfound religious faith, marked a pivot also in the wider landscape of conservative American Protestantism.

Carl F. H. Henry (1913–2003), the Baptist widely regarded as dean of evangelical theologians at midcentury and after, had penned a seminal book, The Uneasy Conscience of Modern Fundamentalism.[1] *Henry would soon become founding editor of* Christianity Today, *the house journal of the evangelical movement, established under Billy Graham's patronage a decade later.[2] Also founded that year was Fuller Theological Seminary, of which Henry was a faculty member, in Pasadena, California. A later president of Fuller, Richard J. Mouw, writes that Henry and others "would soon come to be known as the leaders of a 'neo-evangelicalism' . . . concerned that those Christians known as 'fundamentalists' or 'evangelicals'—the terms were interchangeable at the time—were ill-equipped to address the crucial issues of the day."[3] Henry critiqued the rigidity and societal withdrawal of the fundamentalist movement, and helped trigger the reconstruction of theological conservatism that has so influenced American soci-ety in the second half of the century, such that* Newsweek *could proclaim 1976 the "year of the evangelical."⁴ Christian Smith, in* American Evangelicalism: Embattled and Thriving, *writes of the leaders of this midcentury movement: "They were self-consciously drawing on their own nineteenth-century evangelical heritage and seeking to resurrect its temperament and vision—which had grown dim in the early twentieth century. These founders of mod-ern evangelicalism believed that what conservative Protestantism had become in their lifetimes was not the best of what it had been or could be but a sad deviation from a more impressive, respect-able tradition. They were determined to turn things around, to get orthodox Protestantism back on the right track."⁵*

One consequence of Koop's early collaboration with his min-ister and friend Donald Grey Barnhouse was early access to the top table of conservative religious leaders across America. He and Henry became friends, and he soon also got to know the young Billy Graham (1918–2018), then emerging as the focal point of an ecumenical evangelicalism that united conservatives in the mainline, theologically mixed, denominations with those in more conservative groups and independent churches.⁶ Thereafter, the labels "evangelical" (the "neo" was quickly dropped) and "funda-mentalist" began to diverge in significance, which is why the ten-dency of journalists and other commentators to refer to Koop as a "religious fundamentalist," as we noted in the Introduction, is so misleading. Henry had called for an outward-looking embrace of the life of the mind, pressing social issues, and public culture, and that vision was made to measure for the young Koop.

It was February of 1936. Winter Carnival was in full swing, a gala weekend of dances and sporting activities. Since Dartmouth was a men's college, "dates" were arriving in large numbers from out of town.[7] Koop's date was a girl he had known from home, but she soon drifted off and he was left on his own. Meanwhile, a Vassar freshman, Elizabeth Flanagan, all of seventeen years of age, was visiting her boyfriend.[i] Dan just happened to be Koop's roommate, and Koop got to spend time with her while Dan was imprudently taking a nap. It was apparently quite a conversation. As he later observed, "it had a prophetic quality."[8] One week later, Koop sent Betty an "anonymous" Valentine.[9]

Some weeks passed, and in May, Koop and a friend were driving back to campus from New York City. Koop suggested they divert to Poughkeepsie, to "find Vassar College, and visit Dan Barker's girl." "Dan Barker's girl" seemed pleased to see Koop, and they took a stroll around the lake. Koop persuaded her to join them on their drive to Dartmouth. It was the weekend of the "spring parties," another Dartmouth tradition. Back then Vassar women needed family approval to visit a men's campus, so she called her grandmother—and the three of them headed north.

On the drive up, Koop made up his mind that "this was the girl for me." Once they arrived, Barker outmaneuvered him and took Betty out to dinner. Koop waited until late in the evening, and—bold as brass—headed over to the Hanover Inn. He walked up to the third floor, knocked on her door, and Betty let him in.

i Apparently, Koop had been asked by Dan to help him to choose between the photos of two potential dates. Koop had recommended Betty. Confidential interview.

They spent the night together in conversation.[ii] More than half a century later, Koop reflected that "In those few hours, a great many things in my life changed." He crept out at 6:00 a.m. in his stocking feet, and that was that. He called his mom, and told her he was engaged. "Chick works with dispatch!" Betty liked to say.

Two years later, on September 19, 1938, they were married—in the Vassar Alumni House, with Betty's religion professor officiating and only close family present. Koop recalled "stepping out of a quiet family wedding into the wind and rainstorm we later found out was the beginning of the infamous hurricane of 1938."[10]

---

ii   Had this come out at the time, Koop later noted, he could have been expelled.

CHAPTER 1

The Koops

Unlike most only sons, I do not feel I have suffered the usual spoiling.
My parents have applied the necessary discipline and censure that did
not permit of my being headstrong.

—CEK, aged seventeen

The Brooklyn Boy

The census of 1920 finds the Koop family at 216 Fourteenth Street; ten years later, at 489 Rugby Road, Kings, Brooklyn. C. Everett is listed as grandson of John A. Koop, the head of a five-person household. His paternal grandparents, who evidently owned the building, lived upstairs.[1] Family tradition set the Koops within the Anabaptists of the Netherlands in the late 1600s, with the first migrants apparently arriving in Brooklyn[i] in 1690.[2] Koop's maternal grandparents, as well as other relatives, lived in the same street. He was the only child of John Everett Koop (1889–1958), and the former Helen Apel (1890–1974).[3]

Koop's grandfathers doted on him. "My life as a kid was fascinating," he recalled. "I learned a lot from both. We used to wander through the cemetery on Sundays, and they would use the tombstones to teach me the history of Brooklyn." His maternal grandfather, Gustave E. Apel (1853–1941), a keen church musician, "took me to Nova Scotia. He took it upon himself to entertain the lighthouse keepers. . . . He'd sing hymns and play his concertina."[4]

While in Nova Scotia, at the age of ten, Koop learned to drive (there were no rules there in the '20s, it seems). His mother was

---

i Until 1674, New York was formally part of the Dutch colony of New Netherland, with the name New Amsterdam, although the British had occupied and renamed it a decade earlier.

determined to learn also, but feared a veto from her husband, so she took lessons in secret (her mother paid). Koop later recalled her as an abysmal driver. He had to keep helping her out of scrapes, like getting stuck on a level crossing with three elderly ladies crammed into the back seat. On another trip, she was about to hit a drunk staggering onto the roadway; Koop pulled on the handbrake and lessened the impact. She managed to convince the Irish traffic cop that her husband would beat her if she got a ticket! When they finally reached their destination, Grandpa Apel, who had been seated in the back, "decided he had all the driving from my mother he could take," and promptly got a train home. His mother never once drove his father.[5]

The young Koop began at public school but soon transferred to the private Flatbush School, where "he managed to avoid being the science nerd" by editing the school paper, being president of student council, and joining the wrestling, football, and baseball teams.[6]

As Koop prepared for the memoir published after he stood down as Surgeon General, his memory was flooded with boyhood reminiscences. Like the time he was ten, considered to be getting fat, and required to eat buttermilk, which he hated. "I'll starve to death first!" he told his mother. He could recall saloons on every street corner before Prohibition arrived in 1920; and shooting thereafter, including a gunfight outside the Koop home. He recalled Grandpa Koop taking him to the circus. This involved getting up at 4:00 a.m. so they could see "the elephants and the horses erect the big top," watching the parade the next morning, and then finally going to the show. A "tremendously exciting 24 hours in the life of a kid."[7] He recalled Grandpa Koop's wake, his corpse propped up in a corner, his pipe in his mouth.

There were various branches of the extended family around Brooklyn. "He was my mother's first cousin," Dale Alekel told me, "and being an only child and living within a block or two had all these other cousins. They spent a great deal of time together. He was like a brother to my mother. They spent weekends and every holiday together all throughout their growing up." Dale was one of four children, and when they were small they were crammed into a one-bedroom apartment. By the early 1960s, Koop was in a position to help, and wrote a check for the downpayment on a three-story brownstone. When Dale was in junior high she was being bullied. Koop encouraged the family to look for a private school; and when they were able to get her a scholarship, he paid for her books. When she was thinking of public colleges in New York, Koop sent Dale a ticket to Chicago and suggested she check out Wheaton. Meanwhile, he was writing to Wheaton's president on her behalf.[8] "Everett is extraordinarily revered in my family," Dale told me.[9]

The Koops spent summers in an isolated house on the north coast of Long Island that could be reached only by boat. Cousins and aunts and friends would come stay in the ample sleeping porches, the fathers joining at the weekend. "Every morning my mother gave her fish order, and depending on what she had asked for I spent a few minutes or the whole morning to satisfy her fish desires. The possibilities were fish, eels to be speared, chowder clams to be dug, little necks to be dug in eight feet of water two miles away by rowboat or finally the longneck steamer clams in the mud."[10]

Koop retained vivid memories of his maternal grandfather's eccentric cousin, who was a physician and an immigrant from Germany. Otto Henry Risch was "very irascible . . . not an easy person to talk to. He flew off the handle. I knew him as a queer-looking man who other kids laughed at." There was a rather good reason to laugh at Uncle Henry. "Summer and winter—you can imagine a man with a flowing mane of hair like Einstein—he wore white linen suits that were never laundered. Every day he rose from his bed, got on his bicycle, pedaled five miles down to Coney Island, parked his bicycle in the sand and kicked off his sandals and walked into the ocean in his white suit. That not only laundered him, but it laundered his suit. And then he got back on his bicycle and rode to my grandmother's house, where she had German coffee cake waiting for him."[11]

This irascible eccentric had played the key part in what Koop later called "a personal experience that I don't remember."

His mother was in labor, and it was long and difficult. After more than ninety hours, her obstetrician said he could do nothing more for her and left the house. In desperation, his father went in search of Uncle Henry. And "he came in and delivered me at 96 hours by applying forceps to a floating head, which . . . is a pretty risky business. I guess one of the first miracles of my life is that I wasn't born a spastic."[12] Later, when he was at medical school, he asked his mother why Uncle Henry was "such a famous doctor in Brooklyn." She explained that he used to treat people with pernicious anemia, "and nobody else knew how to do that." Koop responded that three people just got the Nobel Prize for understanding pernicious anemia, "so if what you say is true, he was way ahead of his time. Do you know what he did?"[13]

His mother replied, "Yes, after he took his bicycle ride to take the bath in the ocean and went to Mama's house to have coffee cake, he then went to the slaughterhouse, where he bought fresh liver, took it home to his own cellar, packed his own sausages and delivered those sausages to patients who came from far and wide and stayed at one of Brooklyn's two hotels, and they got better and went home."[14]

"My father was an amazing person," Koop recalled years later. "If I asked him a question he didn't know, he'd go to the library and find the answer."[15] Shortly after stepping down as Surgeon General, his heart was warmed to receive a letter from an elderly stranger who, back in 1920, at the age of fourteen, had worked as a bank messenger in New York City. He recalled working with a "J. Everett Koop." Why does he remember him so well, seventy years later? "In my 47 years with the Bank I can't recall another man who was as friendly and kind as was Mr. Koop. He endeared himself to all . . . . [Treating all] with the same respect whether president or porter. . . . Would Mr. Koop be your father?"

Koop replied, "Your estimate of my father was correct. He was a kind and gracious man. . . . He was not only my father, but my best friend, and he is sorely missed. Thank you very much for writing."[16]

College

At Dartmouth, friends began calling him Chick. Before then he was Everett, or Ev, and that's how he would stay to his immediate family.[17]

Curiously, both his father and grandfather had been called Chick when they were children, but dropped the nickname in their teens. When fame overtook him, Koop was still happy to be addressed as Chick, even though some of those he worked with—from FDA head David Kessler to his aide Lester Gibbs who looked after him in his final years—found this familiarity uncomfortable, and stuck with Dr. Koop.[18]

The Koop we meet in college is a young man bursting with enthusiasm, and a self-confidence verging on the reckless that more than once came close to killing him, and certainly derailing the career in surgery on which he had set his heart. We see an impetuous energy, a disregard for risk, and also a disdain for the good opinion of others—traits that would help power, and sometimes imperil, his high-octane career across the decades.[19]

The famed "Red" Blaik was coach, and Koop was an outstanding football pick, but his career in college sports was quickly cut short. A nasty tackle knocked him out cold and left him with what proved lasting injuries. As he staggered to the sidelines, he realized he was seeing double. The next morning it was worse. He had to work on the muscles around his eyes to get them to a single focus. The injury had actually been caused by a brain hemorrhage. Special glasses solved the problem. But "even now," he wrote more than forty years later, "when I put my glasses on, I see double for a fleeting two or three seconds, and when I take them off the same thing happens." He mused that his patients' parents might have had less confidence in him had they known he had double vision! The eye specialist he consulted just happened to have a global reputation, which helped convince Koop to take his advice: Give up football. Coach Blaik thought him a wimp and told him so.[20]

Meanwhile, he continued skiing almost every winter day. One time, in his sophomore year, he was helping pack snow on the ramp of the ski jump, when he fell. He slid down the ramp on his back and was mercifully caught by his friends before he shot off into space. The very next day he was planting flags and helping administer a race. It was extraordinarily cold (Koop recalled a temperature of minus

40°F),[ii] so he dug himself into a foxhole. No one came looking for him, and he was soon panicking, as he couldn't get out! He had to extend the hole to thirty feet in length before he could find purchase on the crust and scramble up. "I had come close to frostbite on my hands, once more risking my planned career as a surgeon."[21]

These hazardous experiences were not, however, enough to put him off skiing. On his first competitive ski jump, he landed on his back. Friends took him to the college infirmary on a sled, but his injury was not well managed. It was Koop's first time as an inpatient, and as he lay there for days, depressed and in pain, with little attention from the staff, he learned some inverted lessons in patient care. He later diagnosed himself as having had a "spinal concussion." And more. "A small part of my ski-jumping injury remained hidden at the time, for I had also sustained a very fine fracture of the neck. That would eventually catch up with me in the eighth decade of my life, nearly bringing to a quadriplegic conclusion my tenure as Surgeon General."[22]

He skied less at medical school but continued to take risks. One Christmas, he broke a leg. It was a bad fracture. "The bone had to be refractured and reset as I hobbled around in a series of plaster casts, with crutches, then with a brace, and finally with a cane." It was eighteen months before he could walk normally again. "It took fifty-two years for my new walk to destroy my right knee."[23]

He had opted for Dartmouth in part because of a program that would allow him to cut a year and go on to medical school early. But in the end he decided to make the most of his time at the college, where he could have his own little lab. He discovered a new species of shrimp, and was tempted to stay, pursue the research, and have the shrimp named *Eubranchipus koopii*. He even considered revisiting his plan for medical school altogether.

"I really had never varied from that career goal at any time in my training except for one period of time, when I was in college. . . . I had two wonderful mentors here, both of them biologists, and they

---

ii   Implausible though this may seem, meteorological records support Koop's memory. In 1934 a temperature of −47°F (−44°C) was recorded, which has only recently been matched. See *New York Times*, February 4, 2023.

said, 'You go ahead and be a doctor because when you are one, you can always back up and do what we're doing, but we can never go forward and do what you're going to do.' It was very good advice and didn't take long to tell me, and I got the picture."[24]

Freshman English offered him his first crack at autobiography. "Confronted with the task of writing the story of my short life at the age of seventeen," he wrote, "I realize the difficulty without that mature aspect usually assumed by an autobiographer." He reckoned his parents had made a good job of things, and in particular ensured that he had not become "headstrong." "Unlike most only sons, I do not feel that I have suffered the usual spoiling. My parents have applied the necessary discipline and censure."[25] He has a "passion for healing," and "great aspirations of being not only a medical doctor but one of the greatest surgeons of my time. . . . I would give all I had to be in the position where I might help my fellow man."

He had no great love of Brooklyn. "Never was there a person born and brought up in the large city of New York that dislikes it more than I. The stuffy streets . . . and hustle of millions . . . puts me in a mood of restless longing for the spots of beautiful countryside and bucolic scenery that I have occasionally lived with on vacation in Maine, Nova Scotia, and Long Island." And that really appeals to him about Dartmouth. "Although I came to Dartmouth College for its scholastic offerings, I am going to enjoy in [sic] these most beautiful, natural surroundings."[26]

And next? He is looking forward to medical school, "the place where I might learn the most about preservation of life."

Young Koop ends the essay with a formulaic expression of religious faith, but one that foreshadows the particular emphasis on God's guiding "for our best" that will be central to his convictions fifteen years later when he redefines himself as an evangelical Christian; and thirty-five years later as he wrestles with the loss of his own college-age son. "It shall be necessary then, as before, to place all my cares in the hands of One whose infinite wisdom guides us for our best."[27]

Family Life

Despite Koop's distaste for the "stuffy streets" of the big city, his hunt
for a residency following medical school took him to Philadelphia,
which would remain home for the Koops for the next four decades.

Like many fathers of his generation, he later regretted that he
had not spent more time at home when his children were small. Yet,
even by the standards of the time, the Koop case was extreme. As a
writer in *US News and World Report* reviewed those early days, "At
home, Betty feels like a single parent, as she patiently explains night
after night that 'Daddy's not here because he has to operate on a little boy.' The children will later regret they hadn't known their father
better."[28] It was not simply the demands of the hospital that com-
peted with family time. Several years running, when the children
were small, Koop would leave home every Sunday afternoon and
spend the rest of the day—sometimes until 1:00 a.m.—supervising
students caring for the needy on Philadelphia's skid row. "I made
a serious mistake in judgment in the tension between family needs
and spiritual obligations," he later confessed. "I did not spend as
much time with my family as I did with the homeless."[29] And this
was Sunday afternoon—"really the only time I was likely to be able
to be home uninterrupted." When in later life stresses emerged in his
relationship with the children, he will not have forgotten that he had
often described his own father as his best friend.[30] As daughter-in-
law Anne reflected to me, long-term problems in these relationships
could be traced far back.[31]

Koop treasured memories of summers from his boyhood, and as
the family grew, he and Betty were eager to find a vacation home.[32]
They considered a 200-acre farm near that of his parents, on the
island of Vinal Haven in Maine. But one night they had a scare.
"Norm, then a toddler . . . had a spot of bright red blood on the
seat of his pants," and they could not get off the island to a hospital
because of fog. So they prudently decided on a mainland location.
"The next day we left and after depositing Liz[iii] and the children . . .

---

iii   Elizabeth Koop was known to friends and family as Betty, but her husband called her Liz.

I bought the Moose Mt. farm. So the whole Maritime future was changed overnight in order for us to be near a medical school." He continues: "That one very simple decision changed the lives of many people. Allen, Norman, David, and the women they loved on Mount Washington."[33]

Koop's view was that the key to his family life was the summers they spent together on the farm in New Hampshire. This was a special time, and they certainly had fun. One summer they rented horses. His mother was visiting, and they got her to squeeze one leg into Betty's skinny jodhpurs for a rather ungainly horseback photo. Come Christmas, Koop purloined his parents' address list and sent all their friends a card with mom on the horse on the front. Practical jokes were evidently appreciated in the Koop households.[34]

He later lamented that, given his doctor's lifestyle, "none of my children wanted to go into medicine," though that was not entirely true. David had started out at Dartmouth "with the thought of becoming a doctor, and spent his first two years in the pre-med curriculum."[35] Then he asked his father "if I would be very disappointed" if he switched to geology.[36] He told David he had his support, though the disappointment was palpable. "I suppose I had steeled myself against that being a disappointment because I realized that nobody, none of my children in their right mind, would want to duplicate the kind of a life I spent with my children. And I don't feel guilty about that because . . . when I did have time with them, I tried to make it extremely important time, and . . . as soon as I was able to do it and was making enough money to be able to stop working for a month, I spent four or five weeks with my kids up here in New Hampshire, and I did anything they wanted to do. I think that was kind of the glue that held our family together."[37]

One granddaughter, Jennifer, did become a physician, and another, Christina (Tina), had wanted to, but was put off. Her father—Norman Koop—told her, "if you want to be a wife and a mother, you won't be able to be a doctor. And if you're a doctor, you won't be able to be a wife and mother." She commented, "Like he just didn't see that there could be any kind of balance there."[38]

In conversation many years later with trainee Moritz Ziegler, Koop told a favorite story. Way back in the 1930s, his wife-to-be Betty was counseled by her mother, the wife of a "really old-fashioned family doctor." She said: "Betty, you know Chick will always put his patients first. And if he didn't, you really wouldn't want to marry him." Koop's comment: "Well, I think that was the keystone of my wife's ability to understand what I was trying to do."

When he was around ninety, he shared the wife-to-be tale with a class of medical students at Dartmouth. "When I told them what my future mother-in-law had said to my future wife, they laughed. They thought it was a joke. It was one of the most depressing experiences I've ever had in teaching."[39] That hurt him, and according to one friend persuaded him finally to stop.[40]

Friends of the Koops over many years have shared candid perspectives. One friend and colleague commented, simply, "I think he had an interesting relationship with the children. Not close."[41] Another: "There was a sense that his profession, his honors, and his success, left them in the back seat of their relationship."[42] A third—a distinguished pediatric surgeon—told me simply: "When my son had a little league game, I just put it in my schedule. It was the only way to do it."[43] A fourth took a more sympathetic view. "One of them played little league. . . . He once said, 'My father would never cancel a speech or work around an operation to come to a little league game.' In their minds, his job was more important than they were." Yet, he continued, "He loved his family tremendously. But his job interfered. It just did. And it was just by virtue of being who he was, and what he was doing . . . I don't think he got a fair shake on that by the kids."[44]

Norm looked most like his father, daughter-in-law Anne told me, and had a measure of his strength of personality. As a child he had constantly challenged him. "When Dad was young, when they were younger, he just looked at them and they would run and scoot. But Norm would be like, What did you say? When he said, Don't jump over that line, Norm would say, What line? And it came out in counseling, they all went to counseling, that Dad was harder on Norm than any of the other children because he saw so much of himself in Norm."[45]

It was very much the medical household. In the fifth grade, granddaughter Tina fell and cut herself ice-skating, and Koop stitched her up in the living room. Koop's colleague Louise Schnaufer had a house by the beach in Maryland where they would often spend time in the summer. "This is a really funny thing, because I thought this was normal, growing up this way. The first rainy day at the beach we had mole day. Louise and my grandfather just removed moles from everybody throughout the house all day. And so every year when we'd go back, we'd be like, Okay, first rainy day, it's mole day."[46]

Koop would sometimes take the grandchildren on trips. One time he took Tina and a cousin to California, where he had speeches to make. While he was busy, they toured a movie lot, and he arranged a limo ride, and had them "dress up and go to a fancy cocktail party where we got to experience his life a little bit. I know my grandmother was behind that, having him connect with us as busy as he was."[47]

Tina recalls one Thanksgiving when the family were at her parents' home, and during dinner the telephone rang. She left the room to answer it, and when a woman's voice asked for Dr. Koop, the "sassy teenager" told her they were in the middle of dinner and hung up the phone. "I didn't even say goodbye." Back at the table she told her grandfather it had just been one of his secretaries. Someone called Hillary.[48]

David

In an extraordinary interview during his final year as Surgeon General, Koop shared with *Los Angeles Times* writer Marlene Cimons a haunting memory from his days at the Children's Hospital. It was the spring of 1968. He had just penned a little article that would find a very wide readership in the *Reader's Digest*, with the title "What I Tell the Parents of a Dying Child."[49] Then it dawned on him that "four members of his staff who had become specialists in each of four pediatric problems each 'had a child born to his wife with that very same problem.' He asked himself: 'What am I famous for?' With horror, the answer came: 'Dying children.' A premonition, which he shared with no one, began to gnaw at him. 'I was convinced I was going to lose one of my children,' he says."[50]

Just two months later, on the evening of Sunday April 28, the Koops were sitting at home awaiting their weekly call from son David away at Dartmouth. Instead, they received the call "that all parents instinctively dread."[51] David was dead. An avid rock climber, the twenty-year-old Dartmouth junior was climbing with a friend "when a rock slab broke off as he drove a spike into it."[52] Roped to his friend, Charlie Eriksson, he had fallen a hundred feet. "Eriksson told rescuers that Koop and the rock slab fell together. When Eriksson climbed down to his companion, he found him semi-conscious. He roped the victim to the mountain and went for help."[53] David Koop's last words to his friend were, "I'm sleepy."[54] He was formally pronounced dead by a physician who climbed up to him with a sixteen-strong rescue party. The local news report notes: "The accident happened about two-thirds of the way up the trail at a point called 'Sam's Swan Song,' about 1,000 feet above the floor of Franconia Notch." It was not far from a spot where two young men had died a decade before.[55]

The Koops' daughter-in-law Anne, then the teen girlfriend of son Norman, recalled the terrible night. "I was there," she told me. "The night they got the phone call. Dad [Koop] called me and I went over because I was only fifteen minutes away. . . . And Dad just gathered the family together and said we need to pray. The Lord has taken our son home, taken your brother home, and he got together the family . . . at that time it was only Norm and Betsy, Mom and Dad, and I came over shortly after . . . and they all stayed together in that living room downstairs of the house on 614 Righters Mill Road." Anne recalled especially Betty's grief. "Mom was, to me, the one that showed more grief as time would go on; she would always say, don't ever tell people they need to get over their grief."[56]

Anne had started dating Norm in her midteens.[57] Soon after, in the fall of 1967, her father, under great stress from business, had taken his own life. So in 1968, weeks after David's death, it was Koop who took her to the daddy-daughter banquet her senior year in high school. And who told her just to call him Dad, which she still does. Anne and Norman were married in December of that year.[58]

Koop also called family friends Joe and Joyce Stein, whose son Andy had died under Koop's care six months before. "So he called and he said, Joe, we have something else in common. And I said what do you mean? He said David was killed on Mount Washington this morning."[59] Joe Stein recalled the occasion to me more than half a century later. "Joyce and I rushed to Betty and Chick's home, sharing out of our faith what we were able to." Koop also called David's girlfriend, Lark; in years to come, Anne told me, "we all kept in touch."[60]

Meanwhile, a new minister, twenty-nine-year-old James Montgomery Boice (1938–2000), was in the process of arriving at Tenth Presbyterian Church.[61] He actually moved into town the very next day. Carroll Wynne, on staff with the church, recalls that "News of their son's death happened the first day the Boices arrived . . . as they were unpacking—Jim had trouble finding his suit before going over to be with the family."[62] Boice's widow Linda recalled to me that "We got a call from the secretary. I can't tell you, such memories. It was stunning for the church, for everybody. And it put a whole different light on our first weeks and months at the church. Jim said, I think I should go visit the Koops. And he'd never had to do anything like this before. And Chick was famous even then, you know, he was certainly famous in Philadelphia. . . . And so I made a simple fruit jello. Do you know, Nigel, for years, for years, they would bring up how Jim came out to visit them. And so our lives were woven together in a much deeper way."[63]

The following Sunday, Paul Brand (1914–2003), distinguished physician and longtime friend of the Koops, was scheduled to preach at Tenth Church on medical missions. He later recalled to writer Philip Yancey that as he walked to the pulpit he could see the whole Koop family, seated in the front row, dressed in black. When he met with them afterward, he remembered their "enormous personal discipline," their "stiff upper lip," their "resolve," and he also used the word "repressed."[64]

Three months later, Koop and Betty were aboard the liner *S.S. France*, returning from a trip to the UK. They sat down together to write a little book about David and his death.[65] Once they were home, they sought publishing advice from well-known evangelical writer Frank Gaebelein.[66] But the children were unhappy with the prospect of this very intimate exposure, and publication was postponed for a decade. [67]

In *Sometimes Mountains Move*, the Koops write of "the outworking of a sovereign God's particular plan for a particular family . . . as He[iv] takes them through an experience that both shatters them and blesses them."[68] A decade later, the wound had healed to a scar, but the book is still raw.[69] "Your gentle son, presumed dead, tied to the face of a cliff hundreds of feet above the valley floor, the temperature below freezing, and the only person who could possibly shed any light on the matter lying under sedation in a hospital."[70] They reflect: "We believe that from the beginning of time God's plan called for David to climb . . . to become expert at it; and to die in that particular, awful way—for a number of reasons we think we can see, and probably for an infinite number we'll never have the human vision to understand."[71] Son Norman would reflect, at Koop's own funeral nearly a half-century later, that David's death "took us ten steps deeper" into Christian faith.[72]

Much of this small book is taken up with the detail of the accident and what followed.[73] There is curious comfort in the report of the expert climber who finally recovered the body. "I feel a high measure of respect for the two participants. They had all the equipment necessary for the climb, and every item that could be felt desirable for any conceivable contingency. . . . I went through Koop's pack and was quite impressed." To the Koops he wrote: "While I can give you no effective condolence or sympathy, you have my deepest respect, as did your son."[74] A memorial service in Dartmouth Chapel was followed by one at Tenth in Philadelphia.[75] The church was filled. The Koops received more than one thousand letters and cards of

---

iv   It is less common now, but many evangelical and other Christians used to capitalize pronouns referring to God as a sign of respect.

sympathy, many from the parents of Koop's patients shot through with the terrible irony that he had saved their child but lost his own.[76]

As Easterbrook writes in his essay *Surgeon Koop*, "Koop and his wife . . . tried to accept the news coolly. After all, they had three other healthy children, Allen, Norman, and Elizabeth. But soon the surgeon, who in the course of his work so often had to bear the distress of death at an early age, could not even mention David's name without sobbing. . . . Often Koop would sit grieving, repeating in despair, 'I'm never going to see him again.'" Easterbrook quotes long-term friend and fellow pediatrician at the Children's Hospital, Patrick Pasquariello: "David's death was a turning point in Koop's life. One of the joys of his life was gone forever. . . . After his son's death, religion may have become even more important in the life of this already religious man."[77] Twenty years later Betty Koop would tell *Los Angeles Times* writer Marlene Cimons, "I told my husband it would better enable him to deal with parents. It would give him more insight into their grief and loss. When he would say, 'I know how you feel,' they would believe it." Yet, writes Cimons, "the loss of his son—which he calls the most profound event in his life—drew him into the grief of his young patients' parents, and his professional detachment disintegrated. He says it took him a long time to get it back."[78]

Lost children can haunt their families, and David Charles Everett, the namesake, haunted his. Kenneth Larter, friend and pastor who would spend much time with Koop in his final years, shared with me that "as I thought about our conversations, the family member he spoke to me most about was David."[79]

Another friend shared how distraught Koop remained many years after the death, as he continued to reflect on his son's loss. "We talked for hours one time," said Michael DellaVecchia. "I think, you know, I could see that affecting his relationship with his other sons, because he had this great relationship with David and it just vanished."[80] The *Los Angeles Times* describes the "lovely, almost ethereal black-and-white photograph" that "hangs above Koop's desk in his office in the Department of Health and Human Services and on a living room wall in his home on the campus of the National Institutes of Health."[81]

More than a quarter-century later, Koop bequeathed "the black and white photo of David C. E. Koop on Mt. Adams that hangs over my fireplace in Hanover" to his daughter Betsy.[82]

Betty

Koop's son Allen stressed to me the enormous importance of his mother's role through the years, as quiet confidante and sage adviser to her flamboyant and often impetuous husband.[83] "Mom was the backbone to Dad," recalled daughter-in-law Anne, Norman's widow. Family and friends alike speak of her modesty, simplicity, and kindness. Norman and Anne's daughter Christina (Tina) retains vivid memories of her grandmother. "She was the glue that kept everybody together. She was the easiest person to get along with. I have memories of her playing Little Red Riding Hood with me as far back as preschool. She was the on-the-ground-playing-with-the-grandkids person. And she was happy to be that, but then would support my grandfather and put on her cocktail dress and go to the parties."

Yet, "she was very simple, you know; she had the money to be extravagant, but she was in no way extravagant.[84] She had a very limited wardrobe. She loved not to stand out if she didn't have to. She went for comfort over style. And she was never afraid to laugh at herself. Because we would do things to try to embarrass her and she loved it." She "did what she needed to do to keep the family constantly in contact, reaching out to her kids and grandkids. And I mean, in college, I got lots of handwritten letters from her just supporting, encouraging. She was a great letter writer. But every night she had to watch Peter Jennings and have her cheese and crackers."

The grandkids called her Gommy. "One cousin couldn't pronounce her name and it just stuck."

A Life of Faith

The Koops' lives had been upended by their religious conversion back in 1947.[85] Koop, like most Americans of his day, had been raised to attend church, but—as he later explained—it was without much thought or personal commitment.[86] All that changed when nurse colleague Erna Goulding suggested that he and Betty sample the preaching of the minister at Tenth Presbyterian Church just a few blocks from the hospital. She told Koop she thought he might appreciate his intellectual approach.

The minister's name was Donald Grey Barnhouse (1895–1960), one of the most influential religious leaders of his day. Koop was very much impressed. "Dr. Barnhouse was a great bear of a man," he would later write.[87] "His authoritative voice held my attention, his physical appearance was arresting, and his preaching was teaching of the highest intellectual order. . . . I always marveled at the simplicity of the faith of this very intelligent and learned man."[88]

Around twenty years his senior, Barnhouse, like Koop, was tall, broad-shouldered, witty, and self-assured; "cocky, sometimes brusque, full of boyish enthusiasm."[89] In temperament, with deep wells of energy and drive, and also somewhat in looks, they were much alike. Both stood over six feet tall[v] and had large, powerful, frames, to match their egos.[90] Throughout their professional lives, they traveled relentlessly, and made daunting use of the latest dictation technology to maintain voluminous correspondence ("I am rather compulsive about writing letters," said Koop).[91] Perhaps most curiously, in their later years both would be awarded the high French distinction of the *Légion d'honneur*.[92]

It's plain that alongside being father to a young family, and starting out in his career as a pediatric surgeon, Koop had been exploring matters of religious faith. During a recent summer, while he and Betty and the toddlers were visiting his parents at their summer home, he had done something rather remarkable: he had read through the entire New Testament, twice over. That's the context for Goulding's suggestion that he and Betty might like the preaching at Tenth Church. The following Sunday, he later recalled, "I made my rounds as was my custom at 8:30 and these rounds usually lasted until well after 11:00 and

---

v   Koop was six-one; Barnhouse six-two-and-a-half.

attracted members of the house staff, medical students and some visiting physicians in the community.[93] On this particular Sunday for some reason I finished early and felt impelled to go up the street from the hospital to the corner of 17th and Spruce Streets to the Tenth Presbyterian Church of which Miss Goulding had spoken. I slipped in the back door, went up the stairs in the vestibule into the balcony and sat down in one of the back seats. . . . He was talking about the Scripture he was about to read and was explaining in the tenth chapter of Hebrews, who Melchizdek[vi] was."[94]

Koop's initial response was curious. "I was annoyed by the whole affair." Despite his summer reading of the New Testament, he could not recall this name at all! And he found the notion of Jesus Christ being called a "priest" confusing. He adds: "As a youngster I had lived across the street from a priest," a Father Gresser, "and inasmuch as he played poker every Saturday night and vomited out of the front window when he was drunk, it didn't seem right that the Bible would say that Jesus Christ was a priest. I therefore made up my mind to go back the next week and prove that Dr. Barnhouse was wrong."[95]

"Well, of course, I did not find that he was wrong."

"I began going to the evening service as well as the morning service, and after each of these I would go home to my wife who was not able to accompany me to church because of her pregnancy and her two toddling boys and repeat the whole sermon to her. Naturally, we would look things up in the Bible and she came along in understanding just as fast as I did."[96]

Koop's recollections of his developing religious convictions are not always clear. He remembers a crucial discussion he had with Betty. "I cannot recall the time that my mind changed on this matter, but I think it was in October 1947 when I had gone to Atlantic City to deliver a paper to the American Medical Association meeting. . . . I drove down with my wife and children and we were walking along the boardwalk talking about spiritual things without any flashes of

---

vi   *Sic.* Normally written, today, Melchizedek. The reference is actually to Hebrews, chapter 7 verse 17: "Thou art a priest for ever after the order of Melchisedec." (King James Version.) It is a very obscure passage.

lightening, or other supernatural phenomena."[97] He later confirmed in an interview with *Philadelphia Inquirer* medical writer Donald Drew that it was indeed in 1947 that he and his wife had come to their new faith.[98]

"I do not know whether my wife and I really straightened it out with each other that day, but from about that time on, both she and I recognized that we were indeed Christians and were this by the grace of God and could indeed say that we had been born again."[99]

CHAPTER 2
At Tenth Church

On September 12, 2008, Tenth Presbyterian Church in Philadelphia, Pennsylvania, dedicated the Elizabeth and David Koop Memorial Organ—a four-manual digital Aeolian-Skinner. . . . "To commemorate the life of my recently deceased wife and the life of our own third son, David, who went to his heavenly home in 1968."

—World Reformed Fellowship Blog

To the Koops' consternation, friends and colleagues responded warily to their sudden enthusiasm for religion. "Our old friends thought we had really lost our minds, they stuck with us as long as they could but gradually . . . disappeared and the Lord provided us with a series of new friends."[1] One of those new friends, with whom they quickly struck up a close relationship, was Dutch missionary Cornelius Vanderbreggen. "Cornie came to us at our home and taught us. He taught us while driving . . . . We went off to New York on a simple retreat with him, just Betty and I. . . . After a period of time he began to teach a periodic Bible class in our home and it was my great pleasure to go around and find the parents of my patients and the parents of other physicians' patients who were unoccupied on Thursday nights and take them to our home for Bible studies. After Cornie stopped teaching classes, I began to teach them."[2]

The Koops were forced to confront the social implications of their decision to associate with Tenth Presbyterian Church. Even though it was a relatively open community when compared with the legalistic "fundamentalism" that still defined much midcentury conservative Protestantism, among their "new friends" there were certain expectations. "Some of these things were easy to understand, like drinking and smoking and certainly gambling. But mowing the lawn or reading the newspaper on Sunday did not seem to be prohibited by anything that we saw in Scripture. They were confusing times for us . . . we would probably have to go along with all of these other things. We knew particularly, of them all, drinking an alcoholic beverage was probably that behavior that was most taboo."[3]

Donald Grey Barnhouse

This may help explain the Koops' reluctance to become formal members of the congregation, which did not happen until May of 1952.[4] Koop makes much of the fact that Barnhouse, who would say from the pulpit that he never pressed anyone to join, finally broke his rule. "Dr. Koop, it has been my custom . . . never to ask anyone to join Tenth Church but I am asking you to do that now, because I believe that there are many things that you could do that would be of benefit to our church, and we would like to have you there."[5] He clearly saw Koop's value not simply as a convert but as an ally. He immediately invited him to aid him in an evidently controversial plan to acquire a new organ for the church. He arranged a debate at a congregational meeting, with Koop making the case for purchase; it was approved 148–79. Amusingly, Koop was such a newcomer that the recorded minute of the discussion lists him as "Dr. Coop."[6]

The alcohol issue proved a slow-burning fuse. When they went to social events associated with the university, the Koops would drink ginger ale. "There were joking comments about this . . . and eventually we found that we were talking to ourselves at these affairs." Things came to a head in 1957, when Koop had been in New York City reading a paper at a meeting of the American Medical Association (AMA). "My excuse for being there was the paper but my real reason was because Billy Graham's first crusade was taking place in Madison Square Garden. I went each night I was there." On the Friday, he took the train back to Philadelphia in time for the "annual surgical banquet given by Dr. Ravdin." Arriving midway through the cocktail hour, he tried to slip into the ballroom unobserved. But Ravdin,

the mentor and boss with whom he had a complex and sometimes
fractious relationship, had seen him slip in, and decided to put him
on the spot. Ravdin raised his hand for silence, and announced to
the room: "There comes this member of my staff who was in New
York ostensibly to attend the AMA meetings but instead was attending the Billy Graham meetings each night. Not only that, but he was
sitting in a box near the podium while my wife was sitting in the
balcony as far away as one could get." He turned to Koop: "What will
you have to drink, Chick?"

"I said, 'Bourbon on the rocks.'"[7]

Shortly after Koop's conversion, "I had a young lady referred to
me with what was obviously acute appendicitis.[8] Her mother was
distressed that the child's father could not be here to help make
the decision about the need for an operation. As I was going to the
operating room with the child, a telegram was received for her and
given to me. . . . The telegram was simple. It said, 'I will be thinking about and praying for you. Do not forget that underneath are
the everlasting arms,' and it was signed Daddy." Daddy was Francis
Schaeffer.[9] This chance meeting sparked a friendship with one of the
formative figures of twentieth century American religion that would
last until Schaeffer's death from cancer in 1984.[10] Characteristically,
Koop immediately engaged with the Schaeffers and their ministry.
He later recalled that he was "privileged to be part of their decision
to leave the country and go to Champerey, Switzerland, and later in
their decision to go from Champerey to Huemoz which became the
home of the now world famous L'Abri Fellowship."[11]

The Koop family, parents and children alike, became deeply
involved in the congregational life of Tenth Church over more than
three decades. Koop later encouraged his parents to join in Barnhouse's weekly meetings in New York City, and in due course both
they, and Betty's widowed mother, joined them in their newfound
evangelical faith.[12]

Early on, Koop was generous, establishing his own foundation,
Light of Life, with friends as trustees, as a vehicle for his own charitable giving—mainly to medical missions—although others would

contribute.[13] His main focus, over many years, was the Tarascan Indian tribe in Mexico, where he established several small clinics.

Thomas Getman remembers the family well. Back in the 1960s, when the Koop kids were in their teens and early twenties, he was a minister in Philadelphia working with Young Life, a faith-based outreach to high schoolers. Years later Getman met Koop again, this time as a staffer on Capitol Hill. Getman spoke to me about the Koops he got to know, "the kind of modesty the family practiced, then how they were concerned for others." What he found most impressive, he told me, was that "Chick was a stage-setter." What he did "spawned lots of other things."

"I got to meet all the kids. And I remember David especially. . . . And [after his death] watching how that family coped had a huge impact on me. Because even when they were still grieving, they invited me into their home to encourage me in the work I was doing. And so to have somebody like young Betsy, who was a minister in her own right. I mean, she really cared for people." Getman told me he "can still picture the house I would walk into. And I distinctly remember sitting at their dinner table, and having them not share so much their concerns and griefs, but share their love for other people."[14]

Koop first saw Barnhouse in his pulpit, but Barnhouse was much more than a parish minister. After stateside military service in the latter stages of the First World War, he had volunteered as a missionary in Belgium and France between 1919 and 1925. After serving another church in Philadelphia, he was called to Tenth in 1927. In 1931 he founded *Revelation*, a religious magazine that would be widely read across American evangelical churches.[15] Meanwhile, he was developing a nationwide speaking ministry, for which from 1940 the church formally released him for six months of each year.[16] Perhaps most significantly, he was America's pioneer radio preacher. As early as 1928, he became the first religious leader to purchase time from a radio network—a $40,000 contract with the Columbia Broadcasting System (CBS) to broadcast his Sunday evening "vesper" services across the nation.[17] In tandem with his broadcasts, his extensive speaking ministry led one historian to judge that, before the advent of evangelist Billy Graham, Barnhouse "spoke personally to more individuals than any other Protestant religious leader of his generation."[18]

Barnhouse was an extraordinarily active man. "In 1955 he remarked that for three decades he had preached an average of six nights a week, often seven, a total of approximately 12,000 sermons."[19] He was a man of strong and decisive opinions, on everything from Roman Catholics (he opposed Kennedy's election as he feared that Canon Law would determine his policies) to Joseph McCarthy (he opposed him too). Through the course of many controversies, he managed to fall out both with his colleagues within the wider presbyterian church, and also with more theologically conservative critics, who could not understand how he could stay within a mainstream denomination that included many with liberal theological views. In a fine biographical essay, C. Allyn Russell sums him up like this: "Disliked by both liberals and some fundamentalists, the response of the relatively 'lonely' Barnhouse was his own multifaceted ministry—his one-man Bible conferences, his radio broadcasts, and the national and international work engendered and conducted by his own Evangelical Foundation. Theological intransigency, ceaseless activity, and the endeavor to correct others where they were wrong, constituted familiar trademarks of Donald Grey Barnhouse."[20]

His first wife Ruth had died of cancer in 1944. For some years thereafter, the younger Barnhouse children were homeschooled by their maternal grandmother. "Each morning they would put on their coats, bid goodbye to their grandmother, walk around the block and come back to the house, greeting her as 'Mrs. Tiffany' and starting the day's work. They were not allowed to play with other children."[21] The Barnhouse household was unusual in other ways. They would often speak French at home.[22]

Decades later, when Koop was Surgeon General, Barnhouse's younger daughter Dorothy wrote to him out of the blue. "We met only briefly back in the '50s," she begins, "but I remember how often and how warmly my father . . . spoke of you. When I see you on television or read about you, my heart warms and tells me, 'yes—that is a man my father would have valued as a friend!' Thank you for your work."[23]

This is the man whom Koop deeply admired, and who had an enormous influence on his new life as an evangelical Christian. As he was stepping down as Surgeon General, four decades later, Koop reflected on his time with "Barney." "To work with him for all those years was phenomenal."[24]

The Evangelical Foundation

Barnhouse and Koop bonded immediately, and from 1952 Koop served on and later led Barnhouse's "Evangelical Foundation," the nonprofit that hosted his various projects outside of Tenth Church itself.[25] The foundation was a substantial effort, and must have drawn significantly on Koop's energies as he freed up Barnhouse for his itinerant ministry. Established in 1949, at one point it employed no fewer than fifty-three staff.[26]

In addition to his role in the foundation, Koop was appointed in 1953 to serve on the "session," the church's leadership group, as an elder,[i] and soon to chair key committees. He rapidly became the most influential member of the congregation, where he and his family worshipped until he moved to Washington, DC in 1981. Because of Barnhouse's unusual relationship with the church, this frequently led to tension between them, as Koop felt himself duty-bound to represent the interests of the congregation, and Barnhouse increasingly saw his role at Tenth Church as simply one among his various efforts.[27] On February 8, 1956, a year that saw several clashes, Koop wrote to a physician friend who had treated Barnhouse in the University Hospital that, "This man is one of the most remarkable I have ever known." To which he added: "To know him as I do is to love him although at times I do not necessarily like what he does."[28]

---

i   In presbyterian churches members of the committee of leaders, often called the "session," are ordained in much the same fashion as are ministers. In most other Christian traditions Koop would be referred to as one of the leading "laymen" in the church—indeed, he was a leading "lay" figure in American evangelical religion—but that handy term is not strictly available in the presbyterian context.

After a lengthy struggle with diabetes—he was not an especially compliant patient—Barnhouse would die at sixty-five of a brain tumor. His death placed an immediate and heavy burden on Koop's shoulders, as the foundation with its various works depended crucially on the profile and contacts of its founder. Its survival owed much to the energy Koop brought to the task, as the new de facto leader of the ministry.

Immediately after Barnhouse was hospitalized, Koop had laid out the problem to his fellow directors. "Certain things are as obvious to you as I believe they are to me." Every facet of the ministry has been built around Barnhouse's "voice and personality." Of the various foundation projects, "the most likely to survive is the magazine." Somewhat eerily, he asked his colleagues to reflect on these matters as they prepare for their next meeting, scheduled for November 5. That would be the day Barnhouse died.

Shortly before the Koops left Philadelphia for Washington in 1981, Tenth Church, under the leadership of minister James Montgomery Boice, embarked on a lengthy process of departure from the mainstream United Presbyterian Church in the USA (UPCUSA). As a result of long-standing theological disagreements, the congregation had decided to associate with a more conservative denomination. Koop, who had been active in the church's leadership for three decades, opposed the move, and together with a handful of others stopped attending the church in protest. As Boice's widow Linda explained to me, the key congregational vote was taken on March 9, 1980, at a time when Koop had been away for long periods making and promoting the *Whatever Happened to the Human Race?* movies. "Chick hadn't been around for all the agonizing and all the discussion of should we leave the denomination and, you know, all the reasoning that led up to what was really big. So when the vote came, Chick and Betty voted No. And one or two older people, otherwise the vote was overwhelmingly to leave the denomination."[29] This was a very difficult decision for the church, as they risked losing their property—both the church building and the minister's home.

When Koop's opposition became public, Boice found himself having to respond to this criticism in the media.[30]

At the time, Koop was angry, indeed bitter. As he shared with Francis Schaeffer in a lengthy letter, he had been close to Boice, having "served as his confidante," but felt that Boice had over a period of years maneuvered him out of the position of influence he had long held in the church. "I was about the only member of the congregation who would stand up to Jim and disagree in such matters."[31]

Yet, as Linda Boice explained, the disagreement "wasn't totally destructive of the relationships." After a couple of years others had returned, "and it was in the past and then the Koops were there."[32] When, in June of 1990, Boice died of liver cancer at the age of 61, Koop flew to Philadelphia for the family memorial service. At the graveside he sat beside Linda and held her hand.[33]

Nearly two decades later, on September 2, 2008, a widowed Koop would dedicate a new organ for Tenth Church to the memory of his lost wife and son. He cannot have forgotten the role he had been called upon to play in securing another organ for the church, way back in 1952.

The dedication of the four-manual Aeolian-Skinner proved important for quite another reason. Koop first cast his eye on Tenth staff member Cora Hogue, and decided he would like her to be his second wife.[34]

Part II
SURGEON

I have great aspirations of being not only a medical doctor but one of the greatest surgeons of my time.

—CEK, aged seventeen

The medical landscape in which Koop trained was vastly different from our own. In the Brooklyn of the 1920s, surgery was often done at home, and the mother of the family might be called on to deliver the anesthetic. "People who had their tonsils out had them done in the kitchen or the bathroom at home. . . . The custom was to just grab somebody in the family and tell them how to pour the ether over an ether cone, and that was the most risky part of having surgery in those days, for kids, was having it done in your home with somebody who knew nothing about anesthesia at all."[1] Koop recalls the time he had his own tonsils out. His father was actually criticized for his extravagant decision to insist on hiring a professional "anesthetist."[2]

Sir Alexander Fleming had discovered penicillin in 1928, but it would be much more than a decade before antibiotics were in general use to treat infection. Koop later reminisced that in the early 1940s "at one point the entire supply of penicillin for the city of Philadelphia was in the small refrigerator in my lab."[3]

The story of Koop's career in pediatric surgery is substantially the story of the profession in the United States. His decision to focus full-time on children—his boss I.S. Ravdin's idea—set him apart as one of merely half-a-dozen full-time American pediatric surgeons. His six-month stint in the one acknowledged center of excellence, Boston, exposed him not only to the expertise and wisdom of the top practitioners in the country, William E. Ladd and Robert Gross, but enabled him to build solid relationships with these two brilliant but

prickly men as he took on the burden of leading the younger gener-
ation into the professionalization of the specialty. It is very striking
that, as late as 1954, of the forty-five children's hospitals in the United
States, only eight "had surgical services headed up by full-time pedi-
atric surgeons."[4]

"I can't remember a time when I didn't want to be a doctor," he told
his trainee, Moritz Ziegler, looking back from his ninetieth year.[5]
"Shortly after I knew I wanted to be a doctor, I also knew I wanted
to be a surgeon."[6]

While his eventual move into pediatric surgery came as a surprise,
many years later he recalled a childhood experience that eerily fore-
shadowed his future. His maternal grandfather would take him to
Coney Island, where he recalled "an unusual sideshow—a display of
premature infants in incubators, attended by nurses from the New
York Foundling Hospital." The memory haunted him. "Every time I
would go and work on a baby, in the beginning, I'd have these reminiscences of Coney Island, where I first saw them."[7]

His eccentric Uncle Henry was not his sole physician role model.
"Other physicians were very impressive to me as a child. I loved the
awe in which my family held physicians. Most of my experience with
doctors was in house calls when I was a child, either for me or other
members of the family, and I remember the hush that used to fall
over the house when Dr. Justice Gage Wright, our homeopathic physician, used to make his entry."

In a *New York Times* interview many years later he told "a startling story about himself as a high school student, borrowing a white
coat and sneaking into the Columbia-Presbyterian Medical Center
every Saturday morning to sit in the amphitheater and watch surgery being performed from eight in the morning until two in the
afternoon."[8] Koop had got to know a student at Columbia's medical school who showed him how to slip in "as though I belonged
there."[9] Since he was already six feet tall, there was never a problem.
"Nobody else would be there on Saturdays, so the surgeons, all being

showmen, would look up and see me there and describe everything they were doing. No one ever stopped me! I learned an awful lot."[10]

And he would come home itching to imitate what he had just been watching—"as night followed day." So "My grandfather built me a little operating table, and my mother . . . was my anesthesiologist."[11]

On his retirement from the Children's Hospital, his friend and one-time boss, former university provost Jonathan Rhoads, shared the story. "I had thought that we had taught him surgery at the U of Penn Hospital, but it turns out that he began operating while he was in high school. He had a habit that some of you may not approve of—catching neighborhood cats—and being an only child he prevailed on his mother Helen Koop, whom I came to know rather well later, to pour chloroform while he operated on them. Beyond that he would place an isinglass window in the abdominal wall, so that he could subsequently observe what went on inside. After the experiment, the cat was reanesthetized, the isinglass window removed, the wound closed, and in due time the cat returned to its environment in excellent shape."[12]

Meanwhile, determined to improve his manual dexterity, he was practicing tying knots one-handed.[13]

CHAPTER 3

The Making of a Surgeon

I saw a movie about a surgeon. When I saw what he could do—
remaking lives—I never wavered from it.
　　　　　　　　　　　　—CEK, *Los Angeles Times Magazine*

Koop entered Dartmouth College at the age of sixteen. Summers
were spent at the family vacation home on Long Island, and he
volunteered at the St. Charles Hospital for Crippled Children, where
his responsibilities consisted mainly of changing dressings. Surgeon-
in-chief, Frank S. Childs, would sometimes invite him to assist in
the operating room. One morning he had a surprise. Embarrassed
to have turned up late, Koop saw Childs standing at the side of the
table awaiting his arrival. He was about to amputate the gangrenous
leg of a diabetic man. "I saw that he was on the wrong side of the
table, and I thought he was going to take off the wrong leg, and so I
said, 'You're on the wrong side of the table. It's that leg.' And he said,
'Koopie, you've seen me do this a number of times, and . . . I think if
I help you, you could take this leg off.' So I did my first amputation
when I was in college."[1]

The medical student friend who had helped him slip into Columbia to watch surgery had also invited him to dances on campus and
generally helped convince him that Columbia was the only place he
wanted to go. "I felt that I was really slated to be a medical student at
Columbia." Though he did also apply to Cornell, which turned out
to be fortunate.

He was in "fine fettle" when the day came for his interview at Columbia. "I sat around a table of white-coated individuals. I got to know

some of them when I was myself a surgeon later on and they were middle-aged surgeons by that time, and I can tell you that a couple of real stuffed shirts were sitting around that table, making decisions for Columbia." Young Koop did not impress them either.

The following week he was accepted by Cornell.[2]

His rejection by Columbia left him smarting, and he was still smarting decades later when the school invited him to make a speech, and get an award—"$25,000, which in those days was a real bunch of money!" He told them he hoped they "felt a certain sense of guilt for not having let me go to Columbia because if they had, I might have been able to make something of myself. . . . Took my money and left."[3]

When after one term at Cornell he broke his leg skiing, he was impressed by the school's response. "The dean called the class in, told them about my situation, how hard it was to go through the first year of medical school with a broken tibia, and he asked the class to make its own plans but to see that I was kept up-to-date, and those students took a subway over to Brooklyn, which took an hour, and kept me up-to-date until I was able to get back. I never was able to take care of myself because I had a non-union,[i] and my father drove me to work every morning from home in Brooklyn, and they got me through."[4] He would later fondly recall those drives and how they helped him get to know his father better.

He remarked acidly, "I'm sure that they would have thought anybody stupid enough to break his leg didn't belong at Columbia either."[5]

The Hospital of the University of Pennsylvania

As his final year began at Cornell, Koop was searching for an internship—a two-year commitment that would offer a bridge to a residency. The search was not going well.

"I was turned down for the first two internships that I applied for, one at The Brooklyn Hospital in Brooklyn and one at Methodist Episcopal

---

i   A fracture that fails to heal normally.

Hospital in Brooklyn, which I chose not because I lived in Brooklyn but because . . . both of those were considered to be really highly ranked, and both of them asked me the same question. They said, 'Do you think you can do this job married as well as unmarried?' And I said, 'Yes, I do. I think I've already proven that in medical school.'"[6]

But they thought otherwise.

In tandem, he was looking ahead to the residency, and—taking the advice of Cornell faculty—sought out the surgeon he most wished to work with. The search led him to the celebrated I.S. Ravdin at the University of Pennsylvania.[7] Ravdin had him interviewed by a colleague, John Lockwood, and Lockwood turned him down, telling him, "You had best go home to New York because there was no place in Philadelphia for you," as Ravdin later recalled.[8] But Ravdin decided to see him after all. Koop sheepishly admits that he removed his wedding ring, "so that we wouldn't start any conversation based on that," which suggests how the Lockwood conversation had begun.[9]

The Ravdin interview went better, until the famous surgeon spelled out what success actually entailed.

"When could I begin?" Koop asked. "And that was the shocker," because "he said, 'I'm pretty well loaded, but, if you want to come, you'll have to finish your two-year rotating internship. . . . I think you'll probably have four years in the dog lab, and then you can have the job.'"[10] There were actually three concurrent jobs—as Ravdin's surgical resident, as an instructor in surgery, and as a Harrison fellow in surgical research. "So it would be the seventh year after we were talking that I could look forward to working as a surgeon."[11]

Once the interview was over, Ravdin dictated a note to his colleague Jonathan Rhoads, whom he had recently persuaded to rejoin him at the university out of private practice, with a view to running the department in the event of war—"I'm sure, at great financial sacrifice."[12]

Dear Dusty,

I was greatly impressed with young Koop, and have given him all the advice that I could. If he wants to try for a fellowship with me, he will have to qualify by obtaining an internship in a rotating hospital. This is mandatory in the State in order to obtain a license before he becomes a Fellow.

The Pennsylvania Hospital is an excellent place but the appointments are all made by the Board of Managers. I hope you will write to Dr. Francis C. Grant and ask him to speak to Mr. Sydney Clark about young Koop. Dr. John Gibbon is giving him the names of some other Managers whom Koop's father can get letters to.

Rav.[13]

Plainly, a campaign was required to get such appointments through the Board of Managers! It's unclear how Koop's father could help, though he revered his father and had presumably offered his assistance.

Ravdin suggested an internship at one of the Philadelphia hospitals, where Rhoads could "keep an eye" on him. "And so I applied to Philadelphia General Hospital, the big-city hospital, as well as the Pennsylvania Hospital, which was the country's first and oldest. I was accepted at Philadelphia General, and they wanted an answer right away. I was not accepted yet at Pennsylvania, and I couldn't get Pennsylvania to speed up their decision, and I couldn't get the other hospital to slow down theirs, and so I accepted the job at Philadelphia General, only to find out a couple of days later that I was appointed at Pennsylvania, so I wiggled out of that and did go to Pennsylvania, where Jonathan Rhoads was on the staff and where he did keep an eye on me. . . . Meanwhile, the war was getting pretty tough between Germany and the United Kingdom, and my two-year rotating internship was shortened to one year."[14]

Koop's wartime years at the Hospital of the University of Pennsylvania (HUP) were to prove extraordinarily important. Not only did he distinguish himself as a young surgeon, and work on research for the ScD degree (Doctor of Science in Medicine), but he met several people who would be important to him for the next half-century.[15] Jonathan Rhoads, whom Ravdin left in charge as he went off to war, became his boss and soon longtime friend. Erna Goulding, the nurse whom he quickly recruited to the Children's Hospital, was soon a close family friend. Margo Deming would be assigned to work alongside him, serving as the Children's Hospital's first director of anesthesiology and his close partner in pioneering surgeries.

It was also during his years at HUP that Koop built on the heavy work routine he had developed in medical school which helped shape his extraordinary productivity. Back in 1939 he had concluded that the severe migraines he was getting on Sundays were the result of his kicking back and taking the day off. "His solution: Don't relax. 'Tell me I've got a lot to do today,' he instructs his wife as the weekend approaches. Now, Koop works seven days a week."[16]

Meanwhile, he sympathized with the two residents for whom he was responsible, Doris Bender and Ralph Pipes, telling them: "If during the year you find there are times when you are getting too much to do . . . or when you have gripes . . . I wish you would please talk them over frankly with me rather than be unhappy in your work or harbor a grudge about the service." He adds, to Bender, "Please remember that this job is a horrible grind and that you have to rest when the opportunity presents itself."[17]

As the *Washington Post* drily noted in its obituary seven decades later, "Although he was married, and by 1944 a father as well, he spent nearly all his time at the hospital. He estimated that he did as many operations in four years as residents do in 'seven or eight years—there was nobody around to do the surgery.'"[18]

The Children's Hospital

It was December 8, 1941, the day after Pearl Harbor. Koop's wife Betty was working as a secretary in the HUP social service department. She stopped by the snack bar called the Corner Cupboard and overheard a conversation at the next table. It worried her, and once she had called her husband it worried him too.

Koop was actually also in the hospital, but as a patient. He was so alarmed by what Betty had to say that he snuck out of bed, located his clothes, and spent several hours that evening squatting in a parking lot on the running board of a Packard. In the hope of catching the man on whom his future depended.

I.S. Ravdin had also been in the Corner Cupboard, by chance at the next table to Betty Koop's. He had been sharing his plans with his colleague John Lockwood. That night he would fly to Pearl Harbor to help treat the wounded.

So Koop was suddenly anxious to confirm the details of the rather complex career plan that Ravdin had laid out, as Ravdin, and America, went off to war. After absconding from his hospital bed he took the trolley across to West Philadelphia and asked Ravdin's secretary for an urgent appointment. "'I have got to see Dr. Ravdin today.' And she said, 'Dr. Koop, everybody has to see Dr. Ravdin today. . . . Dr. Ravdin can't see anybody today.'" He chanced a further request: "Could you tell me what kind of car Dr. Ravdin drives?" She didn't just tell him that her boss drove a Packard; she told him where he parked it. Looking back, Koop says that he sensed the "hand of God" at work in this sympathetic secretary. He located the Packard, sat down on the running board, and waited. It was early evening and getting dark before Ravdin turned up. "Can you give me a ride downtown?" Koop asked.

Once in the car he was characteristically blunt. "Dr. Ravdin, I know you're going to Pearl Harbor tonight, and I think we ought to settle my future before you go." As Koop tells the story, Ravdin was taken aback that Koop knew his plans; either he had supernatural knowledge or was very well-connected! After a minute or two of silence, Ravdin replied: "Don't sign any papers. I will declare you essential to the University of Pennsylvania for the duration of the war, and you come out here on the 1st of July and assume those jobs I've promised you." "So he cut six years off my training right there, and the rest is history."[19]

Just a month later, Ravdin was back from Hawaii and following up with the paperwork, writing to him on January 15, 1942, to confirm the new arrangements, with the salutation, "My dear Dr. Koop."[20]

By chance, at the next critical juncture in his career, Koop was once again in the hospital as a patient. Four years had passed, and at war's end Ravdin had returned from running a large military hospital in India. "Dr. Ravdin came back . . . and that is when this unusual series of appointments came of surgeons to populate certain specialties."[21]

As the *Washington Post* later reflected, Koop "was among the last survivors of a small generation of American doctors forced by World War II into highly responsible roles at very young ages."[22]

Ravdin quickly made Koop his chief of staff, responsible for the training of all the surgical residents. But the future was unclear. Many surgeons were returning to civilian life, and they were looking for jobs. Koop went back to Dartmouth for a weekend to think things over, and was informally offered a position at Cornell Memorial Hospital, as surgical liaison with what would later become Sloan-Kettering. "So I was somewhat in a quandary on the sleeper back to Philadelphia." He was also sick.

"When I got off the train, I had a pretty high fever, and my colleagues diagnosed a strep throat, put me in bed and started me on an IV, and the next morning about five o'clock I.S. Ravdin came bursting into my room, in the uniform of a brigadier general, and he said 'Koop, what do you expect to do with your life?'"[23]

His surprised response was that he'd like to run the tumor clinic.[24] But Ravdin had another idea, which had actually originated with Rhoads.[25] "How would you like to be the surgeon-in-chief[ii] of the Children's Hospital instead?" Ravdin added: "There are some caveats you should be aware of. First, you give up adult surgery completely. Secondly, you go down to the Children's Hospital of Philadelphia in January. When you've gotten to know them and they've gotten to like you, you go to Boston for a year, where we've arranged for you to work with Dr. William E. Ladd, and then you come back and you make the best possible academic service for pediatric surgery that you can." As Rhoads later recalled, "It was therefore agreed that Koop would go to run the service with the assistance of one resident and the backup of five senior surgeons, all of whom had had some experience in pediatric surgery and had worked at Children's Hospital."[26] At that time, Koop had never operated on a newborn.[27]

Koop continues: "And so I did come down to the Children's Hospital, where I was not the least bit welcome. I arrived on the 4th of

---

ii   The titles surgeon-in-chief and chief of surgery (variously capitalized and hyphenated) tend to be used interchangeably. The Children's Hospital has a surgeon-in-chief.

January 1946, and I was met by the chief medical resident, who said 'Why don't you go back where you came from? You're not wanted here, you're not needed here, and you put four good men out of a job.'"[28]

In fact, these "four good men," general surgeons in the city with a part-time association with the Children's Hospital, had each in turn been offered the self-same job by Ravdin and had declined it, though it's hard to imagine that Ravdin made these offers in good faith; it looks like a political move to ease a difficult situation. No general surgeon with an established practice was likely to agree to forswear all but pediatric patients, and take a year off from his practice to go to Boston!

On the same January day that Koop received his warm welcome from the chief medical resident, he sought out the formidable Dr. Joseph Stokes, chair of the university's department of pediatrics and head of the medical staff at the Children's Hospital. Stokes gave him a tour of the building and explained that "all patients in the hospital were his, that when he thought they needed an operation, he would let me know, and when the patient was returned to him for postoperative care, my position would be that of an observer."[29]

Koop's response took him much by surprise. "That's the way it was up until today, Dr. Stokes. That's what I'm here for. I am going to run a surgical service, and I will be responsible for the patients, for their diagnosis, for their treatment, for their postoperative care and for their follow-up."[30]

Stokes replied: "We'll see about that!" As Koop later recalled, "He went to the phone and called Dr. Ravdin, and I could only hear one side of the conversation. . . . I could hear Rav's voice rising once in a while. I also knew from the way Dr. Stokes spoke on the phone that he was defeated. Rav essentially told him what I had told him, and I guess it was a pretty bitter pill for Joe Stokes to swallow. We eventually buried the hatchet, and things went along much better as time went on."[31]

"We were all flabbergasted by how quickly this young fireball knocked our senior doctor down several pegs," observed Richard D. Wood, Sr., president of the Children's Hospital through most of Koop's time there.[32] On this key issue—the independence of the surgical service, and the surgeon's crucial pre- and post-operative role—Koop was following precisely Ladd's example. When Ladd had been named to the full-time staff of the Boston Children's Hospital in 1937, after a decade as part-time surgeon-in-chief, he had reorganized the surgical service along these lines.

As Don K. Nakayama notes in his review of the history of pediatric surgery, "The assignment of patients to a medical or surgical service . . . was an issue from pediatric surgery's earlier days. In an era when most children were treated in the home, pediatricians supervised care when inpatient care was required, including surgery. They did the workups, made the diagnosis, and spoke with the family. When a child needed an operation, the pediatrician might sometimes assist at surgery or provide anesthesia."[33] Before Ladd went full-time, the Boston Children's Hospital, like the Children's Hospital of Philadelphia, had only a part-time surgical staff.

The context for Koop's unwelcome arrival at the Children's Hospital lay in a crisis. Ravdin, as chair of the HUP department of surgery, had been handed a mandate to shake up the surgical service. In Koop's words, "The beginnings of pediatric surgery at the Children's Hospital of Philadelphia came about through the dissatisfaction of the very well trained nursing staff with the surgical care of children. After one particularly unfortunate incident, in 1944, Miss [Frances] Clyde, the then directress of nurses . . . and a woman trained in the Boston Children's Hospital who had seen the work of William B. Ladd . . . delivered an ultimatum" to Dr. Stokes: "[U]nless you are on the way to building a surgical service with the safety that Dr. Ladd and Dr. Gross have in Boston, I and my staff will quit."[34]

Stokes shared the problem with Alfred N. Richards, then vice president of medical affairs, and he in turn passed it to I.S. Ravdin, the chair of surgery, to resolve.[35] It would involve a young man who, as the *New York Times* recalled upon his death, had already "acquired a reputation for boldness."[36]

Looking back on his choppy beginnings at the hospital, Koop reflected: "Rav said 'When you get to like them and they get to like you, you go to Boston.' Well, they never did like me, and I didn't like them either."

In her review of the history of pediatric surgery, Catherine Muse-meche sets the dispute between Stokes and Koop in context. "The pediatricians were accustomed to being in charge without any full-time surgeons to get in their way. They controlled referrals. . . . The presence of Koop, a full-time pediatric surgeon intent on building a program, threatened their control. To complicate matters further, the party line was that the risk of surgery was prohibitively high in infants and children and should only be undertaken as a last resort."[37] Resistance was related also to financial loss, as physicians were paid for the patients under their care, and to sign their surgical patients over meant losing income.[38]

For an office, Koop was offered a table in the library; and during the spring of 1946 he was largely ignored. "I . . . would spend many dreary days just sitting there; the staff often would not bother to call me to consult on surgical problems that had come into the hospital. As I was being frozen out, several children with surgical problems that were correctable died on the wards."[39]

Meanwhile, he was making other discoveries. Most of the patients were black, since the hospital was located "in the black ghetto." But there was a private floor, which was whites only. "When I first admitted a black patient to the private floor of the hospital, one of the nurses resigned. That is how bad racism was in Philadelphia in 1947. At least I changed that at the hospital, and quickly."[40] As anesthesiologist Peter Safar records in his memoir, at that time there were no African American doctors at all in the entire HUP.[41]

To Boston and Back

The plan had been for Koop to spend a year in Boston with Drs. Gross and Ladd.[42] "That was the mecca, the beginning of it all in pediatric surgery," according to Harry Bishop, who himself had trained in Boston and would be Koop's long-term surgical colleague.[43] In the event the Koops were there for a mere five months, departing Philadelphia in the first week of May and returning in early October. For the family, the timing could certainly have been better. Betty had two-year-old Allen to care for, and had given birth to Norman, their second son, less than a month earlier on April 8.

Koop writes to Ravdin on May 2 that he was sorry to have missed saying goodbye (Ravdin had been out of town), but wishes to renew his thanks "for all of your help and confidence."[44] He writes again, a week later, with details of their less than satisfactory accommodation in Somerville, Massachusetts, and his initial connections with the hospital.[45] They are settled in "a barn of a house" which lacks central heating "and many other conveniences hitherto thought to be essential." In the immediate post-war period, "there was an unbelievable shortage of housing." When he was preparing to move to Boston, Koop had shared his problem with one of the scientists he had worked with on plasma substitutes at the Knox Gelatin Company, who said he could find him somewhere as a colleague owned a house in Somerville. It was on Adams Street, and "looked like the television set of the Addams family." It had not been occupied for more than a decade. They basically camped on the first floor and ignored two more above them.[46] Unsurprisingly, "I was making my plans to leave as soon as I could."[47]

Koop declared to Ravdin that, "From this vantage point Pediatric Surgery in Philadelphia can have a very happy future if cooperation from certain individuals is forthcoming."[48] In any case, "I shall be increasingly anxious to get back and get started." It would not be long.

Ravdin's rejoinder is rather interesting. First he played down Koop's complaint about their housing. "I am delighted to know that you are comfortably settled, even though you miss some of the modern conveniences of living." And then: "make yourself as agreeable as possible, in order that they make everything available to you."[49] Plainly, Ravdin believed Koop to be capable of being less than "agreeable," and that's on display in this correspondence as they argue about money. Before he left for Boston Koop had asked for extra help, since during the time away they would need to retain their Philadelphia apartment. His salary was then set at $2,000 a year.[iii] He asked for an extra $10 or $15 a month to balance their budget.[50] This extra was evidently paid for the

iii   This figure was significantly below the median 1946 U.S. income for a family of four, which was $3,286, per the Bureau of the Census Current Population Report for January 28, 1948. https://www2.census.gov/prod2/popscan/p60-001.pdf A comparable 2021 figure was $70,784; in other words, a rough multiplier of twenty times helps us make sense of these figures. https://www.census.gov/library/visualizations/2022/comm/median-household-income.html 3/18/23 first two months but did not appear in July. So Koop raised the issue again. Ravdin replied firmly on August 15: "In regard to your salary question it was decided in consultation with Dr. Richards that since you are getting money from the University and from the Children's Hospital and since the University salary was in excess of that which any senior resident had previously obtained that no increase would be given this year. I wouldn't worry about the fifteen dollars a month."[51]

Meanwhile, Koop wrote to him of a more general anxiety as to whether he will be able to make enough money as a pediatric surgeon. Ravdin sought to calm him. "Don't worry too much about making a living in pediatric surgery. I am sure that you will."[52] Koop plainly did worry, and money features in quite a few exchanges with Ravdin. For example, he asks if the University will pay some of the cost of typing and binding his ScD dissertation. On June 2, 1947, he sent his account, for $54; and Ravdin scribbled on the bottom "sent ch for 27–00." But not before passing the note to Rhoads, asking "Jon, would you agree to paying ½ of this?" to which Rhoads responds, "Yes or whatever you arranged with Chick." Ravdin is plainly irked. Before Koop's letter was filed, he wrote on it: "ISR didn't 'arrange' anything."

Koop of course was champing at the bit to get back to the Children's Hospital, and reminded Ravdin that his plan is to be "back in the fold" by October 1, though suggested delaying his return to the Hospital until October 15 "when the present consultant's term expires." Ravdin concurred.[53]

Meanwhile, Koop had an unrivaled opportunity to spend time with the giants of the nascent field of pediatric surgery, William E. Ladd (1880–1967), and his trainee and successor Robert Gross (1905–1988). In his survey of the history of the discipline, Randolph baldly states: "Surgery for infants and children in the United States began with Dr. William E. Ladd."

Ladd had joined the staff of the Children's Hospital of Boston in 1910, occasionally performing surgery on children in his early days alongside his general surgical and gynecological practice, though that was to change.

"Ladd and Gross became very good friends and almost a father/son relationship. . . . Ladd was a doctor of the old school. He was the kind of gentleman who . . . wore a flower in his buttonhole when he made rounds. He was—when you got to know him—a very kindly gentleman, willing to share his knowledge with a young squirt like me. But . . . he was a formidable character. . . . I would say he probably had very little flexibility in his relationships with other people."[54]

Gross was known, like Ladd, for his meticulous preparation and procedure. He rose to become in 1947 the second William E. Ladd Professor of Children's Surgery at Harvard (the first, somewhat oddly, having been Ladd himself). His fastidiousness is the stuff of stories. On his operating room wall hung a sign: "If an operation is difficult you are not doing it properly." In a preface to one of his books he writes: "In commonly performed operations, there is no excuse for diddling around; technical jobs which are thought out ahead of time can be practiced . . . [so the] whole operation clicks along in a quiet, rapid and orderly fashion." He chided Dr. Judson Randolph in a memo: "In the dining room, coats should be worn." (Randolph promptly framed it!)[55] His 1952 surgery textbook ran to precisely 1,000 pages. Which made it all the more amusing that, when someone pointed out that there was no chapter on Sacrococcygeal Teratoma,[iv] Gross discovered to his chagrin that the typescript of that chapter had fallen off his work table and was lodged behind a radiator in his office.[56]

Gross's approach was meticulous, but also subtle. "The care of children," he wrote, "requires a certain indefinable something . . . which might well be called the 'art' of pediatric surgery; it cannot be quantitated or characterized any more than one can describe adequately the tints of Titian or the bold strokes of Michelangelo; . . . this 'extra something' is a priceless attribute which is most sought for in members of the visiting and house staffs."[57] One is reminded of Koop's remark to Rhoads about Doris Bender, his first trainee, that "she has a special knack for knowing a sick baby."[58]

Ladd, who was no longer operating, taught Koop the "philosophy" of pediatric surgery; Gross taught him the practice. While he spent most of his time observing, for six weeks he was able to join Gross's

---

iv   A tumor that grows on the baby's tailbone.

surgical team as the "pup" (lowest on the totem pole). "I learned the most from William E. Ladd, although I never saw him operate. Ladd lived out in Natick, and he had a farm, and he'd get up in the morning and be the gentleman farmer. His chores took until noon, after which he went to the Harvard Club for lunch, then to the Children's Hospital where he would sit on an empty crib, his long legs dangling, hoping a member of the house staff would come along for a chat. I tried to meet with him as often as I could."

"Gross never appreciated me as a contender in the field until after I got back to Philadelphia," he recalled. "The first time I returned to Boston, I even wondered whether I should go and see Gross," whom he had found abrupt and unfriendly. Koop goes on to say he could hardly blame him, when he discovered what had been going on.

There had been a serious breach between Gross and Ladd some time before, and things kept getting worse. The initial rift in the relationship had occurred back in 1938, when Gross, Ladd's chief resident, was the first to ligate a patent duct arteriosus.[v] He had been forbidden to do this by Ladd, so Gross waited until Ladd went to Europe on vacation and got permission to proceed from the associate surgeon-in-chief. The child, named Lorraine Sweeney, survived and thrived, and twenty-five years later joined Gross in an anniversary celebration at the hospital. But Ladd was furious, and on his return peremptorily fired Gross (though the hospital insisted on reinstating him).[59]

Back when Ravdin and Ladd had arranged Koop's visit, Ladd was still surgeon-in-chief. Gross had not yet been appointed his successor, and Koop officially reported to Franc D. Ingraham (1898–1965), a neurosurgeon and evidently quite a character. Koop recalled a story that he instructed his secretaries never to open envelopes that addressed him as "Frank" rather than "Franc." And that on the day that Britain declared war on Germany, he was rumored to have gone into Boston to buy two Jaguars, just in case the war lasted for some time and he needed to replace his current model. Koop recalled getting a kick out of that story, "inasmuch as I had no money and no car."[60]

---

v   A heart defect, in which there is an opening between two blood vessels leading to the heart.

Once they got talking, Gross confided in Koop that Ladd had made a series of accusations to the Board of Overseers in an effort to prevent Gross from succeeding him. Koop lists the charges in order. First, he was incompetent; second, he was dishonest in his handling of research funds; and, third, he was Jewish. Koop adds: The Jewish charge was "probably the most ignominious thing that the Ladd and Gross argument ever made Ladd do, and . . . Gross told me this, and so I presume it is true—he said he had to take the train and go to Baltimore and find the Lutheran church in which he had been baptized to get this great big book of the archives and take it to a photocopier and have a picture made of that page, take the book back to the church and then get back on the train and deliver the copy to the board of overseers. . . . Note, this was never public, but eventually the board of overseers said they had chosen Robert E. Gross." On December 5, 1946, Koop sent Gross his congratulations. "Word has come to Philadelphia via the grapevine that you have finally received the appointment to the chair of surgery you so richly deserve."[61] It was of course the chair named for Ladd to which he was appointed, an irony that cannot have been lost on either of them.[62]

After this unburdening, the next time Koop visited Boston Gross greeted him "like a long-lost son" and canceled his appointments for the rest of the day, telling his assistant, "Chick Koop and I have got to talk about a lot of things."[63]

When Koop returned to take up his duties at the Children's Hospital, he already had a residency program in place, having recruited Doris (Dottie) Bender, whom he had supervised at the University Hospital, as his first trainee. She was in post early in the year. In his memoir he recalls her "valiant service . . . especially while I was in Boston." She was the first woman in America to be trained in pediatric surgery.[64]

On the financial front, always a worry to Koop, the year 1946 had begun on a high note. On December 31 of 1945 Rhoads had mailed Koop a gift from himself and Ravdin. "Here is a year-end check to fortify you slightly toward the increase in your family expenses— from Dr. Ravdin and me." He adds: "I do not know just what the financial set-up will be when you go to Children's but please be frank in coming to me if you run into financial difficulties as I am determined that you have the opportunity to develop the pediatric surgical work if you like it. Rav seems to have arranged all the more difficult problems and the financial ones should be soluble."[65]

And at the close of 1946, they sent another check. Koop wrote to Ravdin, from his office on the Fifth Floor of the Children's Hospital, on December 31. "When you spoke to me of a bonus I had no idea that you would be so generous. I am quite overwhelmed and exceedingly grateful. The timing of this very welcome stipend could not have been better: I had just had my overcoat stolen and I was feeling very low indeed."

Koop was capable of feeling "very low indeed." Behind his bravado, he could be prey to severe discouragement. He rarely admits it, and it's a sign of his friendship with Rhoads that he does here. But in a remarkably candid note to self from the mid-1950s he goes further. He is writing of some trouble affecting his colleague, the neurosurgeon Eugene Spitz, who left the Children's Hospital around that time. It's not clear if his departure resulted from a disagreement; Koop refers to it as the "Spitz affair." It has left him depressed (his word), and re-thinking everything. "Practice is falling off," he notes. "Proportionate less income." He's concerned about "financial security," and "retirement." The specialty of pediatric surgery is still "not believed in"—even within the Hospital of the University of Pennsylvania: "only ISR [Ravdin]. . . ." "Essential frustration," he writes, "re fact that this community has repudiated the surgical program at CHOP that has been developed thru my efforts." He summarizes his note: "I feel I have accomplished a great deal—I've built a remarkable faculty for children—but it isn't really wanted and therefore I suppose it really isn't necessary." What to do? "Should I seek a new type of job—Adult surgery—Administrative...[?]" Mercifully, his spirits picked up, and he persevered.[66]

CHAPTER 4

Shaping a Specialty

I was the salesman for pediatric surgery. I have the knack of talking
to an audience and convincing [them] about what I'm saying is true.
—CEK, Heskel interview

The early 1950s witnessed an extraordinary burst of professional activity on the part of the young surgeon, still in his 30s, as the American Academy of Pediatrics (AAP) gave him his head on a series of issues.

Though Koop's career had been directed away from the tumor clinic, his interests had not. In 1951 we find him one of eight members of the AAP Tumor Registry Committee, the goal of which was "to further the study of cancer in childhood." He was tasked with looking into the problem of "Shoe Fitting Fluoroscopes" (X-ray machines in children's shoe-shops, common at the time).[1] Koop played a major role in securing state-level regulation and subsequent prohibition of this dangerous practice.

Soon after, in 1955, he played a leading role as the "surgical member" of the AAP's Committee on Accident Prevention, for which he drafted a protocol for "The Emergency Care of Childhood Skeletal Trauma." This was no small project—the draft required review by the American College of Surgeons, the American Red Cross, and Civilian Defense.[2]

He was tasked by the same committee to report on "handling children hurt in an accident and being transferred to the hospital."[3] As the record of the meeting points out, it was (and indeed is) common for an injured child to be picked up and carried, in a manner no one would think of handling an injured adult.

What's more, Koop has been working on the treatment of burns. At that same meeting, the committee report that Koop "has actually done much of the work that led to this statement on the treatment of burns and the treatment of skeletal trauma." As a result, he "has been invited by the American College of Surgeons to present a paper. This is perhaps the first time that surgeons were addressed by a pediatric surgeon on how to handle childhood injuries." The writer of the minute notes, "Dr. Koop was quite excited over that opportunity."[4]

Meanwhile, he was playing a prominent part in the committee of the Section on Surgery's work—elected, together with his friend Potts, to succeed Gross and Lozoya as they rotated off; and he was active on its Committee on Medical Education.[5]

Seven years later, it was Koop who took the initiative to petition the American Board of Surgery (ABS) for board recognition of pediatric surgery as a specialty. That first approach came surprisingly close to success, but ran into opposition from the Society of University Surgeons and the American Board of Neurology. "Because of their opposition, the American Board of Surgery withdrew their proposal to the Advisory Board of Medical Specialties in 1957." This rather dramatic turn of events muddied the water for some time, though Koop fruitlessly tried again three years later.[6]

Pioneers and Colleagues

In 1946 it was still very rare for a surgeon to specialize entirely in children. There were many "children's hospitals," but—bizarre as this now seems—aside from Boston none of them had a full-time surgeon. At that date, it appears that only three surgeons in the entire United States are known to have chosen to limit their practice to pediatric cases, so Koop was likely the fourth.[7]

The first was Herbert Coe (1881–1968), who deserves the title of first American pediatric surgeon. Coe had chosen back in 1919 to refuse all adult general surgical patients, and at the same time he began to lobby for professional recognition of pediatric surgery, and to encourage friends and associates to join him in the specialty. He had limited success on either front.

He did secure one convert—Oswald Wyatt (1896–1957), who "went 'all in' for a practice devoted to pediatric surgery in 1928." His timing was less than ideal. In 1927 he closed his office and spent time studying clinical pediatrics and children's surgery. H. William Clatworthy later wrote that after the Crash of 1929 Wyatt "nearly starved to death!" But his practice later "became a success as pediatricians . . . preferred his specialized training and his fulltime focus on children's surgery over the general surgeons at the university hospital."[8]

In 1910, William E. Ladd had joined the staff of the Children's Hospital in Boston. Randolph suggests that the reason he went on to focus on children was the terrible 1917 Halifax disaster, though Ladd later demurred.[i]

In 1927 he had been appointed surgeon-in-chief. "Part of Ladd's genius lay in meticulous attention to detail," noted Randolph. "By 1940 . . . a critical mass for the organization of an academic pediatric surgical service had been assembled in Boston at the Children's Hospital." By then, Ladd had "brought about prodigious clinical progress in children's surgery."[9]

Koop knew the actual trigger for Ladd's interest. He "had a series of three newborn patients with malrotation of the colon with midgut volvulus[ii] that neither he nor Dr. [John Lewis] Bremer understood, nor could they fix them and save the babies' lives. That started Ladd's crusade for 'child surgery.' He presented the three patients and his hopes for child surgery to the Boston Surgical Society, and was rebuffed. Ladd then asked the hospital for some surgical beds. They gave him three." So, "the beginnings of child surgery in this country were three beds at the Children's Hospital."[10] He continued to operate on some adults until 1930.[11]

Coe had made repeated requests of the leadership of the American College of Surgeons (ACS) for pediatric surgery to have a specialist

---

i   A US munitions ship had been involved in a collision in the harbor of Halifax, Nova Scotia. After an enormous initial explosion, there were further detonations that sent concussive waves further across the area. Hundreds of children's faces were pressed to windowpanes; terrible facial injuries were suffered as the glass shattered. The American Red Cross sent sixty-five nurses and twenty-nine doctors from Boston, led by Ladd, who rushed to the scene the next day.

ii   A congenital abnormality of the gut.

place alongside ophthalmology and urology and other specialties, but to no avail. He "busily lobbied his friends and contacts in the hierarchy" to such a degree that he earned the nickname "the politician"![12] Yet "the College met Dr. Coe's entreaties with an unyielding brick wall."[13]

Coe secured his first bite of institutional success in 1947, by coincidence the year in which Koop was appointed to the Children's Hospital. The AAP program committee gave him two hours at its general assembly to make his case. As a result, he was appointed to chair "a committee to form a special category of membership in the AAP for surgeons." Coe insisted on tight criteria for inclusion, including a commitment of at least 90 percent of one's time to surgery on infants and children. "Getting Gross on board would add stature to the fledgling organization, so he offered the Bostonian a place on the new group's steering committee." Gross took some persuading, initially "lukewarm" about the whole idea. Coe "appealed to Gross's notorious professional vanity" by referring to "the pre-eminence of your group"—and offering both to waive the joining fee and halve Gross's annual dues.

That was the context for the organizational meeting of the new "section on surgery" at the AAP conference in Atlantic City, on November 21, 1948, with twelve surgeons in attendance. Despite Coe's efforts, the "notoriously moody Gross" decided to skip the meeting, "but Ladd was there and was the likely cause of Gross's absence."[14]

Also present was a young Koop, fresh from his appointment as surgeon-in-chief. And it was Koop who, seven years later, would take the next step and first formally approach the ACS in a bid for board recognition.[15] He was to persist in these efforts for nearly twenty years.[16]

While they were mostly general surgeons with a special interest in children, the early members of the Section on Surgery from Ladd down formed a powerful band of brothers (yes, all brothers) and included several already distinguished and influential figures. We've noted Oswald S. Wyatt, Coe's friend who had forsworn adult surgery back in 1927. Another was Willis J. Potts (1895–1968), who returned from war service having read Ladd and Gross's textbook *Abdominal Surgery of Infancy and Childhood* and became fired up with a vision to devote himself full-time to working with children. At the age of fifty he arranged a fellowship with Gross in Boston, before returning to Chicago to serve as surgeon-in-chief at Memorial Hospital. With the help of a neighbor in Chicago's Oak Park, who just happened to manufacture surgical instruments, he designed a vascular clamp that soon became standard—and crucial to advances in vascular and cardiac surgery.[17]

More than once Koop found himself pushing back against the rampant antisemitism of the period. He tells the story of how he and Potts collaborated to help a Jewish colleague get a job in the face of prejudice. It has an amusing side. "I don't know what was wrong with Bill Potts," Koop reminisced. "Do you know what Bill Potts called me all his life? Chester. I don't know whether he got the C. Everett mixed up or whether he thought my name was really Chester. . . . Anyway, he always called me Chester. It used to drive me crazy." Stephen L. Gans (1920–1994), Koop's collaborator and successor in the *Journal of Pediatric Surgery*, had applied for a job at the Children's Hospital of Los Angeles. When he arrived for the interview, "a young man took him to a room where they were by themselves and closed the door, and he said 'I am here to tell you privately that we have our token Jew. You will never get a job in this hospital because we don't want any more Jewish people on the staff.'" Gans shared this with Potts, and Potts called "Chester" who—forthright as ever—wrote immediately to the hospital board, who told him to mind his own business. But, in the end, Gans got the job.[18]

The Long Road to Recognition

General opposition to pediatric surgery's specialty recognition arose from several causes. For one thing, hardly any surgeons were committed to it full-time. It's plain that for the individual practitioner, in the early days, there was a serious financial disincentive. Adult surgery paid better, as it had many more options. When J.

Alexander Haller (1927–2018), who later became chief of surgery at Hopkins, asked pediatric surgeon Mark M. Ravitch (1910–1989) for career advice, he was much surprised by his mentor's response. "You might not be able to make a living operating only on children. Be a well-trained general surgeon first and let pediatric surgery be your hobby."[19]

Of at least equal significance was the much higher mortality and morbidity in pediatric patients. Koop noted that even Jonathan Rhoads, whom he deeply respected, disliked those occasions when he needed to operate on children. In a retrospective essay, Koop recalled: "In my early days as surgeon-in-chief, I found that none of the correctable congenital defects incompatible with life had ever been successfully treated in Philadelphia except rarely and then by good luck more than good management. The mortality for a simple colostomy[iii] was in the range of 90%."[20]

So the number of surgeons prepared to commit themselves to this novel discipline was small, and that in turn offered a reason why the wider professional communities—within general surgery and among the medical specialties, the two gatekeepers to specialty recognition—were unenthusiastic. Too many saw it, in Ravitch's striking term, as a "hobby."

More broadly, the surgical profession was already under wider pressure to split into specialties, especially after the war—which had, necessarily, advanced surgical skills of many kinds. Whatever the theoretical appeal of focused expertise, general surgeons felt their living was under threat, and their skills challenged, and many were determined to resist this effort to take from them a whole class of patient. In Koop's words, "Pediatric surgery's problem was that we came along and not only said, 'We want to be another splinter, but we've got a special problem, and that is that we think that we can do a better job than the urologist or than the-this or than the-that, who are anatomical specialists if you're dealing with babies that are very small' . . . and we based it on Ladd's principle that a child is

---

iii   A procedure to re-route the intestine through an incision in the abdomen.

not a small adult and the fact that their pharmacological responses, their physiologic responses and their pathologic responses were all different than just percentages of adult weight." So "when I came to Philadelphia I found the hospital hostile, I found the city hostile and I even found the University of Pennsylvania hostile, except for the president, the provost, Ravdin and Rhoads. I even found pediatricians hostile."[21] Koop notes that even Ravdin and Rhoads were initially unenthusiastic about the push for specialty recognition.

Further applications from the Surgical Section were turned down in 1957 and 1961.[22] "While its practitioners felt otherwise, to the broader, medical and surgical communities there were two flaws that had to be addressed. To the outside medical world there was no body of knowledge of pediatric surgery that was independent of the broader disciplines of pediatrics and surgery."[23] And then there was the organizational question. The chair of the ABS, William H. Holden, explained their reasoning to Robert Izant, who summarized for his colleagues: "As long as the Pediatric Surgery organization is tied to another organization, and therefore, not an independent one, the problems with affiliation with the American Board of Surgery would be difficult if not impossible."[24]

These concerns were addressed in 1965 and 1970 respectively. One key step lay in the establishment in 1965 of the *Journal of Pediatric Surgery*, a collaboration between Stephen L. Gans, who took the initiative in setting it up, and Koop, who served eleven years as founding editor.[25] From 1964, Gans had served as chair of the Surgical Section publications committee. Since 1958 the journal *Surgery* had devoted a "small section" to the subject, with Mark Ravitch as editor. "Other journals, such as the *American Journal of Surgery, Pediatrics, Clinical Pediatrics*" and more "published articles on a sporadic basis." But there was "no group image projected by this scattered output."[26] There was, however, plenty of material.

So Gans persuaded the Surgical Section leadership that a new one was needed. "He formed an editorial board before they had anything to review." In an effort to persuade a publisher to take it on, Gans recruited the British Association of Paediatric Surgeons (BAPS) as a sponsor. His next step was to bring Koop on board, because "success required a prominent editor."[27]

As Zeller and colleagues tell the tale, "Koop decided that a message was needed for the wider audience outside the field, especially those that opposed its recognition as a bona fide surgical specialty. For an introductory editorial he prevailed upon Isidore[iv] Ravdin, his chair at Penn and recognized dean of American surgeons." Ravdin, now plainly persuaded of the case, did not disappoint. He wrote: "A new star is on the horizon of medicine. In this country and abroad, pediatric surgery has reached the place where we must admit that it now deserves to rank with other specialties concerned with the particular problems of treating specific types of patients." Gross sent his congratulations: "I think the Journal has done more to advance children's surgery, not only here but around the world, above *anything* else in the last couple of decades.'"[28] High praise for both Gans' vision and Koop's editorial leadership, from a notoriously difficult colleague.

That was also Koop's view. He saw the launch of the journal as "perhaps the single greatest event . . . that enhanced the future of pediatric surgery."[29] It was the same year that the Surgical Section set up its education and training committee, under H. William Clatworthy.

A further run at board certification was rejected in 1967.[30] In response to this further rebuff, and concern expressed earlier about the absence of a separate organization of those in the would-be specialty, the independent American Pediatric Surgical Association (APSA) was established in 1970, in partnership with the *Journal of Pediatric Surgery*, to which conference presentations would need to be submitted.

The first meeting of the APSA was held at Pheasant Run in suburban Chicago. Gross was persuaded to be the first president, and Koop president-elect—neatly spanning the two founding generations of the profession and its two major centers.[31] Strong membership criteria included board certification, an exclusive pediatric practice, and the need for members to be at least two years out of residency. Only

---

iv   Ravdin's first name is spelled variously. Per the University of Pennsylvania Archives, it is properly Isidor.

two hundred of the three hundred members of the Surgical Section of the AAP immediately qualified.[32]

Continued resistance to the emerging specialty is well illustrated by a 1968 exchange between Koop and Rhoads. A prominent Los Angeles surgeon approached Rhoads to help recruit a replacement for surgeon-in-chief of the Los Angeles Children's Hospital, writing dismissively that there will be "a deluge of so called pediatric surgeons seeking this post. However, it is the feeling of many that the man to occupy this post should be . . . primarily interested in general surgery." Rhoads shared the letter with Koop, whose response—as a "so called pediatric surgeon"—was predictably acerbic. "The institution is anti-Semitic and the strifes and envy which exist on the surgical service are considerable. . . . I would not be interested in recommending anybody to that post unless there was a real shake up in philosophy in the entire institution."[33]

Yet, slowly, the climate was shifting. In 1969 the ACS established an advisory council on pediatric surgery. It's no surprise that they invited Koop to serve as chair. And finally, two years later, under the guidance of Canadian surgeon Harvey Beardmore, the ABS was finally persuaded to support a new board examination in pediatric surgery—on condition that it was focused on "newborns and small infants."

Recognition

In 1974, Beardmore, Randolph, and Marc I. Rowe took the inaugural board examination in Philadelphia. The ABS hosted the first general examination for the Certificate of Special Qualification in Pediatric Surgery in April 1975, for which Beardmore and his colleagues had set the questions. Two hundred fifty of the three hundred pediatric surgeons then in practice, Koop included, gathered in a resort ballroom in Puerto Rico just before the sixth conference of the APSA to sit the three-hour exam. Only two of their number, Gross and Swenson, had been grandfathered into board certification.[34]

Beardmore spoke shortly afterward to the conference about the lengthy odyssey to specialty recognition. He concluded with the words:

"Gentlemen, you have your boards." Koop later recalled, "The hairs on my arms stood on end."[35]

James O'Neill, who became Koop's successor at the Children's Hospital in 1981, also entertained vivid memories of the day. "In the front row, there was Dr. Ravitch, and I don't know who else. . . . But they were all there, I mean, the real higher-ups in pediatric surgery. Well, I was about three or four rows back. The people from the board were there proctoring the exam. Within five minutes of the exam starting, Dr. Ravitch pulls out this big cigar and starts to smoke this cigar, with smoke everywhere. People were coughing. . . . I moved to the back of the room."[36]

Like O'Neill, Beardmore later shared an anecdote of the Puerto Rico meeting. His flight to the island was in a small plane piloted by a young woman with striking red hair. He was wearing aviator sunglasses and she seemed to think he also was a pilot. So she invited him to join her in the vacant co-pilot's seat, which he did. His wife, seated in the back, became increasingly alarmed. Beardmore grew alarmed too, when the pilot asked him to keep the wings level.[37]

Meanwhile, there had been a lengthy struggle underway in the background for the naming of the specialty. Nakayama notes that the first textbook in the field was oddly titled *The Surgical Diseases of Children* (1860, by John Cooper Forster of London); that in the first half of the twentieth century "children's surgery" was the most widely used term; and that "children's surgeons" were its practitioners.[38] The Harvard chair endowed for Ladd had duly been named for "children's surgery." The varieties of nomenclature are even more striking in the naming of pediatric hospitals, none of which was actually called "pediatric." There had been a Babies' Hospital, an Infants' Hospital, and a West End Nursery, though as in both Boston and Philadelphia "Children's Hospital" had increasingly become the norm.[39] Amusingly, in the UK it was felt necessary in several cases, such as the Great Ormond Street Hospital for Sick Children, to point out that these hospitals were for children who are sick!

"Pediatric surgery" had been in occasional currency alongside "children's surgery" and "child surgery." Koop found the term "child surgeon" highly amusing. There was pushback in the course of the recognition process from general surgeons, who preferred "pediatric general surgery" as a less specific term, that could imply a more limited range of skills. But the use of "pediatric surgery" for the journal and the American Pediatric Surgical Association for the society helped build momentum. All along, it was Koop who had driven it. It was six years after he returned to Philadelphia from Boston that Koop decided to start calling himself a "pediatric surgeon," and his service the "pediatric surgical service" at the Children's Hospital. "Many people say that I'm the person who invented" the term, he mused. "But child surgery became pediatric surgery."[40] Nakayama states it simply: "C. Everett Koop established 'pediatric surgery' as the specialty that 'pediatric surgeons' practice."[41]

After all that, at Koop's retirement dinner in 1981, the board chair of the hospital introduced him as "the world's leading child surgeon."[42]

The Global Scene

From his early days in the field Koop was active in international professional engagement. The AAP already included Mexican and Canadian members, and the famous picture of the 1948 Surgical Section organizational meeting includes representation from both. There had all along been a close connection between the United States and the United Kingdom, which was acknowledged at key points to have been in lead position. Great Ormond Street was the world's first children's hospital, and Sir Denis Browne, doyen of British pediatric surgeons, has been acclaimed as the world's first full-time practitioner.

Koop was first introduced to the BAPS back in 1954 during a visit to Philadelphia by one of its leaders, Peter Paul Rickham, and two years later Koop attended the BAPS annual conference for the first time. "It was also my first trip to the United Kingdom, where they were understandably a lot slower regaining their prewar status than the United States. So, going to London was like stepping back a decade, and going to the BAPS was to me like entering a fantasy land that I never even thought might exist." He was fascinated by their pattern of brief presentations followed by much discussion in place of the overstuffed lengthy lectures and slideshows of such events in the United States. In his retrospective review of BAPS on its fiftieth anniversary in 2003, he reflected that it "has come from a small coterie of people with a sincere desire to improve the welfare of children in surgery, who knew each other, worldwide, by their first names, to a preeminent organization that has provided a home for international pediatric surgery."[43]

Meanwhile, Koop encouraged his British friends to network with US colleagues, and in turn asked them to aid the British in their own push for recognition within the very formal ranks of medicine in the United Kingdom. On September 5, 1963, he invited the Ravdins to the Koop home to meet distinguished visitors from the UK.[44] Koop followed up a few weeks later: "Dear Rav: The pediatric surgeons from Great Britain whom you met at my home are striving for recognition of pediatric surgery in the British Isles where such recognition is much more important." Ravdin readily offers his aid. "If I could do anything in the way of writing some of my friends in Great Britain, I would be overjoyed to do so. Do let me hear from you about this matter."[45]

Koop returned to the BAPS conference almost every year until his retirement from the Children's Hospital, and for eight of those years served on the Council of BAPS as its first foreign member. As we have noted, BAPS, in turn, had been recruited as a sponsor of the *Journal of Pediatric Surgery*. BAPS conferences were sometimes held outside the UK, and it was after one convened in Rotterdam that on the train home—gathered on boxes and bags in the baggage car!—a group of members including Koop decided to begin the International Society of Pediatric Surgery, to bridge the various national networks.[46] It is small surprise that, among his many honors, he would in due course hold Fellowships in no less than four of the British medical and surgical Royal Colleges, and in 1980 received the prized award of the French *Légion d'honneur*.[47]

Koop's global networking yielded signal friendships with like-minded pediatric surgeons that would last over many decades.

Peter Paul Rickham (1917–2003), as we have noted, first introduced him to BAPS in 1954.[48] Back in 1939, as Peter-Paul Reichenheim, he had managed to escape first Nazi Germany, and then internment in the UK.[49] When the *Journal of Pediatric Surgery* was established, Rickham was made British editor.[50]

Robert Bransby Zachary (1913–1999), a leading British pediatric surgeon, in 1953 was one of the founders of BAPS. Celebrated for his pioneering work on spina bifida, he campaigned for pediatric surgery as a specialist discipline. Zachary was a practicing Roman Catholic. He suffered from a serious spinal deformity.[51]

Leading French pediatric surgeon, Michel Carcassonne (1927–2001), became a particular friend, in part since he shared Koop's evangelical Christian faith and its Reformed tradition; Carcassonne's forebears had been Huguenots.[52]

Doyen of Japanese pediatric surgeons, Keijiro Suruga (1920–2023), and Asia editor of the *Journal of Pediatric Surgery*, was also a personal friend over many years.[53] Like Carcassonne, he was a deeply religious Protestant Christian. Koop made many visits to Japan, and in 1960 helped found the Japanese Society of Pediatric Surgery. He so stressed the importance of anesthesia, that "fifteen years later I was introduced at a Japanese meeting as the Father of Japanese Anesthesiology."[54]

Strategic Transformation

Much has happened since Koop and his colleagues took their board exam in Puerto Rico. Pediatric Surgery remains a specialty of the ABS—one of seven; the American Board of Pediatrics, meanwhile, offers twenty more specialties of its own. Koop and his colleagues had wisely resisted the suggestion of the Board of Surgery to use membership in the Surgical Section of the AAP as an alternative to certification. His "principal concern—and it was shared by others—was . . . we were indeed very pediatrically oriented, but we were surgeons, and we deserved to have recognition among surgical specialists," surgeons with special pediatric skills, not pediatricians trying their hand at surgery.[55]

It was Koop who led his colleagues to build on Ladd's pioneering work and establish pediatric surgery as a specialty. Ladd had been born in 1880; Koop, born in 1916, led the next generation. Rhoads and Ravdin saw Koop's gifts and potential and provided him with an extraordinary opportunity. The Surgical Section gave him his head, when he decided the time was ripe for the first approach to the ABS. Colleagues would trust him and turn to him for advice and aid—like Potts confiding in him that Gans was facing antisemitism, and Gross baring his heart to the young man back in Boston. Meanwhile he became likely the fourth American surgeon to specialize exclusively in children, served as first editor of its journal, and led the repeated charge for institutional recognition. When he passed the baton to Beardmore and it was finally attained, he was credited with securing the term "pediatric surgery." All in addition to innovative and exemplary surgical practice as he built out his team at the Children's Hospital, to which we now turn.

CHAPTER 5

At the Children's Hospital

I am looking forward to a brilliant period in the history of surgery at
the Children's Hospital.

—I.S. RAVDIN to Koop, June 29, 1948

The year of Koop's thirty-second birthday, 1948, would prove
decisive for his professional life, and for that of his specialty. He
was duly confirmed in the position of surgeon-in-chief, and joined
the storied Atlantic City charter meeting of the Section on Surgery
of the American Academy of Pediatrics (AAP) that set in motion the
push for specialty recognition that Koop would spearhead.

Writing to Koop in the mid-1950s, I.S. Ravdin cast his mind back
to 1940, when they had first met. "A great deal has been accomplished
since sixteen years ago when John Lockwood told you that you had
best go home to New York because there was no place in Philadelphia
for you. It is one of the joys . . . that I reversed the decision the next
day and that you have been able to accomplish what you have."[1]

But Koop's first years at the hospital had not been smooth. Koop
went without an office for his first months, before being assigned a
cubicle in the upper floors of the facility. Immediately on his return
from Boston in the fall of 1947 he was eager to get to work, and filled
his first day's schedule with a list of thirteen operations. The staff, he
reports, unaccustomed to such a heavy load, promptly quit.[2] He was
then still in an acting capacity—a full appointment came only after
he passed his boards in surgery.

Koop and Ravdin

Isidor Schwaner Ravdin (1894–1972), doyen of American surgery mid-century and Koop's boss at the University of Pennsylvania, deserves a substantial slice of the credit for what Koop accomplished at the Children's Hospital.[3] [i] The plan to have Koop devote himself full-time to surgery on children had been his; and he provided substantial administrative and political support that were crucial in the early years.[4] Theirs was a complex relationship, between two driven individuals with matching intellects—and egos. It was not always smooth.

At Koop's retirement dinner nearly forty years later, Jonathan Rhoads, Ravdin's deputy during the war years, reflected that after Ravdin returned from war, "It became evident to me rather soon that he and the Professor were not going to mesh too well." So he suggested Ravdin send Koop to the Children's Hospital and was relieved when he took his advice.[5] From the start, there was tension. In his memoir Koop recounts how, after challenging his chief one time during rounds, Ravdin looked him in the eye and said—loud enough for others to hear—"Boy, someday you will push me too far."[6] Moritz Ziegler recalled to me Ravdin's reputation for "irascibility" in the university hospital community.[7]

Along with unstinting professional support, Ravdin gave Koop more advice than he had wished; even at arm's length, "meshing well" could prove a problem. Koop ran papers he was writing by Ravdin, who—ever candid—responded with edits and critical remarks. On July 12, 1950, Koop shared a paper on diaphragmatic hernia in children.[ii] Ravdin's response: It is "well worth publishing, but I think you ought to work it over again. You will see that I have done a bit of

---

i   I've opted not to use the mildly amusing acronym CHOP for the hospital, though it is now widely employed, including in some signage around the building—noting that Koop's long-time surgical partner Harry Bishop objected to it. "I rarely use the word 'CHOP.' The connotation is not good for me." See Ehrhart/Bishop, 4. The first use of "chop" dated from a snack bar, named the Chop Shop as a result of a competition. Betty Koop had worked there. Remarks to the Children's Hospital Alumni Organization, May 20, 1988. HML CHOP Box 79 11–12. The hospital is a separate legal entity from the university, though the university makes its academic appointments. Shirley Bonnem, head of public relations, had occasion to chide Harry Bishop for describing the Children's Hospital as "of" the University of Pennsylvania. Bonnem to Bishop November 20, 1980. HML CHOP files, Bishop, Harry C.
ii   A hole in the diaphragm that separates the chest and the abdomen.

changing of the first few pages, but many of your thoughts are excellent. The writing is a bit obtuse. It would be unfortunate for the first of your papers after several years to be written in a form that was not of the highest caliber." And he continued: "I hope you will read it over carefully and rearrange it and make it just as short as possible; but at the same time, make every sentence just as clear as possible."[8] A month later, he actually wrote Koop twice on the same day, May 8, about different papers. On biliary atresia,[iii] Koop could state his conclusions "a little more clearly;" on cryptorchidism,[iv] "Here and there you could brush up the English."[9]

Fees were also a concern to Ravdin. On December 3, 1952, Koop followed up a conversation with a summary of the fees he has charged over the previous year. Apparently Ravdin had accused him of over-billing. Yet, he says, he has had only sixteen patients billed more than $200, the highest being $350; "so that I think there can be no question about the fact that I am a 'fee gouger.'"[10] On March 9, 1955, Ravdin informed Koop that a patient on whom he will operate for a hernia is the grandchild of a "long supporter of this hospital," and continued, with a degree of exasperation: "For goodness sake, keep this in mind when you think you have to send him a bill."[11]

Somewhat wearily, Ravdin persisted in seeking to persuade Koop and his team to be more collegial and join in "grand rounds"[v] at the University Hospital. "Each year," Ravdin writes, "I have written to you saying that you and your group ought to come to Grand Rounds, and this year I am going to say the same thing. What you fellows do is to sit yourself down in the corner and keep yourselves away from the mother-tree of all surgery—general surgery." His closing is quite the put-down. "I know how busy you fellows think you are, and I would be happy to exchange positions with you for one month and you probably would be but a slip of your former self—if that much."[12]

This acerbic note came hard on the heels of an unpleasant exchange about another matter. Ravdin had been upbraiding Koop for failing to train surgeons who will work in the community rather than academic

---

iii A condition that damages the liver.
iv When one or both testes fail to descend into the scrotum.
v Grand rounds are case conferences.

departments. He closed, "If you have any feeling about this matter, I wish you would come out and see me." Koop's response, dated the following day, is emotional. "My unhappiest days in surgery during the past seven years have come with the realization that on repeated occasions when you have heard accusations leveled against me, you have without determining their accuracy assumed their truth and then proceeded to reprove, correct, or instruct me. . . . I will be out to see you in reference to your letter because I am not only hurt, but quite discouraged."[13]

Koop both appreciated Ravdin's attention and found it irksome. While sometimes addressing his boss as Rav, Koop tended to default to more formal styles. In response to one "Dear Dr. Ravdin" missive Ravdin retorts, "I have your letter regarding Dr. Bieber. Don't be so stuffy in writing to me."[14] In the 1950s Koop generally returned to addressing him as "Dear Professor."

In 1955 Koop sent a gift for the development of the university's I.S. Ravdin Institute, and Ravdin responded: "Everything I have ever done . . . you fully deserve. It has been wonderful to watch your progress at the Children's Hospital."[15] For his part, Koop's gratitude, admiration, and affection for his boss, which survived many sharp encounters, was not uncritical. He later wrote that "Rav could be a bear in the operating room. . . . During long operations I watched him berate and criticize his first assistant, then the senior resident, then the junior resident, and then any medical students who happened to get caught in the crossfire. Even though the surgery might have been a great success, everyone in the operating room would be in utter dejection."[16]

Somewhat curiously, from time to time both men comment on the importance of their relationship. So Ravdin wrote to Koop in January of 1958: "It was good to see you at Grand Rounds yesterday. I wish you could come more often. Come and see me anytime, or drop over at my house and see me. It is not good . . . to drift apart." Koop responded (after a delay of nearly a month): "Dear Professor, I am sorry that you have any feeling that we are drawing further apart. There are many times when I would appreciate your counsel and advice and many other times when I would enjoy your fellowship. However, I realize the demands that are made on your time and have a reticence about increasing the burden in any way."[17] Three years later, Koop ended a letter with "I . . . will never be able to express adequately my gratitude for the many things you have done for me and in my behalf."[18]

Koop's letter of June 11, on the occasion of the dedication of the university's Ravdin Institute, began by quoting Saint Paul's Second Letter to Timothy: "And the things that thou hast heard of me among many witnesses, the same commit thou to faithful men, who shall be able to teach others also." Koop continued: "Your influence on American surgery, not only in surgical management but also in surgical ethics, comes to mind whenever I read this verse. Your imprint will accordingly be left upon many surgical generations in days to come. . . . I count it a privilege to be one of the 'faithful men' and will endeavor to hold up my end of the bargain."[19]

By December, he is back to "Dr. Ravdin" again.

Meanwhile, Koop had been trying to interest Dartmouth, his alma mater, in awarding Ravdin an honorary degree. On October 18, 1956, and February 6, 1957, he updates Ravdin on meetings he has had at Dartmouth to press his case. He tells Ravdin that this is a highly political process, that there is a committee that includes several members who support Ravdin, and that nominees are often reviewed over several years before there is a decision, up or down. Koop is plainly seeking to mend fences with his boss in a big way. Ravdin seems to have been embarrassed by the whole business. He is "pretty sure this thing will not go through," and then later he is "deeply grateful," but "I wish you wouldn't work too hard at this."[20] In the event, despite Koop's considerable efforts, Dartmouth was not interested.[21]

On June 16, 1962, Ravdin replied to another Koop letter:

"Dear Chick:

"Your letter of June 11th will be treasured by me all the days of my life. I have never had a nicer one come to me. I count myself a very fortunate person for having helped in a part of your training."[22]

Which makes yet more stunning the fact, of which Koop knew nothing, that that same year Ravdin gave a lengthy memoir to Columbia University, following up an earlier series of oral history interviews, all sealed until his death. In the memoir of more than five hundred pages there are references to one hundred sixty physicians. Koop is never once mentioned.[23]

Yet a few years later, in February of 1966, it was to Ravdin that Koop went for the opening editorial of the *Journal of Pediatric Surgery*.

While Ravdin did not share Koop's evangelical Christian faith, he understood it better than Koop might have guessed. One of the more surprising facts we learn in the unpublished "Reminiscences of Isadore [*sic*] Ravdin" is that in his youth his family would summer in a Chautauqua[vi]—with the famous evangelist Billy Sunday as a neighbor. The young Ravdin "got to know Billy very well." So well, that when he was apprehended for smoking, and hauled up before the Chautauqua elders, he went to Sunday for help. Sunday asked what other sins he had committed in the Chautauqua, and he admitted he had been dancing. "My God, you ought to be fried," shot back the evangelist. But then it emerged that he had actually been dancing in the home of the elder conducting his trial! "And that was the end of my troubles, at Winona."[24]

Koop and Rhoads

Jonathan Rhoads (1907–2002), the tall and mild-mannered surgeon Ravdin had recruited to run the surgery department, was, like Koop, a young man handed an outsize job.[25] Ravdin had a reputation for sizing up young talent. He had actually chosen Rhoads, just a year out of his residency, to operate on his own gall bladder![26]

Rhoads was a Quaker, and therefore a conscientious objector. On Ravdin's return, he stayed on at the university for the remainder of his long career, later rising to be provost.

Rhoads and Koop got to know each other well during the war, and a friendship blossomed that would last more than sixty years until Rhoads's death at 94 in 2002. He offered the young Koop family much

---

vi   Now widely forgotten, the Chautauqua was a hugely popular movement a century back, with Methodist roots in the 1870s; it combined summer camps and other leisure and cultural activities. Teddy Roosevelt was said to have described it as "the most American thing in America." It continues at its home base in Chautauqua, New York. See chq.org.

encouragement and practical aid. It included use of the Rhoads's vacation cottage, which the fastidious Koops were horrified to find infested with mice, something Quaker Rhoads seemed to regard as normal. This is Rhoads who was famous for saying that he couldn't think of anything better to do with money than to save it, and who once bought a Christmas tree on the day after Christmas.[27] Koop's relationship with these two celebrated surgeons offers a study in contrasts. There is an ease in his dealings with Rhoads that never emerges with Ravdin.

One time he confides that "I feel myself so unwelcome in the department of surgery these days that I find myself longing for the good old days where there were only your feet . . . to trip over." It's too bad, says Koop, that Rhoads missed a grand rounds where a colleague had recounted his experiences in Boston. "They should have passed out emesis[vii] basins as door prizes . . . one of the most nauseating ass-kissing orations I have ever been forced to listen to. You're the only one I know who might have gotten the same reaction that I did." Meanwhile, work was slow at the Children's Hospital. "The planning committee has ceased to plan and everybody is porked about that but nobody makes any move to correct the situation. My practice could be sold for $100 at a handsome profit. Enough of my gripes, Jon, and thanks for reading them."

Rhoads's response is genial and sympathetic but ends firmly: "It is important to maintain unity of purpose—and as the department gets larger it takes more effort."[28]

Koop and Deming

As soon as Koop started work at the Children's Hospital it was clear that his major challenge was anesthesia. Nearly half a century later, he would write: "When I first encountered these problems, the [operative] mortality rate was 95 to 100 percent." And why? "The chief reason surgeons avoided children was the primitive state of anesthesia.

---

vii   Emesis is a term for vomit.

Doctors were afraid to put children to sleep, because they weren't sure they could wake them up."[29] Only after "making anesthesia safe for newborns" could the focus shift to correcting congenital defects.

A parallel move within general surgery was leading to the increasing professionalization of anesthesiology. Ravdin had been responsible for Robert D. Dripps's (1911–1973) move from his department of surgery to chair the separate department of anesthesiology at the HUP.[30] So just as Ravdin was recruiting Koop to go to the Children's Hospital, there was a related conversation about anesthesia, which had been in the hands of nurses. Dripps was described by Peter Safar, one of his trainees in the early 1950s, as "the undisputed leader of our specialty at that time," leading its top academic center.[31] He was also "liberal, tolerant, and cosmopolitan," with evidently quite a sense of humor ("his humorous poems became legendary").[32] Dripps took the opportunity to revolutionize the Children's Hospital's approach to anesthesia. So just as Ravdin picked Koop to become the first full-time surgeon, Dripps picked Dr. Margery (Margo) Deming (1914–1998), who had in fact been the first anesthesia resident at the University of Pennsylvania Hospital itself.[33] Safar knew her well, and characterized her as "dynamic, a clinical wizard, outspoken . . . and tenacious."[34]

Like Koop, she was chosen for her star qualities. As Selma Harrison Calmes, a founder of the Anesthesia History Association, explains, Deming had an "unusual residency, spending a great deal of time in research and producing four research papers on such topics as oxygen toxicity, postoperative atelectasis and drugs to raise blood pressure during spinal anesthesia." She and Koop knew each other at the hospital. Just as Ravdin sent Koop to spend a year in Boston with Ladd and Gross, so Deming was tasked with a year at the Children's Hospital of Los Angeles, under pioneering pediatric anesthesiologists M. Digby Leigh and Kay Belton. "Both arrived back in Philadelphia in November 1946 and began working together. . . . Dr. Deming was the first director of the Anesthesiology Department, and Dr. Koop was the first full-time surgeon."[35]

The situation was no easier for Deming than for Koop, "due to the political environment, the lack of knowledge and the lack of

equipment. The nurse anesthetist was married to a powerful surgeon. . . . There was resistance to Dr. Koop, which must have had a
'splash' effect on Dr. Deming. There was little knowledge of pediatric
physiology, and Dr. Koop was pushing to do more difficult operations. In spite of the difficulties, Dr. Deming made some critically
important contributions."[36]

Or as Koop later wrote, "She was tireless in her efforts to improve
techniques. It was she who in the United States made safe the technique of endotracheal anesthesia. This is where a flexible tube is
placed directly through the vocal cords of an infant into the wind
pipe . . . putting the breathing of the child under the care of the
anesthesiologist."

Deming had faced many challenges. After childhood polio left her
with a "severely damaged right arm that would later make intubation
difficult," during medical school she contracted tuberculosis and
was forced to spend a year in a sanitarium.[37] Yet she shared Koop's
passion—not simply for pioneering pediatric surgery, but for every
pediatric patient. "In the first several years we used these homemade
endotracheal anesthesia techniques on twelve hundred small babies,
and we never lost one. We had our share of scares, and there were
many nights when Margo Deming and I sat up with a small infant
whose windpipe had been traumatized, just in case the developing
croup might call for a tracheostomy.[viii] Fortunately, in all those early
experimental procedures, we never had to do one."[38] "People then
did not believe it, and even now some refuse to believe it," Koop said
later. "We sat up with some kids all night, but we never did a trache."[39]

Koop was reluctant to publish their results, for fear that other
surgeons would seek to follow and yet be less careful.[40] This curious
decision cannot have aided Deming's career, but she is lauded today
as one of the founders of pediatric anesthesia.[41] Calmes concludes
that "Dr. Deming laid the groundwork for the outstanding pediatric
anesthesia to follow her at the nation's first children's hospital."[42]

---

viii   Tracheostomy: an incision in the windpipe to facilitate breathing. The tracheostomy is
the hole; the procedure is called a tracheotomy. The short form "trache" is pronounced "trake."

Deming was concerned about her own health, and her mother was sick. In 1954 we find Koop seeking help from Ravdin, as Deming was speaking about moving elsewhere. Ravdin recommended that Koop get her a raise, which, in the event, Dripps declined to approve.[43] Deming left the Children's Hospital the following year, "to join her good friend Eugene Conner, M.D., at Philadelphia General Hospital."[44]

Koop later recorded his indebtedness to Margo Deming, "an utterly selfless person and one of the great workaholics of all time. She took an entire category of medicine that was not then acceptable and transformed it into a field with intellectual respect."[45]

Four decades later, after stepping down as Surgeon General, Koop wrote warmly to his former colleague. "I have thought so much about you in the past several years as I was writing my memoirs and then as I travel around and people recall incidents of the old Children's Hospital and even of HUP [the Hospital of the University of Pennsylvania] before that." What's more, Betty Koop has not forgotten Margo Deming's critical role in the birth of their first child. "You will remember that you took over and got her to the delivery room in time."[46]

Armed with the early techniques he and Deming had pioneered, Koop was able to make a rapid, dramatic leap in improving surgical survival rates for infants. "I lost a few patients," Koop later recalled, "but really, only a few. This built in me a great sense of outrage. Back then anytime you visited a hospital to do grand rounds or attend a mortality conference you'd find an anesthesia death for something as simple as a tonsillectomy, and the surgeons would act highly insulted if you called that an outrage. Which I frequently did."[47]

Koop later recalled that "one of his first arguments with Dr. Ravdin" was over his determination to operate on very young children. At the time, the custom was that "no child . . . was ever operated on electively until the age of three." Ravdin turned up one Sunday morning to find Koop "had operated on six infants under the age of four months on the previous morning and was going to send them home less than twenty-four hours after their operative procedure."

Ravdin "hit the ceiling," but was talked around as "all the things that we did in order to make the procedure safe" were explained.[48]

Meanwhile, Koop remained deeply concerned about his income. In these early days he was finding it hard to get enough work to pay his way. "I had been in practice for fourteen months before I cleared my office rent in any given month." The chief medical resident, then Andrew B. Hunt, a former medical school classmate, asked Koop to fix an inguinal hernia.[ix] Koop operated, and discharged the child the following morning. As the child was on his way home, Hunt called the referring physician, a Dr. S. Emlin Stokes—as it happened, brother of Penn pediatrics chair, Joseph Stokes. Emlin Stokes was upset. He was unable to provide the follow-up care that was needed. They should have kept the child for a further two weeks. Hunt assured him that no special follow-up care was needed. The next week, Stokes asked Koop if this was an exception, or could he do more? Stokes had a large practice and therefore a "large backlog" of infants needing surgery. "Very gingerly he tried me out on another one and then another one." Then he began to "unload his tremendous back log of hernias." Koop adds: "It is safe to say that without those hernias I would not only not have been able to support my family but it is entirely possible that I might have gotten so discouraged as to leave the developing field of pediatric surgery."[49]

Koop and Rappaport

As Koop was struggling to establish himself at the hospital, one incident stood out: his clash with Milton Rappaport, a smart and influential colleague who was also "huge." Koop greatly esteemed "Rapp," but the esteem was not returned. In fact, "he hated me." Matters came to a head in what Koop later called the "shoot out." There had been disagreement about a patient, and the case was slated for discussion at a case conference. Rappaport put it about that if Koop recommended surgery, "it is the end and Koop will go." In his

---

ix   Inguinal hernia: a bulge of the contents of the abdomen through a weak abdominal wall.

view it was a simple case of empyema,[x] to be treated by pulling out the pus with a needle. Koop suggested that Rappaport had misread the X-ray. The patient in fact had a congenital cyst. Up stood radiologist Dr. Bromer. "You know, Rapp, he's right." The following Monday morning the amphitheater was packed to watch Koop operate, and the dynamic within the hospital began to shift.[50]

Koop and his Trainees

Between 1946 and his retirement in 1981 Koop took on nearly fifty trainees, beginning with Doris Bender that first spring.[51]

Koop proved a striking supporter of women in the early days of pediatric surgery, at a time when there were very few female general surgeons.[52] From 1946 onwards, he took on a fresh resident every year, generally for a two-year period. Three of the first seven were women; there were five women in his first ten years: Doris Bender, his very first surgical resident, 1946–48; in 1949, the celebrated Rowena Spencer; then Mary Marlene Schwab-Jones, likely 1951–52; Gretchen Bieber (Wagner) from 1952; and from 1956, Louise Schnaufer.[53]

Koop and Ravdin shared an interesting exchange on the subject. In considering Gretchen Bieber, initially in December 1948, Koop wrote to Ravdin that "I . . . would like not to have two women at the same time under any circumstances." And he expressed concern that the program would become known as one that takes only women as trainees! Ravdin responded: "I can't have two females at a time either."[54]

Curiously, after Schnaufer in 1956, all Koop's trainees were men. Many years later, Lesli Ann Taylor, a fellow at the Children's Hospital after Koop's retirement (from 1988–1990), recalled joining a reunion of Koop fellows at an APSA conference in 1992. "After the presentations we gathered for a picture. . . . Dr. Koop pulled Dr. Schnaufer and I over to him, and put his arm around each of us, and said, 'I'm sorry that I didn't bring more women along,' or something to that effect."[55]

---

x   Koop defines empyema as "pus in the cavity that contains the lung."

Bender returned to the HUP, and Koop soon after asked Ravdin to release her to supervise her successor residents, Rowena Spencer and a Dr. Barker, during his summer vacation in 1948.[56]

Spencer (1922–2014) returned south to her native Louisiana, as the state's first female surgeon, where she spent many years on the faculty of the University of Louisiana Medical School.[57] She had come to Philadelphia after graduating from Hopkins in 1947, where she had also completed her internship. In a brief notice after her death in 2014, *Hopkins Medicine* notes that she was a student of surgeon-in-chief Alfred Blalock, who "only grudgingly accepted her presence in the department." Spencer credited Blalock's African American technician, the remarkable Vivien Thomas—who had only a high school education—with being "her mentor and most influential instructor in surgical techniques."[58]

Rowena Spencer "called all of her tiny patients 'my babies.' 'She was dedicated to her babies to the nth degree,' observed her nephew, retired Brig. Gen. Lewis Spencer Roach. 'She would fight for them like a tigress.'"[59] Somewhat curiously, given her later prominence in the profession, not least in the matter of conjoined twin separations (on which she wrote a textbook), Koop makes no mention of her in his memoir; they were evidently not close.[60] The significance she gave to her time at Hopkins may help explain that fact. Later Koop trainee Moritz Ziegler, who helped coordinate many gatherings for Koop alums, writes that "Rowena Spencer left quite a reputation at CHOP," but he never saw her at a Koop event.[61] She was not present at his retirement dinner.[62]

When asked about "the most satisfying part of her work, Spencer answered, 'Holding the babies. I love babies more than a mule can kick.'"[63]

Koop, Bishop, and Schnaufer

Harry Bishop (1921–2009) worked with Koop for a total of thirty-seven years.[64] On his death, Koop wrote that "Philadelphia and the surgical world lost a warrior and I lost a close friend and surgical partner when Harry Bishop died this week."[65] Another Dartmouth grad, Bishop had trained with Gross in Boston, so they had much in common. Koop recruited him in 1954, and Bishop worked with Koop until his retirement. Ziegler remembers him well, as he had the office next door. He was "a master surgical technician," though "seemed to personally avoid himself dealing with the complex patient if at all possible"—in other words, he was more risk averse than Koop. He was an energetic sailor, on several occasions inviting Koop and Schnaufer to join him in his boat in the Caribbean; he had named it *Heaven*. A family man, he was also known among his friends as a skilled amateur electrician and plumber![66] Bishop liked to take a nap in the afternoons and would station his secretary near the door to make sure he was not disturbed. He was also not above poking fun at Koop. Discussing the medals that bedecked the Surgeon General's uniform, he quipped "I don't know which store he goes to."[67] Unlike Schnaufer, Templeton, and some other colleagues, Bishop was not an evangelical Christian. "I think I will get to heaven as soon as they will, [but] I don't believe it the way they believe it."[68]

Louise Schnaufer (1925–2011) first joined the Children's Hospital as a resident in 1956, before spending more than a decade at Hopkins. In 1971 Koop invited her to return and serve as his "chief surgical assistant." She leaped at the chance, and would spend the rest of her long career at the hospital, adding to her remarkable surgical skills a pivotal social role within the hospital community, as den mother to the younger staff.[69] Ziegler recalls her as "the backbone of the surgical service" and "the busiest surgeon by far of the faculty."[70] She also became a close friend of the Koop family. Koop later recalled that "I don't think our kids knew she wasn't related to us until . . . they were fairly old."[71] She was also close to Erna Goulding. Like Goulding and Koop (and also trainee and later colleague Jack Templeton), Louise Schnaufer was a member of Tenth Presbyterian Church. But she kept her faith "pretty private," noted James A. O'Neill, Jr., Koop's successor as surgeon-in-chief (who served from 1981–1994).[72]

Bishop later reflected, "It's been a very close personal relationship and I've enjoyed knowing her. . . . We, as a group of people, got along extraordinarily well. Usually there's a lot of competitiveness, arguing back and forth amongst people who worked in the same institution, but we never had that." One reason, he suggested, was "Dr. Koop's ability to select the right people to work with him. With the group, not [just] with him, but with the group."[73]

Like Goulding, Schnaufer remained unmarried, and she threw her life into that of the institution and—again like Goulding—into the Koop household. O'Neill reflects that Schnaufer "was a very human person and taught people that you have to have a personal life as well."[74] She constantly encouraged others to spend time with their families. "She would say to the residents: 'Are you taking your wife out?' . . . something I didn't do. I was 'the taskmaster.' She'd throw them out of the hospital, make them go home, make them be with their families." She "set a human standard at CHOP . . . because people like me, and certainly Dr. Koop, were all business. There was nobody more fun than Louise!" The residents came to call her "Auntie Louise," and this even caught on with some of the patients' families. O'Neill recalls one parent calling to tell him "Oh, we love Dr. Schnaufer, we love Aunt Louise, my wife and I." A person of very small stature (Ziegler suggests four foot ten), she famously needed to stand on stools as she operated.

Her original recruitment is recorded in a laconic exchange between Koop and Ravdin in 1955. He asked Ravdin to approve Schnaufer and another resident. "These were the best of the applicants," Koop wrote, as he passed on the c.v.s. Next day, Ravdin responded, "They seem perfectly adequate."[75] Many years later, Koop reflected that "Louise had a surgical personality, which is being very inquisitive. . . . She was very much at home in the operating room surroundings" and "she had very remarkable manual dexterity."[76]

In 2014, three years after her death, the Children's Hospital would inaugurate the Louise Schnaufer Endowed Chair in Pediatric Surgery.

"It was not only a professional relationship, but it was a relationship of big friends," Bishop reflected.[77] Schnaufer herself kept a sailboat on the Chesapeake and would invite colleagues to sail with her. Nurse

Marie Melhuish, interviewed years later for her memories of Schnaufer, recalled the many times they went sailing. "We used to go usually every summer to . . . sail. . . . So it was a fun life." Asked "why do you think so many surgeons are into sailing?" Melhuish replied that they can afford it, and "I think it's because they're in control of this boat . . . they really are the captain of the ship."[78] She shared her insight into the social life of the hospital, and Schnaufer's special role. "I was pretty good friends with Louise. . . . For many years we would go out to dinner, we had tickets for the Walnut Street Theater for probably five or six years. . . . She would invite us to her house on the river down there in Maryland. A couple times a year three or four of us would go with her to her home on the river and just spend the weekend together and go antique shopping. She's a fun person to be with."

Then Koop and his brother-in-law George, together with Louise, decided to buy a boat together and keep it at Tortola in the British Virgin Islands. At his wife Betty's suggestion they came up with the name *Chicken George*—or "Chick'n'George"—a play on the character in the TV series *Roots* that was showing at the time. Then someone said, but what about Louise? So they named the dinghy *What about Louise?* "She's a good sailor," said Koop looking back. "Most of my sailing's been done in the Long Island Sound or Montauk Point. I think four or five times she's gone down in the winter for very hard sailing in the Grenadines."[79] Ziegler remembers that when Louise retired she gave her boat to one of the new residents, so "it continued into the legacy of the CHOP surgical family."[80]

At Christmas, Jack Templeton and his wife Pina (an anesthesiologist at the hospital) would host a party in their home. Lesli Ann Taylor recalls: "I was only there for two Christmases, but they had a tradition where Dr. Bishop would dress up as Santa Claus, and Dr. Schnaufer would dress up as Mrs. Claus at the Christmas party for the department, where the surgeons' children would come and they'd get to see Mr. and Mrs. Claus."[81]

Many surgeons who trained at the Children's Hospital "became future leaders in their field," as Michael Gauderer and Moritz Ziegler note in their Koop obituary for the *Journal of Pediatric Surgery*.[82]

Reflecting the quality of the relationships established at the hospital, "These men and women remained markedly true to Dr. Koop and the support, mentoring, and friendship was always reciprocated."[83] Ziegler himself went on to be Gross Professor of Surgery at Harvard; Michael W. L. Gauderer, to be Chief of Pediatric Surgery at Case Western Reserve University, in Cleveland, Ohio; and Martin Eichelberger, to be Professor of Surgery and Pediatrics at George Washington University and the Children's National Medical Center in Washington, DC.

While his manner among colleagues was businesslike, and could be brusque, Koop placed a great deal of emphasis on the quality of his relationships. When asked to list his criteria for hiring residents, he answered that he looked for young people "who would be trainable, compassionate, innovative, loyal and fun to work with."[84] This led to his concern for the well-being of their families. Work relationships would readily spill over into social activities and the growth of friendship.

Koop later reflected: "Harry does everything just a little differently than I do. Not a significant difference, but just a little differently. . . . Many chiefs . . . would say, 'I want you to do it my way.' [But] I never dictated to a competent surgeon that was trained differently than I was that he had to do it my way. I think that was one of the things that made our fellowship of surgeons sort of a happy circumstance."[85]

Koop's focus on fun and friendship went way back. Early in his time at the university hospital he had once dismissed the nurses so they could go to a dance, then "smuggle[d] them in and over the fence" when they got back after curfew. They thanked him, with a "ceremony where I lit Nightingale's lamp and received a cape."[86]

Yet his relations with the other pediatricians were never entirely cordial. Many years later Koop reflected that they "liked the prestige I brought to the hospital, but not the prestige I had within the hospital. I believe I never had the approval of some until I had succeeded as Surgeon General."[87]

Koop and Goulding

Erna Goulding (1921–2012) played a key role in several dimensions of Koop's life. She was a nurse whom he had first got to know at the HUP. He recruited her to the Children's Hospital, where she served in several capacities and spent the rest of her career. In 1961 she was head of the social service department. Later, as chief nursing officer, she was key to the establishment of the pioneering full-scale NICU[xi] in 1962.[88] Her role four years later in the development of a broader PICU[xii] is noted in the standard *Roger's Textbook of Pediatric Intensive Care*.[89]

It was Goulding who, in 1947, had encouraged him to hear Donald Grey Barnhouse's preaching. And she quickly became a close friend of the Koop family and a mainstay support to Betty Koop in her management of the household during her husband's absences—in the candid words of one friend, a "quasi nanny."[90] As close as an outsider could be, she became a "de facto member of our family."[91] At Goulding's memorial service in December, 2012, less than two months before his own father's passing, Koop's oldest son, Allen, paid this tribute: "She became the babysitter for the Koop children. Whenever our parents were out for the evening, or away for days, or even weeks. I think she always thought of herself as my babysitter. My sister Betsy . . . also thought of her as her second mother. Erna became a member of the Koop family, she was always around spending most weekends at our home in Penn Valley and driving with us to and from our summer vacation home in New Hampshire. She had a bedroom in our house. . . . Erna took the Koop kids everywhere, to the orchestra, the zoo, football games, dinner, the movies."[92] In retirement, she spent twenty-four years volunteering one day a week for the AIDS ministry Harvest USA, which had been spun off from Tenth Church.[93]

Almost as close to the family, in later years, was surgeon colleague Louise Schnaufer.[94]

---

xi   Neo-natal Intensive Care Unit
xii Pediatric Intensive Care Unit

Ravdin was much displeased when Koop poached Goulding from the University Hospital, news he heard while scrubbing in for his first case of the day. "He was infuriated," stamped his feet, and said: "I want to see Chick Koop succeed but not that much."[95] He sent him an angry note, to which a chastened Koop responded on January 31, 1947, "quite distressed to think that I have been the cause of any embarrassment to you." Koop explained that Goulding had been planning to move elsewhere in any case, and enclosed a copy of his letter to Goulding which fortunately began: "Marie Barnes has told me of your plans to leave the University Hospital and go back to Trenton."[96] Three days later, concerned that he had not heard back from his chief, he had copies of the letters in his pocket when he bumped into Ravdin at 4:00 a.m.—a time when his boss would often be doing his rounds, and Koop just happened to be in the hospital. As Koop approached him, "I heard Dr. Ravdin begin to explode before I was fifteen feet away from him and I said nothing except that I handed him the carbon copy of the letter." Ravdin found a light, read the letter, handed it back wordlessly to Koop, and went on his way. It finally did the trick. "Dr. Ravdin was never wrong but Dr. Ravdin was always prompt," Koop acidly observed. Ravdin mailed back Koop's original letter, with "Dear Chick, All is forgiven. Sincerely, I.S. Ravdin, M.D.," typed at the bottom of the page.[97]

Years later, in notes for an unwritten book on leadership, Koop recalled the Ravdin/Goulding incident under the heading: "Jealousy is the Enemy of Leadership," noting that Ravdin's support for his protégé "didn't extend to taking a nurse from HUP to CHOP."[98]

Koop and his Patients

At the time of Dr. Koop's retirement *Festschrift* [xiii] in 1981, former surgical trainees from the Children's Hospital characterized what they termed the "Koopian Method," an operative approach that included "do what you do best; simplify rather than complicate diagnostic

---

xiii   A celebratory academic publication.

and operative procedures. Do an even better operation for the hand-icapped child, as they deserve and need it. Maintain a sensitive respect for the patient and their family, and enter difficult and complicated procedures with both physical and mental preparation for the job at hand." Fastidious attention to organizational detail was a core trait of this "method."[99]

Ziegler summed up Koop's "pro-life" orientation by drawing a contrast with the practice of some other pediatric surgeons, including a team at Hopkins known to have treated a Down syndrome patient "by putting him off in the corner of the NICU and not giving him any nutrition and allowing the baby to die." In Koop's regime, "with Louise [Schnaufer] especially having been there at Hopkins, we would have treated that Down's patient completely differently and would have recommended operation immediately after birth. And we would have, quite frankly gone to any measure necessary to get that operation done. And what I mean by that is, if necessary, getting a court order to do the procedure. And in my experience, I did that several times at CHOP, getting a court order and never ever did I find that the courts denied my ability to proceed with an operation if we deemed it important and necessary, whether the baby was Down's or anything else that was associated with abnormality." Ziegler reflected that Koop's longtime partner, Harry Bishop, "would have probably continued in the same vein as that, but he would have done it with some reluctance and he would have also probably said a few things behind the scenes."[100]

"My secret—if you want to call it that," said Koop, "is to form a bond with your patients, to confide in them in the way you want them to confide in you, to respect them for being what they are: sensitive, decent, intelligent human beings." Which is why, Koop later reflected, he had never been sued for medical malpractice.[101] There could be no better example than that of Joe and Joyce Stein, parents of a patient, who became lifelong friends.

At Koop's retirement dinner, Joe Stein had this to say: "We have been proud to know Betty and Chick for more than twenty years. In fact so proud that at a dinner party in our home while extolling the accomplishments of Dr. Koop, Joyce once told the guests we had a son who died under his guidance. Now, that is some testimony. When we met Chick for the first time, it was a time of crisis. Our second child had just been born with anomalies that were incompatible with life. Chick, crewcut and no beard at that time, saw Andy that first evening and the next morning I delivered our son into the hands of Chick and that very special family of personnel who make up the body of Children's Hospital. Through periods of Chick's uncannily correct diagnoses and plans of action, through the days of hope and despair."[102]

Years later, Koop looked back on a fundamental fact that drove his approach to surgical practice: the incredible love parents have for their kids, handicapped or not. Of course, all parents are not the same. "I've had people . . . who'd say, 'Don't show me that child. I wanted a perfect child. I haven't got a perfect child. Don't show me that child.' And I have taken that child, and I've taken it away, and these things so troubled me that I founded an adoption agency and a child service agency to take care of those kids when I was first in pediatric practice, and it still exists under a different name."[103] But: "You can't look at a child and say, I feel so sorry for her family that I'm going to kill this kid. That's what it amounts to. . . . I don't think that that's our function."

He told this poignant story. "Well, I walked in, and the mother just bespoke poverty. I mean, she was a poor, woebegone thing. Her clothes didn't fit her. She had pins holding her coat together. And she had two little kids who were hanging onto her skirt with one hand and sucking their thumb with the other. And on the table in the examining room was a child who people would call a gork. He was obviously retarded. . . . The woman looked at me and pointed her finger at me as though she was scolding me, and she said, 'Before you examine my child, don't tell me that because he is what he is that he shouldn't be operated upon. Let me tell you that that child means more to me than these two normal children do. And I want everything done for him that you would do for these children.'" Back then, "it was the custom . . . in many of the hospitals in this country to take a child with Down syndrome and just put it in the corner."[104]

With the kids themselves, he would be practical, respectful, and relentlessly optimistic. "My method of dealing with children who have big, serious problems is not to talk to them as though they had big, serious problems but to talk to them in a very flip manner, as though it really weren't a terribly important thing and why should I expect to be given special this or special that to take care of it?" So, "let's say I have a child whose leg I removed because it was a useless extremity. It was five times the size and weight of a regular leg. . . . Well, my way of dealing with a child like that in my office was not to say, 'I was so sorry we had to take your leg off. I'm sorry you have to go through life with that burden.' I'd say, 'Here comes that one-legged kid again. Do you want some special attention? What are you looking for? Oh, by the way, when are you going to build that theater you wanted to build?'"[105]

Three Patient Vignettes

The Sweeneys

In 1965 Lucy Sweeney gave birth to a baby her doctors said would probably not survive, and "will certainly never lead a useful life."

"Koop examines the tiny Sweeney baby, inspects the cleft palate, the facial deformities, the haywire intestines. 'Your son has a lot of problems,' he finally tells the parents. 'But they're all repairable.'" Koop would go on to operate on Paul Sweeney no fewer than thirty-seven times, out of a total of fifty corrective surgeries.[106]

It's 1981, and teenage Paul Sweeney is being prepped for surgery. More than forty years later he told me the story. "I was sixteen, and knew I was in bad shape, and it was the first operation I had had without Dr. Koop, because by this time he was in our nation's capital serving as Surgeon General. Well, by the time the day for the surgery came, I was waiting for the call to go down to the operating room, and I was expecting to see the normal orderly I'd seen many, many times. But instead, in comes Dr. Koop, in his full Surgeon General's uniform, with his hat under his arm. And he asked if he could give me a ride to the operating room."[107]

The Kelsos

It's 1973. Back in 1971, Jane was eight years old and experiencing pain in her leg. Koop diagnosed her with a tumor. Despite surgery, the tumor returned two months later; and despite chemotherapy, it kept getting worse. "Koop was her constant visitor. They often read the Bible together or played board games." Jane's mother Karen tells Gregg Easterbrook, "I know she talked to Dr. Koop about some things she never talked to me about . . . it meant so much to her that she had a friendship and private secrets with a famous man." "Once," reports Easterbrook, "she soiled the hospital bed just as Koop was walking in. Thinking her daughter would be mortified, Karen Kelso tried to shoo the physician out of the room. Instead, Koop shooed her out. Listening at the door a moment later, the mother heard her daughter giggling happily. Looking in, she saw Koop cleaning up the mess, all the while making jokes to distract Jane's attention."

In the final year of Jane's life, Koop gives her mother his private number and his schedule so she can find him any time. He visits Jane at home one evening, shortly before her death. "Coming down from the little girl's room," Karen Kelso told Easterbrook, Koop "sat on the sofa and wept." Over and over he repeats in his tears, "Why is it taking her so long to die?" It takes two more long days. Karen later reflected, "Koop had buried his own child, so he knew some parts of life are unbearably awful."[108]

The Lingles

In July 1976, a Koop family friend, Carl Lingle, and his wife are expecting a baby. They had previously lost three in succession to miscarriage and stillbirth. She called her husband to tell him the baby was coming—this time, eleven weeks premature. Koop had told them to call him at any time. He had also referred the Lingles to the High-Risk Pregnancy Unit at the university hospital, and his colleague, Dr. Maria Papadopolus, who was in charge. Lingle called Koop, but he had just left town to give a lecture. He called Papadopolus. She was on vacation.

Lingle arrived at the hospital at the same time as the ambulance, and he prayed a silent prayer—"Lord, please don't give us another dead baby." Then a woman walked in wearing sweatshirt and jeans, and Lingle snapped, "Who are you?" (expecting her to be a psychologist or something such). "I am Maria Papadopolus—Dr. Koop called me back from vacation—he said you needed me." She held his wife's hand and said, "Don't worry, I will stay with you the whole time and when your baby is born I will take care of it." Lingle left the room for some fresh air, and as he walked down the hall he spied walking toward him "the trademark bowtie and beard of Dr. Koop." "I thought you were on your way to New Hampshire." Koop replied, "I will stay with you until we are sure that your baby does not need me." Twenty-one years later, Carl Lingle shared the story. He was introducing Koop, now retired as United States Surgeon General, at Messiah College in Mechanicsburg, Pennsylvania. The Lingles' little girl—born that day at 3 lb., 6 oz.—was a student in the audience.[109]

"What I Tell the Parents of a Dying Child"

At the close of his famous *Reader's Digest* article, Koop shares his practice with dying children in the Children's Hospital. He gives parents the choice of having the child stay in the hospital or at home. They usually want their child at home, but there may be special circumstances—such as younger children—that lead them to decide to leave the child in the hospital. In that case, Koop says, "I will be in the hospital when the child dies. This often means spending nights there, but this is of little importance when balanced against the comfort it gives to parents to know that their child hasn't been abandoned."[110]

Just two months after this article appeared, Koop's son David would die alone on a New Hampshire mountain.

The First NICU

Koop was determined to develop a specialized unit to care for very sick babies, but it was an uphill task—there were reasons why none of the nation's children's hospitals had them. Reviewing the problems,

Mark C. Rogers of Hopkins notes the financial challenge. "Reimbursement for time devoted to intensive care was virtually nonexistent" in the 1950s and 60s. Equally significant was the personnel challenge. "Nursing was the next barrier. . . . The skills, both technical and psychological, required to deal with critically ill and dying children comprise such a special set that it would be impossible to rotate nurses from regular wards in and out of the ICU."[111] In her review of the history, Briana Ralston writes that "CHOP publicly delineated particular characteristics" that were needed, including nurses "with no other responsibilities elsewhere in the hospital" who could "devote themselves to the expertise of this particular patient population," working with "the same patients over the course of the patient's stay."[112]

Despite its being a "very difficult sell to the hospital," Koop eventually succeeded in getting "a cadre of nurses assigned solely to the care of newborns with surgical conditions." He "emphasized that postoperative care was just as important as good surgical technique."[113]

There is some confusion as to when Koop's NICU was actually initiated. The statement on the website of the APSA that "In 1956 [Koop] helped open the first neonatal intensive care unit in the U.S. at CHOP with the assistance of a grant from the U.S. Public Health Service" conjoins two developments.[114] In that year Koop began keeping careful records of mortality and morbidity that would enable him to make the case for grant funding, and in the "forerunner to the formal infant intensive care unit" set aside three incubators "along a wall in one of the children's units." These beds were staffed by private duty nurses.[115]

Then on October 23, 1961, Koop reported to Rhoads:

> I thought you might like to know of the conclusion of my negotiations with the Children's Bureau in Washington and the Bureau of Maternal and Child Health, in Harrisburg. The Children's Bureau is providing Federal funds by a grant to the Commonwealth for the establishment of a pilot program to prove that neonatal surgery undertaken in a special unit where particular attention is given to surgical technique, anesthesia, nursing and ancillary care reduces mortality and morbidity. The contract will run for five years and the hospital will be paid a per diem. . . . The nurse to patient ratio is never to drop below 1:4. The

Children's Hospital has built a modern unit for such care in the middle of its Baby Ward and we should be under way by mid-November. Funds coming in about January 1.[116]

Ziegler and Gauderer write: "Dr. Koop began, with the help of federal support, the first intensive care unit devoted entirely to the care of the surgical neonate, a unit associated with such an improvement of neonatal morbidity and mortality that it ranks as his greatest early achievement."[117]

John J. Downes (1930–2021), for many years chief of anesthesiology at the hospital, notes that the unit initially had twelve beds. Looking back, Koop reminisced to his friend Bill Clatworthy: "The original neonatal unit in Philadelphia was purely surgical, and I ran it. . . . When the medical people who had not been enthusiastic at all about intensive care for newborns saw our success, they began to ask to have their babies admitted."[118] So there was soon the parallel development of a general pediatric intensive care unit, which Downs directed from 1967.[119] Downs notes that these two together "established the concept and proved the value of having a discrete area for providing special care to critically ill patients," with ramifications throughout the world of children's hospitals. "In January of 1967, the PICU [Pediatric Intensive Care Unit] opened and was immediately full. We cared for over 600 infants and children that first year."[120]

The Twin Surgeries

Years later, in a detailed unpublished history of the Rodriguez separation, Koop reflected on the challenge that twin separations present to surgeons—as when climbers feel the need to climb mountains: Because they're there![121]

It was Koop's operations to separate conjoined twins that first brought him into the public eye. Twin babies born with their bodies fused are still often referred to as "Siamese" twins, after Chang and Eng Bunker—a celebrated Siamese (Thai) pair who found fame as curiosities in the nineteenth century. The Bunkers married a pair of sisters and fathered a large number of children, before dying within hours of each other, still conjoined, at the age of sixty-two.[122]

Koop and his team would separate several pairs of twins, of which three became well-known, in 1957, 1974, and most dramatically in 1977.[123] "Separating Siamese twins really isn't nearly as difficult as a lot of other things that we do, but it's spectacular," he later reflected.[124]

"The most important thing about Siamese twins is the dress rehearsal. Because you get fifteen people doing something they're going to do once, and the most important thing is to get two living children, and it's very difficult to get two living children, and there are all kinds of problems that happen that you don't expect to happen. And if you go through with everybody that's going to be there, and you do it say, maybe three times, and say, 'If this happens, do this, if this happens, be sure you don't do this.' Again, you have to have a ringmaster . . . . But that's the kind of pre-planning that makes a successful surgery."[125]

Koop's twin surgeries would take him to a wedding, to a funeral at which he gave the eulogy, and to a play that focused on the searing ethical dilemma at the heart of his most challenging case. Of the three cases that hit the headlines, each would end with sadness. "All of my experiences with Siamese twins have been tragic ones. I have separated three sets with no difficulty surgically and in each instance lost one through no fault of my own and from problems unassociated with the separation."[126]

Pamela and Patrizia Schatz, October 6, 1957

These little girls, from Long Island, were nine days old when they arrived in surgery. Koop became an international sensation when he separated them. One had a weak heart, which actually stopped during the separation surgery before being massaged back to life; she would die nine years later during another surgery. But "the second thrived, and Koop has said that his most prized possession in life is a picture of himself with the twin on her wedding day."[127]

Clara and Altagracia Rodriguez, September 18, 1974

The Rodriguez girls were born in the Dominican Republic and separated at the age of thirteen months. They spent nearly three months in the NICU, making an excellent recovery before returning to their family. They shared a crib for the first few weeks so they would not be lonely.[128]

The family's trip to the United States was made possible by a local woman who had read of them, and raised funds through her church to bring them and their mother to Philadelphia. Their father stayed behind with three sons and two foster daughters. Neither the hospital nor the surgeons charged any fees.[129]

The precise moment of separation was 12:37 p.m. that day: "A time we'll all remember," observed Shirley Bonnem, the public relations director of the Children's Hospital, who was being kept busy. "It was a week before I had a solid night's sleep again—we were being called from all over the country at all hours of the day and night."[130] Altogether, "it took a total of 26 doctors and nurses eight hours to do the surgery. After an 82-day inpatient stay, the healthy twins returned to their home in the Dominican Republic."[131]

Two years later, Alta choked to death eating beans. A sorrowful Koop flew to the Dominican Republic and delivered the eulogy at her funeral.[132] To his great pleasure, Clara grew up, married, and in 1994 became the mother of a baby boy.

Koop was deeply affected by the whole experience of the Rodriguez surgery, not least how it thrust him into the global spotlight. The Rodriguez separation led to more than five thousand newspaper and magazine articles being written about him.[133] It led also to new relationships in the Dominican Republic. He developed a lasting friendship with the Rodriguez's parish priest. And he decided to write a book.

The friendship with Father Luis Quinn (or Lu, as Koop sometimes addresses him) continued over more than a decade and drew Koop into support for a water development project the priest was leading. Koop purchased pumps and other equipment in the United States, and his nonprofit Light of Life Foundation played a part. He was soon sending sermon tapes from his son Norman to the Father and a group of religious sisters who were also supportive of the Rodriguez family. Koop is first "Dr. Koop," then "Dr. Chic," and finally "Chic." Betty also is writing, and Louise Schnaufer. There is much banter. "Will be looking forward to Norman's tape," writes Father Lu, in fluent English but haphazard typing. "I hope he doesn't get into the

trouble I do. the sermon last week had some people up in arms. . . .
My love to Bette and Louise. Hasta pronto. . . ."[134] Then, "I had a dia-
logue with one of our Bishops the other day. . . . he proceeded to let
me know in no uncertain terms that . . . I was a flop—I have according to him been neglecting my catechetics. . . . I managed to hold my
cool and keep respectful but I was burning. . . . But then he should
know because in the Catholic Church bishops have a special in with
the Holy Spirit (at least the one that talks and directs bishops). . . . Do
you think I could get a job in Philadelphia building country roads or
canals you know something along my line???"[135]

Two sisters with a single heart, October 16, 1977

In both of the earlier twin separations we have discussed there was a
reasonable expectation that both babies would survive and flourish.
That was not so for the third. These little girls were conjoined at the
heart; only one could survive.[136] Left conjoined, they would soon both
die, since their one heart could not sustain the two bodies. "One child
had to be destroyed to save the other," Koop bluntly put it to the *Los
Angeles Times*.[137] "He adds, his expression grim: 'The nurses couldn't
believe it. Here was pro-life Koop about to kill a child.'" But: "As soon
as he examined the twins, Dr. Koop knew that had to be done."[138]

It was a remarkable case, later captured in a play by the writer
Donald Drake whose moving account in *Pennsylvania Magazine*
had been nominated for a Pulitzer.[139] To add complexity to the tragic
circumstances, the twins' grandfathers were both Orthodox rabbis.
They insisted on a lengthy Talmudic debate before they would sign
off on the surgery. It took eleven days. "I'm glad I had that time to get
ready," Koop would say. "I needed it to prepare emotionally." But it
was almost too late. "They were already in heart failure when I began
the surgery."[140]

Koop later said it took him not eleven days but less than ten minutes to decide to go ahead.[141] To him the ethics of the situation were
obvious. God had already made the choice that only one of the girls
could live, by bringing twins into the world with a single heart.
Koop's job was to ensure that the one who could live, did live.

"This was the hardest day of my professional life, but only because of what I had to do, not for moral reasons," Koop has said. "The morals of the situation were clear. We had to choose between two deaths, or one death and one life. We chose life."[142]

Koop himself clamped off the carotid artery that was feeding blood to the weaker baby, and she died immediately.

"'But,' Koop says quietly, 'The other one lived 47 days and died of hepatitis, probably contracted through a blood transfusion. That was a real low point for me.'"[143]

Donald Drake continues the story:

Since this ethic implies that all human life is equal—that one life is worth no more or less than another—would he consider it moral to kill Baby Girl A so that Baby Girl B could live?[xiv]. . . . Soon Rabbi Moshe Feinstein, dean of Tifereth Jerusalem seminary in New York City, was called in.

No less a man could be called upon to try to solve the dilemma confronting the parents of the twins. So Rabbi Feinstein agreed to consider the question.

Word spread through Children's Hospital that surgeons were planning to sacrifice one of the Siamese twins. . . .

The Catholic nurses, of whom there are many, were particularly concerned that the surgeons might be doing something that violated the teachings of their church. . . .

So the nurses were very disturbed by the prospects of beginning surgery in which it was already known beforehand that one of the patients would be taken out of the room dead. . . .

By 1:30 it was all over, and Dr. Koop flopped down on a seat in the operating room lounge to fill out the death certificate.

"Cause of death," he said, reading aloud to himself . . . "hypoxia (lack of oxygen) due to operation to separate Siamese twins. . . ."

Baby Girl B was back in the intensive care unit, alone this time, in stable but critical condition.

And the body of her sister was in a vehicle speeding home for burial before sundown.[144]

---

xiv   The twins' anonymity was maintained at the time; various press accounts assume they were girls.

Life at the Hospital

Skin Like Shoe Leather

A newborn orangutan in the Philadelphia Zoo had a congenital anomaly, one "common in children, not in orangutans," according to Josephine (Pina) Templeton, anesthesiologist wife of Koop's surgical colleague John Templeton.[145] The mother had abandoned two other babies, who had died. This time a vet at the zoo took the baby home and had it sleep with her for warmth. She was friendly with one of the hospital secretaries, whose boss Dr. George Peckham was at the time in charge of the neonatal ICU. Peckham was persuaded to admit the patient to Koop's service.

Ziegler, chief resident at the time, recalls that Michael Gauderer, the junior resident, was on call. "So he for whatever reason arranged for the baby to be sent to the hospital. And he had the baby in a bassinet just outside of newborn intensive care unit. . . . And Michael called me at home about probably 3 a.m. in the morning and said I've got to come and see this. So I came into the hospital and the orang was in a bassinet. And about that time, Mike got a page from Erna Goulding, who said: 'Get that animal out of this hospital!'"[146]

Meanwhile, Pina Templeton recalled, "the pediatric residents decided to have fun with the surgical residents, and called them and said, 'We have a new baby that has some strange anomalies. We don't know what they are, but I do think that he has an acute abdomen. . . . [H]e has reddish hair, and he has long, long fingers, and his toes look almost like fingers.' So you can imagine the poor, tired, surgical residents . . . the first looks at him and goes, 'He almost doesn't look human.'"[147]

Koop remembered how he heard of the new patient. He would hold a staff meeting at 6.30 in the morning at the McDonald's in the hospital atrium, and was lining up at the counter when Gauderer came alongside him and "began to tell me the pertinent events on my service since we last touched base. He came to the end of a long recitation of triumphs and problems with 'we admitted a 2-pounder a couple of hours ago with apparent intestinal obstruction. Vomiting since birth, has been offered glucose and can keep nothing down.' He droned on and on, and finally, 'the only thing unusual about this admission is that it's an orangutan.' Even at 6:30 in the morning it registered." Koop's response was: "Any complication [in the hospital] in the next months will be blamed on that orangutan."

But he relented. Two hours later, "with the agreement of a co-conspirator in the X-ray department," she was still in the ICU, and a diagnosis had been confirmed.[148]

Then the chief vet from the zoo turned up, and asked if Koop would operate, and the scene shifted to the veterinary hospital. "That afternoon in the company of Dr. Louise Schnaufer and Michael Gauderer, I had one of the most unusual experiences in surgery. Four cases were going on in the same operating room at one time. I don't recall two of the subjects, I think a dog and a sheep perhaps, but I know one was a parakeet, and then our patient the orangutan. The time came for the incision on the upper shaved abdomen. . . . I drew the knife across . . . and nothing happened. In a newborn baby, the skin is so easily cut, that the weight of the scalpel is sufficient pressure. . . . Not so in the baby orangutan. It was like cutting through your shoe." Further surgery was needed several days later, but the baby did well and was eventually moved to the Memphis Zoo. Someone suggested she be named Chick in honor of Koop, but it was pointed out that she was female. So, Chickie. Koop ended his recollection, "She has never stayed in touch."[149] Some years later, he took the initiative and went to visit.[150] As of this writing, Chickie is still alive and well.

Vodka from the Children's Hospital

"Do you know anything about Bison grass?" Koop asked his interviewer. "The name in Polish for a bison is Zubrowka and just like cats love catnip, bison love Zubrowka grass. It gets the name because they like it, and whether it's dry or fresh, it has a very pungent aroma. They make a kind of vodka in Poland called Zubrowka. So there's the same name for three things: vodka, grass, and a bison, all called Zubrowka."

He continued:

What you do is you get a bottle of the cheapest vodka you can get—in Poland it costs about 60 cents a quart—and put about a teaspoon full of sugar in that and one blade of grass. Put the top on. And after three or four days, you have a very pungent-flavored drink. . . . Well, I did a lot of things in Poland. We trained the surgeon-in-chief of the children's hospital in Krakow and then we trained the anesthesiologist. It so happened that the surgeon-in-chief, the guy we trained, was a boyhood friend of another guy in Krakow, Poland, who got to be the Pope, the one who just died. So I came back from Poland one time with a sheath of Zubrowka grass. I used that all up, and then I found that there was a nursery in Ridgefield, Connecticut, where you could buy Zubrowka grass, and so Louise, having a nursery right in her office,[xv] we had a pot with Zubrowka grass growing in it. So one Christmas I decided that that'd be a nice Christmas present, so I got a lot of bottles and cheap vodka and then I had a label made. I made it myself and then had it copied. It showed a bison, and it said 'Made with Zubrowka grass grown in the sun-drenched windows of the Children's Hospital of Philadelphia."[151]

Harry Bishop said it tasted awful.

A Special Patient

Koop was sick, "coming down with hepatitis but I didn't know it," and had vertigo, when a colleague "insisted I come in and do an appendectomy because he had promised the father I would." It was a request he knew he could not refuse. He dragged himself into the hospital, but ended up passing out and sleeping on the floor of the operating room while others did the work. Fortunately for all involved, the operation was a success, and Koop recovered from his hepatitis. The father of the patient, it emerged, was Philadelphia's mafia godfather.[152]

Professionalization

Koop's pivotal role in the development of pediatric surgery may best be summed up as one of "professionalization," in two distinct respects.

---

xv   Schnaufer's office was a veritable greenhouse.

In the previous chapter we reviewed his role in the achievement of professional recognition for the specialty—professionalization, as it were, on the outside.

What began in January of 1946, and occupied the thirty-five years following in Koop's life and within the Children's Hospital of Philadelphia, may best be seen as the process of professionalization on the inside. Koop pioneered the development within the institution of a culture of surgical practice that built on the vision of Ladd and Gross—and took it substantially further.

"During this time . . . he realized . . . his vision of a multispecialty surgical team of excellence . . . achieved by his recruitment of faculty that led and provided care in urology, cardiac surgery, neurosurgery, otolaryngology, plastic surgery, ophthalmology, and orthopedic surgery."[153]

In the early days of pediatric surgery, says Koop, "a pediatric surgeon was a surgeon of the skin and all of its contents. . . . When I first went to Children's Hospital, I would work in the skull, I would work on the head and the neck, I worked on the chest, in the belly, in the pelvis, and I worked on the extremities, and I did fractures. I did everything. I did cleft lips and cleft palates. I did various kinds of plastic surgery. I did reconstructive urologic surgery." Yet, "I knew that, from the point of view of physiology and pharmacology, I could provide those patients better care than an urologist or a plastic surgeon or a thoracic surgeon who dealt with adults. But I didn't think that, from a purely technical point of view, my results were as good as—when I did a cleft lip and a cleft palate, it was not as good as when [plastic surgeon] Andrew Ivy did it."[154]

Looking back, he outlined these two fundamentally different approaches. Koop's concept of pediatric surgery was that it required "two different kinds of skills"—the pediatric focus, "what Ladd and Gross contributed physiologically and philosophically," but "now in the hands of an anatomical specialist." It seems curious, looking back, but "there was a long time when it kind of hung in the balance whether you'd follow Great Ormond Street and Children's Hospital [Boston] or whether you'd go the Philadelphia way." Finally, "every single one of the adult surgical specialties has come to recognize the need for an anatomical specialty for children in their own realm. Child surgery in the Boston manner was understood as 'surgery of the skin and its entire contents.' For those of us trained in general surgery it was pure heaven."[155]

But there was a better way.

Koop first identified neurology and urology as fields where he needed to know more—and where the respective experts could be recruited on the same terms that Ravdin had originally recruited Koop: "You give up adult urology and you'll become the best pediatric urologist around. You give up adult neurosurgery, and you'll become the best pediatric neurosurgeon around." So he recruited them. The overlapping surgical and specialty establishments that dragged their combined heels for decades needed to be persuaded of one thing at a time, as also did Koop. "I set my mind to this task: to build the most comprehensive group of pediatric surgical subspecialists in sufficient depth so that no child who came to the oldest children's hospital in the land would ever have to be sent elsewhere for a surgical procedure. I accomplished my goal after more than 30 years and announced to the board of managers when I had 28 surgical subspecialists in nine divisions that included dentistry and oral surgery."[156] Looking back, Koop reflected, "I think that's the biggest contribution that I made."[157] It had been his "lifelong ambition," Koop told the *Los Angeles Times*, "to have the most competent group of pediatric surgeons in the country under one roof. It took me 33 years to do it."[158]

It's all there on his letterhead. On September 16, 1949, he alone is listed in the department of "Surgery of Infancy and Childhood." By October 15, 1980, "Pediatric Surgery" lists the names of thirty-one surgeons, spanning general surgery and seven specialist groups, in addition to that of the surgeon-in-chief.[159]

"Legendary" is how the *Journal of Pediatric Surgery* described his vision and his recruitment of a "multispecialty surgical team of excellence."[160] The evolution of the profession has essentially followed the model of the Children's Hospital of Philadelphia, which in turn followed the model inside Koop's head.

Retirement

"This is a very strange year for me," Koop wrote to his old friend Francis Schaeffer in late summer of 1980, "because I realize that on a yearly calendar basis, everything I do I am doing for the last time at the Children's Hospital." Schaeffer replied: "Chick your last paragraph touched me immensely. . . . This gave me some emotion and I can only say that I walk with you in prayer at this time."[161] To another old friend, Peter Paul Rickham, he declared, "There is no doubt about the fact that I really am a has-been in U.S. pediatric surgery because of the great tendency in the United States for younger people to rise to the top. . . . It is quite unlike the European system where age, experience, and judgment still count for something."[162] He later agreed with Rickham that the government appointment "would be a very nice way to handle the emotional problems I would have in leaving this institution after thirty-five years."[163]

Well before anyone—aside from the Koops and assorted Washington functionaries—knew he was being considered for Surgeon General, Koop's colleagues at the Children's Hospital were preparing for his retirement, originally scheduled for June of 1981.[164] As early as October 15, 1980, Harry Bishop shared their plan with Jonathan Rhoads. There would be an informal dinner on Sunday April 26, for current and former residents and out-of-town visitors; then, on April 27, a formal affair at the Union League Club, for 350 guests.[165]

Hospital chairman Richard D. Wood unveiled a newly commissioned portrait of Koop. "My shoes won't be hard to fill," Koop quipped to his chosen successor, handing a pair of baby shoes to Vanderbilt surgeon James A. O'Neill, who to general surprise and displeasure was an outsider. O'Neill did not find the going easy during his first years at the hospital, which had not hired a surgeon trained elsewhere for many years. But Koop "was wonderful," said O'Neill, and gave him a great deal of friendly advice—including a one-hour cassette tape of it, which he still had a quarter-century later![166]

Among international guests was the distinguished French pediatric surgeon Michel Carcassonne (1927–2001), who had prepared his own retirement gift a year earlier—by lobbying for Koop to receive the high French award of the *Légion d'honneur*.[xvi] After the presentation at the *Assemblée Nationale* on June 4, 1980, Carcassonne had hosted a dinner at the oldest restaurant in Paris, *La Tour d'argent*,[167] where they feasted on catfish, served with Porto; roast duckling; and strawberries with pistachio ice cream.[168]

Another European guest was Koop's old friend, German refugee Peter Paul Rickham (1917–2003).[169] He hailed Koop: After Ladd and Gross, "[o]f the second generation you undoubtedly have been the leader, you have done more than anyone in developing the science and art of pediatric surgery." And looking ahead to his confirmation as Surgeon General: "I cannot think of anybody more fit to carry this resounding title, and think of all the fun you will have writing orders on all the cigarette packets in the United States."[170]

Koop's March 1981 appointment as deputy assistant secretary for health truncated his final responsibilities in Philadelphia by several months. "My last operation" was "on the last Friday before I came to Washington."

That final day, he dipped his finger in soap, and "wrote on the glass wall of the operating room . . . the closing lines of T. S. Eliot's poem 'The Hollow Men.'" "This is the way the world ends/Not with a bang but a whimper."[171] A curious thought, perhaps, since his career as a pediatric surgeon was concluding with something much more akin to a thunderclap!

---

xvi   By coincidence, as we noted, an earlier American recipient of the *Légion d'honneur*, back in 1954, had been Koop's old friend, pastor and mentor Donald Grey Barnhouse. Barnhouse had worked in Europe in his early days, spoke fluent French, and he too had influential friends in France. See Chapter 2.

Part III
CAMPAIGNER

Everything he believes in, he believes in fiercely.
—STEPHEN C. GEORGE, *New Physician* magazine

Opposition to abortion has become such a distinguishing mark of American evangelicals that many are surprised to learn they made scant response when, on January 22, 1973, the Supreme Court declared that it a constitutional right.[1] *Most evangelicals at that time twinned abortion with contraception in their thinking and saw them both as "Catholic issues."*[2]

Three striking examples illustrate how late they came to the party.

First, in 1968, the benchmark evangelical magazine Christianity Today *convened a conference with the (evangelical) Christian Medical Society to discuss abortion and related matters.*[3] *The result was, in retrospect, astonishing: A consensus statement that fetal life "may have to be abandoned to maintain full and secure family life."*[4]

W. A. Criswell, former president of the Southern Baptist Convention and pastor of the huge First Baptist Church of Dallas, Texas, spoke for many evangelicals: "I have always felt that it was only after a child was born and had a separate life from its mother that it became an individual person, and it has always therefore seemed to me that what is best for the mother and for the future should be allowed."[5]

Second, the Chicago Declaration of Evangelical Social Concern, *which on November 25 of that pivotal year 1973 brought together a broad spectrum of representative leaders from the church and the academy to summon evangelicals to broader social engagement. It addressed issues such as racism and poverty but failed to make any mention of abortion.*[6]

Third, on the political front: Given the growing importance of abortion in Republican circles, it is stunning that, as historian Randall Balmer told me, "as late as August 22, 1980, when Reagan addressed 20,000 evangelicals in Dallas, Texas, he talks about creationism, he rails against the Internal Revenue Service for going after segregated institutions . . . but he does not once mention abortion."[7]

Koop had become friendly with his younger contemporary Harold O. J. Brown (1933–2007), who served for a period as assistant editor of Christianity Today,[i] and who with Koop's aid and encouragement went on to found the Christian Action Council in 1975.[8] We have already seen his first chance acquaintance with Francis Schaeffer (1912–1984), who would prove one of the most consequent American evangelical leaders of the late twentieth century, as he performed routine surgery on Schaeffer's daughter Priscilla in 1948. It would be their collaboration on the Whatever Happened to the Human Race? *movies on abortion and euthanasia in the late 1970s that made Koop a celebrity in socially conservative Republican circles, and finally led to his nomination as Surgeon General.*

Koop's relentless campaign against abortion and euthanasia in the 1970s offers a precursor to the series of campaigns that would absorb much of his energy in the following two decades—against smoking, against AIDS, to revitalize the Commissioned Corps, and, in what he dubbed his "final crusade," against obesity, with his nonprofit Shape up America!

---

i   It was Brown who penned the (unsigned) *Christianity Today* editorial when *Roe v. Wade* was handed down.

CHAPTER 6

Advocate for Life

C. Everett Koop . . . who taught evangelicals to hate abortion.

—Christianity Today obituary

Wheaton, 1973

Six months after the Supreme Court handed down its judgment *Roe v. Wade*, Koop found himself on the stage of American evangelicalism's most celebrated institution, Wheaton College in Illinois.[1]

The Koops' daughter Betsy was graduating that year, and the college had persuaded her celebrated surgeon dad to address the graduating class and receive the conventional honorary degree—in this case a Doctor of Humane Letters. But Koop's speech on June 4 of that year to the Class of '73 was anything but standard commencement fare, which he summed up as: "look up, live up, and lift up . . . the latter being accomplished by a firm grasp on one's boot straps." He started out by telling the graduates: "I do not intend to say these things."

The focus of the speech was on the impact of Roe, as he laid out an argument against abortion based on both reason and religion. "I hereby make a plea for the right of the unborn child to life."

"There are a number of episodes in the recent history of man of which we are all ashamed. Indeed we would act in an entirely different way were the opportunity given again. Yet at the time not only were these things legal, but they were accepted by the people and were even proved to be logical to the few who complained."

He continued: "Jews were considered to be non-persons in Nazi Germany. Indians were not thought to be persons in the United

States. The same Supreme Court . . . in the Dred Scott decision in 1857 declared Negros to be non-citizens. They would have been more honest if they had said non-people. Lieutenant Calley expressed the opinion that the Vietnamese were not human. And now the Supreme Court tells us that unborn babies are still not persons in our society.

Not only did Wheaton College fail to publish his speech; neither did anyone else.[2] But Koop had launched the evangelical pro-life movement.

He followed up the speech with two further strategic initiatives.

Koop had called on his hearers at Wheaton to take action, specifically political action. So two years later, on August 14, 1975, Koop and other evangelical leaders convened a meeting at Billy Graham's home in Minneapolis, to found the first national Protestant organization to oppose abortion, the Christian Action Council. The council would be led at first by his friend, theologian and seminary professor Harold O. J. Brown.[3] Graham's wife Ruth was among the luminaries listed as "founding sponsors," enabling Graham to give the movement patronage without his own direct participation, as were Schaeffer's wife, Edith, and celebrated evangelical speaker and writer Elisabeth Elliot.[4]

Despite these famous names, evangelicals at large had not enough interest in the matter to fund the project. Robert Case, Brown's successor as director, explained that "while the new council drew its distinguished members from the evangelical ranks, it drew its funding from the Ad Hoc Committee in Defense of Life, Inc. . . . a Roman Catholic creation."[5] In the end, Case was forced to resign. "I just can't support my family. No Protestants are willing to fund us." We find Koop in October of 1977 struggling to get funds in support, fearing that the organization will otherwise close.[6] Case was succeeded by another pastor, Curtis Young, a "protégé of Joe Brown's" at the seminary, who proved a more successful fundraiser and "took the organization to prominence."[7] Young led CAC into a focus on caring for pregnant women and the seeding of hundreds of "crisis pregnancy centers" around the nation.[8] Brown also brought onto the board another protégée, Melinda Delahoyde, who later served as chair, and then president. She remained close to him over many years.

The following year, Koop wrote his cri de coeur to fellow evangelicals, *The Right to Live; the Right to Die*, which sold 100,000 copies in its first year. "One Saturday in 1976," he later recalled, "we'd just taken three premature babies, all of whom had something incompatible with life, corrected it and given them a seventy-year life expectancy. . . . Yet infants like them, *with nothing wrong with them physically*, were being aborted all over the city the same day. . . . I went home and wrote *The Right to Live; The Right to Die* in a day. After that, I could never turn back."[9]

The book takes its departure from the Wheaton address, exploring its argument at greater depth. Yet to Koop's considerable annoyance—and in illustration of the evangelical situation—the book was not as widely welcomed as he had expected. *Christianity Today*, house journal of evangelicalism, did not even review it, a slight that Koop did not leave unremarked. He wrote in barbed terms to the editor, Harold Lindsell, reminding him that "we share space on the letterhead of the Christian Action Council in Washington DC." And he concluded: "I write at this time to suggest that it should have more interest to your readers than a review of Jeanne Dixon's book subtitled, *How Astrology Can Help You Find Your Place in God's Plan*." There is no record of any response from Lindsell.[10]

It was clear to Koop that even the prestigious platform of the Wheaton commencement, and a book issued by a leading evangelical press (Tyndale House), were not sufficient to gain evangelical attention. It would not be long before opportunity arose to seize more powerful megaphones.

The Ladd Speech

Meanwhile, Koop had been awarded the Ladd Gold Medal, the highest honor in pediatric surgery, which offered him a further platform, at the 1976 conference of the AAP. Awardees typically use their acceptance speeches to share surgical research, though in October 1976, Koop's mind was elsewhere. In the faded grandeur of Chicago's

Palmer House Hotel, he warmed up his audience by sharing possible titles for the speech that he had considered and discarded.

"The Camel's Nose is in the Tent," perhaps? What camel's nose? "[The] thin edge of the wedge in reference to euthanasia." He had their attention. What about, "Dominoes to Dachau"? Not even that will capture the "dynamic situation which can accelerate month by month until the progress of our downhill momentum cannot be stopped." So to his final choice: "The Subtle, Slippery Slide to Auschwitz." And, in dramatic form, the self-same argument, from Wheaton, and *The Right to Live; The Right to Die*. Abortion leads to infanticide leads to euthanasia, and we're already slipping.

The fundamental issue, he continued, was best framed by Raymond S. Duff and A. G. M. Campbell, in their celebrated and remarkably candid 1973 *New England Journal of Medicine* article, "Moral and Ethical Dilemmas in the Special-Care Nursery," where they let the cat out of the bag.[11] Babies born with congenital malformations would often die soon after birth; they would die because that was what had been decided.

"CEK was in his moral outrage persona that day," recalled Ziegler, "to the point that the pediatric surgical community in aggregate were insulted by his attack on those not holding to the same Koopian philosophy about preserving life." There was polite applause, and the crowd melted away.[12] And, despite Koop's having authored hundreds of professional articles, the text of this speech found publication only in a journal with an avowed pro-life orientation, *The Human Life Review*, the following year.[13]

Turning the Evangelical Tide: Koop, Brown, and Schaeffer

Koop's crusade against abortion is best understood in the context of friendships he had developed with two other highly influential evangelicals, Harold O. J. Brown (1933–2007), and Francis A. Schaeffer (1912–1984). As Allan Carlson, head of the conservative Howard Center, wrote after Koop's death, "These three men made opposition to abortion a defining characteristic of late twentieth-century Evangelicalism."[14]

Brown and Koop had first met at a conference in New Orleans in 1975, where Koop was sharing another iteration of his Wheaton speech.[15] As we saw, Koop had first met the Schaeffer family as far back as 1948, when he treated their daughter, Priscilla. By coincidence, it was also through Priscilla that Brown first met the Schaeffers. She was walking by the lake in Geneva, Switzerland, in 1959, when she fell into conversation with another young woman, who had lost her way. It was Brown's sister, Judy, then a student at the University of Lausanne. Priscilla invited her to spend the weekend with her family at their chalet in the village of Huemoz, where Schaeffer had built an evangelical religious community called L'Abri.[i] The weekend "would change Judy's life," as her discussions with Schaeffer "led to her reconnecting with the Christian faith."

Judy told Schaeffer, "You need to meet my brother. He's in seminary. I think you and he believe the same things." Schaeffer made a dismissive remark when he learned that "seminary" was actually Harvard. But after Brown visited L'Abri for the first time in 1961 he and Schaeffer became close.[16]

Carl F. H. Henry (1913–2003), dean of midcentury evangelical theologians and founding editor of the house journal *Christianity Today*, said Brown was the smartest man he had ever met.[17] Henry and Koop were friends, and it was Koop who persuaded Henry over dinner in his home, likely in February of 1970, to take a stand against abortion.[18] But Henry's approach remained more flexible, and in 1979 we find Koop tackling him for permitting abortion in cases of rape and "exceptional deformity."[19]

Brown offered theological heft to Koop's thinking on the issue of human life. Indeed, it has been claimed that it was Brown who convinced Koop not to permit "Christian compassion" in "hard cases," but instead to take an "absolute stand," an argument Koop would

---

i L'Abri is French for "shelter" or "refuge." Begun by the Schaeffers in 1955, the organization continues, now in five chalets, still centered at Huemoz in the Swiss canton of Vaud, with several other centers around the world. See labri.org.

then press on Henry.[20] Brown was no more a hostage to garden variety "social conservative" attitudes than Koop proved to be in office.
He shocked Robert Case by telling him that, "if it would save lives,
save women, high school kids, from having abortions, he would
hand out rubbers in every high school in Northern Virginia. And it
absolutely flabbergasted me that an evangelical would say 'I would
basically promote sexual intercourse among high school kids, if they
didn't have babies, if we could save the babies.' I had to be schooled
by Brown to understand that kind of realpolitik."[21]

Time magazine paints an engaging picture of Schaeffer as "Missionary to intellectuals," and community life in Huemoz in Switzerland. It captures the Schaeffers' story. Originally dispatched by
their small and very conservative denomination to spread the gospel
in post-War Europe, in 1949 the Schaeffers had established a "small
Protestant oasis in the solid, stolid Roman Catholic bishopric of
Valais," in the small town of Champéry. As the *Time* writer puts it,
they "attracted too many adults who were ripe for churching;" and
the cantonal government forced them to relocate. So they moved a
few miles to the neighboring (predominantly Protestant) canton of
Vaud. Since then, they had turned the thirteen-room Swiss chalet
into "one of the most unusual missions in the Western world."

> Each weekend the Schaeffers are overrun by a crowd of young men and
> women mostly from the universities—painters, writers, actors, singers,
> dancers and beatniks—professing every shade of belief and disbelief.
> There are existentialists and Catholics, Protestants, Jews and left-wing
> atheists; the 20-odd guests this week include an Oxford don, an engi-
> neer from El Salvador, a ballet dancer and an opera singer. . . . Sandy-
> haired, sad-faced Francis Schaeffer, 47, and his handsome, mission-
> raised wife, Edith, 41, call their house L'Abri. . . . The talk may begin
> with any subject, from skiing to spaceflight; Presbyterian Schaeffer,
> Bible in hand, trades dialectic with the best of them, as the air grows
> blue with cigarette smoke.[22]

After his initial encounter with Priscilla and Edith, Koop and Betty
had developed a growing friendship with the Schaeffers, and Koop

helped with medical care for their children, especially son Frank[ii] who had had polio.

"Francis Schaeffer and I had been through a lot together, and he had become a strong friend, although our paths had not crossed for about fifteen years," Koop writes in his memoir. Then suddenly, in the mid-70s, those paths did cross. Koop was lecturing to a group of theological students at Canada's York University when a member of the audience pointed out that Schaeffer was speaking elsewhere on campus—and suggested that perhaps the two should collaborate. Koop made his way over after his session was done. "He spotted me walking down the center aisle and leaned down from the platform so that we could embrace. I repeated what the student said and proposed that we get together on my next trip to Switzerland. Little did I realize that I had taken the first steps on the path to Washington."[23]

Soon after, Koop heard from one of Schaeffer's assistants. "The Schaeffers are most anxious to have you here. . . . They very much enjoyed their time with you in Toronto." A two-day visit was arranged for June of 1977.[24]

Whatever Happened to the Human Race?

Schaeffer's son, writer Frank Schaeffer, who survived both polio and his English boarding school, has moved on from the set of religious and political commitments that characterized his early adult life, and the movie project that occupied Koop and his famous father for several years. He has written extensively of his disenchantment with his parents' values and beliefs, and his embarrassment as he looks back at the role he played in helping to promote them.[25] But he retains a fond regard for Koop, with whom he was still in touch many years later, and a vivid memory of that evening when Koop first arrived at Huemoz.

Frank was living with his young wife and little girl in a basement apartment in one of the chalets. When Koop arrived, he joined them

---

ii Frank Schaeffer went by Franky as a child and when he worked on the movie series with Koop. He now goes by Frank.

for the evening, and together they brainstormed the project that would become *Whatever Happened to the Human Race?*, a five-part documentary movie series, with accompanying book.

Frank had just finished working with his father on an earlier project, the book and accompanying documentary series, *How Should We Then Live?*[26] He recalled to me that when Koop saw these movies he had decided to reach out to Frank. "He met with me, because I had produced the series. And he said, you know, the next thing you want to do is to take on this issue alone, the life issue. . . . Chick was very involved, to the extent that he was already working with Roman Catholic bishops and others after *Roe v. Wade* . . . . And essentially, he was the person who suggested to dad and I, that we do a whole series of subjects." In fact, "Chick first suggested I do a series with him. And I said, Well, that's going to be tough to do because no one's heard of you in the circles that we're moving in, in terms of Francis Schaeffer's followers and people who are reading his books. So in the end, that became a joint project that I produced."[27]

In Koop's words, "Late that evening we sat in front of his fireplace and scribbled down the scenario for five motion pictures and the outline for a book. . . . Together, the Schaeffers—father and son—and I determined to awaken the evangelical world—and anyone else who would listen—to the Christian imperative to do something to reverse the perilous realignment of American values on these life-and-death issues."[28]

When they began to make the movies, Frank spent a total of six months working with Koop at the Children's Hospital. He stayed at a hotel nearby and scrubbed in with him in the operating room. They would review takes of the films as they progressed, and they would talk. In reflecting on how Koop had come to his pro-life position, Frank said to me, "I don't think it was a theological view at all." Koop would say: "Look, this is a 26-week-old fetus that has a chance to survive. And we'd go out, and he would walk me down across the street to the pathology lab of the Penn State Hospital . . . and then look, you know, right here in the morgue. Here's one that was aborted of exactly the same age for fetal anomalies and so forth. Look, can you see any difference? And, you know, it was basically nothing to do with the big theological position of when babies have souls or the Bible says this or God says that."[29]

The first in the series is titled *The Abortion of the Human Race* and opens with Koop at work at the Children's Hospital arranging for the emergency treatment of a newborn baby. Then he turns to speak to camera. Few people would kill a newborn. "But would you have killed it a minute before that? Or a minute before that? Or a minute before that? Or a minute before that? You can see what I'm getting at."

The series is punctuated with unforgettable images. One thousand life-size baby dolls float in the Dead Sea, as Koop intones that this was the site of Sodom and Gomorrah, Old Testament cities notorious for their evil.[30] A factory production line, in which imperfect dolls are mechanically discarded. A family picnic with young and old sitting at a table in a meadow of wild flowers. Then the elderly family members eerily disappear. A cartoon sequence in which the nine robed justices of the Supreme Court dance as they sing "Anything Goes."

Brown recalled the impact of the series. "Shown in churches, schools, and homes around the country, [the films] so thoroughly aroused viewers that the term evangelical has come to be synonymous with anti-abortion."[31] James Risen and Judy L. Thomas in their history of "the American abortion war" *Wrath of Angels* put it simply: "Their lecture tour became the event that finally got fundamentalists engaged on an issue that had previously been seen as an exclusively Catholic concern."[32]

As with his previous volume, Koop mailed copies of the *Whatever Happened to the Human Race?* book willy-nilly to friends and professional contacts. A choice reply was received from one Frank E. Ehrlich, MD, of Seattle, Washington. "Enclosed is the copy of your recent book. . . . I am not certain as to why a copy of this book was sent to me. It serves as a reminder that a man having established himself with great brilliance in one career should not attempt to step beyond the limits of that brilliance."[33]

The film-and-book tour was noticed by the *New York Times* of September 29, 1979, under the title, "Two Fundamentalists[iii] Crusade against Abortion in 20 Cities."[34] Nadine Brozan writes: "The mood seems aimed at arousing evangelical Christians to action in a cause that in the past has been associated in the public mind with the Roman Catholic Church." Schaeffer and Koop are "not part of the mainstream right to life movement."

Brozan watched the films in a two-day event in the Felt Forum at Madison Square Garden in New York City. Around 1,000 people attended, mostly paying $28, although students were admitted free of charge. The report's style is distinctly arch. Writing of Schaeffer, Ms. Brozan notes that "his followers call him 'doctor' because of an honorary title" conferred by a theological seminary. Koop is described (inaccurately) as "surgeon in chief of the Koop Surgical Center" at the Children's Hospital. When she asked him why he has become "so involved with this mission," he replied, "One day when I was operating on three newborn babies, I realized that less than 100 feet away in the Hospital of the University of Pennsylvania, they were destroying babies. Knowing what we can do with abnormal children, to know that we're destroying one million normal babies a year just drives me crazy."

The significance of the effort is well summarized by Richard Meagher in his essay on the Republican "new right:" "Abortion originally was almost the sole concern of Catholic groups until the anti-abortion book and video production of theologian Francis Schaeffer and future Surgeon General C. Everett Koop helped bring the issue to evangelicals in the late 1970s."[35]

Fast forward to Koop's take on the pro-life movement after nearly nine years in public office, during much of that time being criticized by a slew of pro-life leaders for his failure to address abortion. At a forum back at evangelical Wheaton College he reflected on his long-time opposition to abortion, under the title, "Ethics of Activism,

---

iii   We discussed the lazy journalistic use of "fundamentalist" for every conservative Protestant in the foreword. Despite the misnomer, the *Times* report captures the message and its context rather well.

Protest, and Dissent." He began, "If I seem critical" of the pro-life movement, "put the shoe on only if it fits."

First off, he clarified—as indeed Frank Schaeffer suggested—that "my opposition to abortion came, not from my theology—certainly not from any political philosophy—but from my medical practice."[36] Koop's own thinking about abortion had developed over many years. In an extensive *Los Angeles Times Magazine* profile published in 1986, Marlene Cimons writes, "even Koop's detractors have begun to realize that his intense feelings on abortion were not lifted verbatim from a right wing primer. Rather, Koop seems to have developed them—and his views on handicapped children—over more than three decades as a pioneer in children's surgery."[37]

Koop continued: "I think the pro-life movement—at times it may be better to call it the anti-abortion movement—has made two critical mistakes. The first mistake has been the sanctioning of extremists," by which he means the shrill rhetoric of those who will not accept any kind of compromise. For example, "the Baby Doe controversy made me see the self-defeating quality of some pro-lifers' absolutist frame of mind—their all-or-nothing mentality." He had been denounced for writing regulations that would offer protection to 97 percent. "Certain pro-life leaders wanted 100% or nothing. I thought 97% was better than risking getting nothing. In a pluralist society, political compromise does not equal ethical compromise."[38] So, why don't "anti-abortion groups and abortion-rights activist[s], while agreeing to disagree on the right to an abortion . . . work together to reduce the number of unwanted pregnancies. A small step, but also a big one," he asked.

"The second wrong turn taken by the pro-life movement was to become worldly. . . . The anti-abortion movement has made a very large tactical error for the last twenty years by concentrating on legal and constitutional issues, when the issue is really moral or ethical. . . . The pro-life movement, maybe even the evangelical church, began to act like just on more political group. . . . Abortion is a moral issue, not a political one." He concluded: "If there is a future for the pro-life movement, it will be one of spiritual ministry, of moral suasion, and of practical results."[39] Yet he continued to be quietly active on the pro-life front. As Richard Doerflinger, over many years the Catholic bishops' key architect of pro-life policy, told me: "Going through the old material reminded me how active he was, and how often he worked with my office, on pro-life issues after completing his term as Surgeon General."[40]

Koop's final impact on the evangelical perspective on abortion was remarkable, though as *The New Republic* notes in its perceptive obituary, "even before taking office Koop's views diverged from the radical conservative [*sic*] of the day. Koop had no interest in using abortion as a political wedge issue. His anti-abortion activity was not part of a broader political agenda. . . . Koop worked against abortion in the same spirit that he worked with MAP International—a Third World medical relief agency—or with Philadelphia's Evangelical Family and Child Service.[41] Koop distrusted the right-wing anti-abortion lobbies. 'He was really suspicious of ideology,' [Harold O.J.] Brown explained, 'so where you have a political ideology that is being presented as a sort of necessary consequence of a theological position he was very suspicious.'"[42]

Another Commencement

Back from filmmaking, and in between trips to hawk the series around the planet, Koop was on a roll. Invited to give the commencement address at the Philadelphia College of Osteopathic Medicine, on June 3 of 1979, he once again departed from the tried-and-true formula of "look up, live up, and lift up." This time he must have left a lot of young people scratching their heads. Without a trigger warning, he projected himself twenty years into the future: "I consider it a privilege,—more than that,—an almost supernatural gift to be able to address the class of 1999. I will say what I should have said by way of warning twenty years ago."

By 1999, the world had undergone dramatic, indeed apocalyptic, changes. Koop looks back on his 1973 Wheaton speech, finally published in the *Human Life Review*. "I don't think I was responsible for the police smashing their presses in 1982, but who knows? Wheaton only lasted five years longer. . . . Some of you may remember that I brashly sued Planned Parenthood because they had not planned a single parenthood in years."

Then he turns to the Supreme Court, whose approval of voluntary euthanasia had "led to the compulsory euthanasia decision . . . in 1995 for the infirm, the senile, and finally for those over eighty who failed the comprehensive test for longevity. I am eighty-two and a little more efficient this year than I was at eighty-one a year ago, but they don't think so."

He concludes: "But I do have the last laugh. You see, I got my notice to report to the Suicide Center before June 30th. If I don't, you know the consequences. I will be taken to Byberry,—that was a hospital for the insane when I was your age. There I will undergo the demise provided by the compulsory euthanasia rule. I hope it is quick and that I am not experimented upon. However, if my Christian faith is what I think it is, I will be in heaven soon."[43]

To Washington

Driven by his outrage over the maltreatment of handicapped newborns, and his fears that Roe, by "de-humanizing" human life, would lead to infanticide and then the killing of the sick and the elderly, Koop had sprung his abortion crusade. That same sense of outrage over threats to human life would power his years in the Surgeon General's office, eclipsing bureaucratic and political efforts to silence him or sway him. To which we now turn.

Part IV
SURGEON GENERAL

I can remember a debate in Ed Meese's office, between Senator Hatfield and [Senator] Jesse Helms. And the Reagan White House began to understand the Surgeon General's deeper understanding of what pro-life really was, it wasn't just before birth, it was after birth too.

—THOMAS GETMAN, Hatfield staffer, interview

The city that worships at the gray altar of ambiguity found there was room for a man of black and white.

—MARGARET CARLSON, *Time* magazine

This is not the man the right wing thought it was getting.

–*Mademoiselle* magazine

He basically was recreating the role of Surgeon General.

—ADMIRAL EDWARD D. MARTIN, chief of staff,
interview with Fitzhugh Mullan

In the November, 1980 election former actor and California governor Ronald Reagan swept up 489 of the 538 electoral votes, and 50.7 percent of the popular vote, turning Jimmy Carter into a one-term occupant of the Oval Office.

We have followed the shift of evangelical Christians into a pro-life stance during the course of the 1970s, a radical move in which Koop played a leading role. In parallel, the Republican Party was being reshaped by a growing focus on social issues, of which abortion was one, as operatives like Paul Weyrich worked to increase support for the party from Christians, particularly conservative Protestants.[1] *The overlapping terms "New Right" and "Christian/Religious Right" have been used to describe the fruit of this process, the transition from Nixon's "silent majority" to the Jerry Falwell-led coalition, the Moral Majority, founded in 1979. As Daniel K. Williams notes in his author-itative* God's Own Party: The Making of the Christian Right, *religious broadcaster Pat Robertson summed up evangelical sentiment in his declaration, that same year, that "We have together, with the Protestants and the Catholics, enough votes to run the country." More specifically, "Evangelical leaders such as Jerry Falwell and Pat Robertson saw that conservative Christians had the prominence to . . . force the Republican Party to begin paying attention to evangelicals' stances on abortion, gay rights, and the ERA."[iv] They "transformed these single-issue campaigns into a comprehensive political agenda that they made part of the Republican Party platform."[2] And they succeeded. "The rest is history," writes Richard Meagher; "the Moral Majority . . . and other religious associations helped deliver the evangelical vote to Reagan and the GOP. . . . The New Right electoral strategy—paying attention to single issues, especially social ones—became standard operating procedure for the GOP."[3]*

This was the party that brought Reagan to power in the 1980 presidential election, though many would be disappointed with the administration that resulted. Immediately after the election doubts were already being expressed among conservative Republicans as to whether moderates, including major figures from the Ford administration, would dominate the government. "The American people didn't vote for moderation," said John T. Dolan, executive director of the National Conservative Political Action Committee. In the event, religious conservatives were "denied all of the key appointments in the administration," so for Koop to be picked as Surgeon General was "a plum for the Christian Right."[4] As William Martin notes in another narrative of the religious right, With God on Our Side, *"The expectation that Koop would launch a crusade against abortion was shared by both his supporters and his critics, with good reason."[5]*

John D. Lofton, writing in activist Richard Viguerie's Conservative Digest, *confessed that "There are even moments when I wonder how much of a hardcore Reaganite Reagan is."[6] As an insider told me, the Reagan White House that resulted was "a house divided," with top appointees drawn from both moderate and conservative wings. As we*

---

iv The federal Equal Rights Amendment.

see in our discussion of AIDS policy, even the social conservatives were not all of one mind.

The Reagan who puzzled Lofton back in the fall of 1980 has proved something of an enigma to historians since. Even Edmund Morris, his authorized biographer, found unprecedented access to the President and his diaries "was of little use, since Reagan devoted most of their conversations to tired anecdotes, tall tales and evasions." Morris's "biography," Dutch, ended up a "partly fictionalized account narrated by an imaginary contemporary of the former President," which historians as well as Reagan fans see as an embarrassment. It was wryly deemed "a book unique in the annals of serious biography" by the New York Times.[7]

It has been conventional to discount the significance of Reagan's own religious convictions, but though they were unconventional they were not simply a political ploy. Paul Kengor's God and Reagan: A Spiritual Life *explores his religious childhood and documents the manner in which his political speeches were speckled with religious references, which had great resonance with evangelical voters.*[8]

The origins of the "Christian Right" lie not in abortion, on which as we have noted most evangelical leaders were essentially disengaged at the time of Roe. One major factor lay in controversy over efforts to deny certain religious institutions tax exemption, notably the segregationist Bob Jones University. In Bad Faith: Race and the Rise of the Religious Right *Randall Balmer quotes conservative leader Grover Norquist: "The religious right . . . . Started in '77 or '78 with the Carter administration's attack on Christian schools and radio stations." And another, Richard Viguerie: The IRS action "kicked a sleeping dog. . . . It was the episode that ignited the religious right's involvement in real politics."*[9] *Balmer traces the growing effort by conservative Republicans to use abortion to their political advantage in the 1978 mid-term elections and after; see his Chapter 7. In* God's Own Party, *Williams writes: "The GOP was a minority party in the 1970s. In order to win, Republicans had to siphon votes from the Democrats, and the Republicans' political strategists believed that a shift to the right on social issues would be the easiest way to do that. . . . But what began as a temporary political ploy proved irreversible, and the party found itself increasingly controlled by the Christian Right."*[10]

The Reagan administration's selection of America's most famous pro-life physician for the largely symbolic job of Surgeon General was politically adroit, since it pleased the many pro-life groups, as well as broader social conservative networks, while risking little. Koop seems not to have recognized the political dynamic, and perhaps he never did. For him, it was the start of a whole new career in public health, and a career he was beginning at the very top. So he felt free to step away from the abortion agenda, and while this did not please his pro-life backers, the administration as a whole seems not to have cared.

When Koop finally took the oath of office on November 17, 1981, after nine months of intense, personally distressing, and very public, controversy, he inherited a job that was barely there.[11] What had once been the top federal position in medicine and bioscience had been whittled down into a role so minor that during President Clinton's second term he never troubled to appoint anyone to play it.[12] As a recent history of Surgeons General puts it, the office "has been sinking for more than half a century." The tenth Surgeon General, William H. Stewart, in office 1965–69, "was stripped of his oversight of 150 federal programs, 38,000 people, and a $2 billion budget, and reduced to a glorified health educator."[13]

Then it got worse. Three weeks before Koop took the oath of office, the system of marine hospitals that had originally birthed the office of Surgeon General, and were staffed by the Public Health Service Commissioned Corps, were shut down or passed to other agencies, victims of the incoming administration's cost-cutting agenda.[14] Then the budget knives were out for the six thousand members of the Commissioned Corps that remained.

Koop walked into a job that mattered little, and made it matter very much indeed. Helped, ironically, by all the controversy—which focused on his lack of qualifications in public health, thought it was powered by his very prominent views on abortion—a man known merely in surgical and religious circles was now well-known to the readers of the *New York Times*. Though not initially a popular one, he had already become a public figure.

In the following eight chapters we look, first, at the confirmation controversy and Koop's re-engineering of himself for his new role. *Welcome to Washington* sets the scene for what comes next. *Bully Pulpit*[v] gives an overview of Koop's time in office as Surgeon General, his routine efforts, and some of the keys to his success—as deputy assistant secretary for health, the post he was appointed to in tandem with the confirmation process, then Surgeon General, and then also as director of the Office of International Health, which was added to his portfolio in spring of 1982. Next we drill down and examine the five major controversies in which he was embroiled during those years. First, *Saving Baby Doe*, when national debate suddenly focused on the fate of a handicapped newborn, and Koop's second career unexpectedly overlapped with his first. Second, his quest for a *Smoke-free Society?* and remarkable success in deploying arguments to alter public attitudes to tobacco in place of the governmental authority he did not have. Third, *Confronting AIDS*, on which the President requested a report on the growing healthcare crisis; it had dramatic implications. Fourth, the Commissioned Corps of the PHS remained under budget threat. Together with key colleagues at HHS Koop took drastic steps toward *Revitalizing the Corps* to fend off its critics in the administration. Fifth, *Abortion Again*. Koop had surprised everyone by saying soon after he came to Washington that he did not plan to address the issue. Six years later, the President asked him to write a report on its health impact on women.

---

v   The term "bully pulpit," popularized by Teddy Roosevelt in respect of the presidency, is often misunderstood to imply that the pulpit occupant "bullies" people. The word "bully" actually has two quite different meanings in English. Roosevelt meant by "bully pulpit" an *excellent* pulpit from which to make a case to the American people, an older meaning that survives in the phrase "bully for you" meaning "congratulations." Of course, it's perfectly possible to occupy a bully pulpit and bully people at the same time.

In 1985 Koop had been re-appointed by the President, without controversy, to a second four-year term. It was his most productive time, though his critics on the right had become increasingly vocal; and, no doubt in part for that reason, the incoming administration of President George H. W. Bush showed no interest in retaining him as Surgeon General, let alone elevating him to the cabinet office of secretary of HHS, to which he aspired. So began the uncomfortable process of his *Stepping Down*.

CHAPTER 7

Welcome to Washington

God plucked me out of Philadelphia and dumped me in Washington.
—CEK

In a 1982 interview, Koop recalled when he was first approached about becoming Surgeon General. It was the summer of 1980, and he had just finished a speech to a pro-life group in Washington, DC. In the audience was Richard Schweiker, his home state senator from Pennsylvania. Schweiker was close to Reagan—he had been his running mate in Reagan's unsuccessful 1976 campaign—and would soon be named Secretary of Health and Human Services in the incoming administration. Schweiker "called him aside and asked if he would consider accepting the Surgeon General post."[1] Various calls followed, notably from the office of Senator Jesse Helms, whose staffer Carl Anderson would join the administration and for a period become close to Koop.[2] "Finally on Valentine's Day," Koop later told Moritz Ziegler, "I did become designated as the surgeon general."[3] Apparently there had been other options. In mid-November of 1980 he had told his attorney somewhat vaguely that he might have a "top echelon position" in HHS.[4] On January 6, 1981, he wrote to Billy Graham that he was being considered for a joint appointment as Surgeon General and assistant secretary for health.[5] Evidently, both Graham and Reagan's pastor at Bel-Air Presbyterian Church, Donn Moomaw, had been pressing his name.[6]

Whatever triggered Schweiker's original approach, once the election was decided there was pressure from the community of pro-life organizations for Reagan to appoint Koop. One activist recalled that beginning in January of 1981, President Reagan would host key leaders of the movement from across the country at the White House on the occasion of the annual March for Life.[7] The March is a Washington rally dating back to 1974, held every year on or close to January 22, the day in 1973 when *Roe v. Wade* was handed down. It is the biggest event of the pro-life calendar.[8]

Accordingly, on January 22, 1981, just two days after Reagan's inauguration, the pro-life elite were gathered in the Cabinet Room with the President; and they asked for Koop.[9] While his nomination was not formally announced until September 16, since the matter of his age had first to be resolved through legislation, they soon learned they had got what they wanted.[10] Just twenty-three days later, on Valentine's Day, February 14, Koop got a call to confirm that he would be the President's nominee.[11] He was swiftly appointed deputy assistant secretary for health, a position that did not require Senate confirmation and was devised to give him an office and a salary so that he could immediately move to Washington.[12]

"Of course, the President knew him, they knew of each other and had crossed paths," I was told by a White House aide who was involved in the recruitment process. "And the President was obviously delighted to have him be part of the team."[13]

A Diminished Office

When Koop was first approached in the summer of 1980 he believed that the office of Surgeon General was a cabinet position that held far greater governmental significance than actually remained to it.[14] The history of the "Surgeon General of the Public Health Service" is a narrative of the United States government's increasing involvement in health care and bioscience, and therefore of burgeoning budgets, rising political significance—and the survival of an alluring but increasingly misleading job title.[15]

Back in 1798 the young republic first established the Marine Hospital Service, a government health service for seamen, funded by a tax levy on the master of every American ship arriving from a foreign port. It was placed under the authority of the secretary of the treasury, where it remained until 1939.[16] The service expanded to include early versions of what later became the CDC and the NIH. In the aftermath of the Civil War, the energetic Dr. John Woodworth, who had served as Sherman's chief medical adviser, was appointed in 1871 as the first US Surgeon General (the original title was Supervising Surgeon).[17] He supervised a cadre of physicians, and in 1889 Congress formally established the "Commissioned Corps," to be run along military lines and have a particular concern to prevent the entry of infectious disease into the United States—especially much-feared cholera and yellow fever.[18]

As the federal investment in medicine and related scientific efforts grew, the Surgeon General continued to supervise the entirety of the ballooning PHS, which came to include the NIH and CDC, and reported directly to the secretary for health, education and welfare (HEW).[19]

Luther Terry was the last Surgeon General to serve out his full appointment as head of the PHS, back in the early 1960s. His successor, William Stewart, while retaining the title "Surgeon General," lost almost all of his authority mid-term.[20] Less than seven months after Stewart's appointment as Surgeon General, on April 25, 1966, HEW Secretary John Gardner issued a directive transferring all of the Surgeon General's statutory responsibilities to himself, a move supported by President Johnson to facilitate fundamental reorganization in the light of higher budgets, new federal initiatives, and a sense that the PHS Commissioned Corps, whose officers had hitherto been required to fill all the senior PHS positions, were not up to the job.[21]

The Surgeon General was downgraded to an advisory status, save some vaguely defined continued responsibility for the Commissioned Corps—a responsibility that recognized that most Commissioned Corps personnel were by then integrated into the various federal agencies, working side by side with standard civil servants.[22] Political scientist Eric Redman aptly "likened the position to a once-powerful European king who had been reduced to a figurehead."[23]

What then remained of the position of Surgeon General in 1981?

Misunderstanding was rife. Senator Arlen Specter announced to a hearing that, "The Surgeon General has four major areas of responsibility: first aging and care of the elderly; second, care of the disabled; third, administration of the public health services; and, fourth, negotiation of bilateral health treaties with nations of the Third World."[24] Almost none of that was actually true. What did remain? An office on the seventh floor of the Hubert Humphrey Building in downtown Washington, DC. An official house at 4 West Drive on the campus of the NIH, in Bethesda, Maryland. A tiny staff of fewer than half a dozen. A travel budget. A three-star rank. A uniform—should the Surgeon General be interested in wearing it. And barely any actual formal duties, beyond signing off on an annual smoking report. In his essay on Koop as a public administrator, James S. Bowman sums up the job like this: "When out of town, the surgeon general was expected to give speeches to conservative groups; when in town, he was supposed to stay in his office, sign documents, and write his annual smoking reports."[25] However, the Surgeon General did not actually write them; he merely introduced them. The tobacco control department of HHS was not a part of his vastly diminished office. Even Bowman, in his otherwise excellent analysis, did not understand this.[26]

So it is perhaps understandable that the assistant secretary for health to whom Koop would report, Edward Brandt, "did not . . . help him get confirmed, because he saw the post as an anachronism."[27] Even Secretary Schweicker, Koop's former home state senator who had backed his nomination, feared that "he was effectively disenfranchised by the grueling confirmation hearings."[28] Another top official observed that "it wasn't clear how he could help us," except to aid the agency in warding off the "political far right." Stobbe, in his history of the job, remarks that when he first arrived at HHS, "Koop was isolated both by his own ignorance of how the department worked and by PHS veterans who deemed him unfit for such a historically important, science-based office."[29] Koop said those days in limbo proved pivotal to his later success. "Out of those tough months I made a number of very important friends in HHS who believed in me, believed I was being given a raw deal, who did think I was credible, who did think I was able, who did think when I had an idea and the ability to do something with it, I would be successful."[30]

Bowman notes that Koop openly complained to visitors that no one returned his calls or invited him to meetings, although this picture of his solitude—reflected in his memoir, *Koop*—is much overdrawn.[31]

For example, "Shortly after I arrived in Washington," he wrote to the assistant secretary for health on May 4, "I got deeply involved" with a committee representing handicapped employees of the PHS.[32] Presaging his appointment on May 3 of the following year as Director of the Office of International Health, in May 1981 he spent three weeks in Geneva as part of the US delegation to the World Health Assembly, in his capacity as deputy assistant secretary for health.[33] He was much involved in a White House Conference on Aging.[34] On October 9 he briefed the HHS chief of staff on his travel schedule for the following three weeks. Before his departure for Paris and Madrid he will be in San Francisco, Chicago, and Boston. After Europe, he will be in San Antonio.[35] Koop shared at a Senate hearing that "in the six months that I have functioned as Deputy Assistant Secretary of State for Health . . . I have been asked to oversee a number of bilateral health agreements between the United States and foreign countries. I feel very comfortable in this role, knowing the health leaders of many of the countries involved."[36] At the end of October, after visits in Asia, he was back in Europe to meet with French officials in Paris and Marseille, and to represent the United States at a World Health Organization regional meeting in Madrid.[37]

He was not exactly idle.

Buzz-saws

The Koop confirmation hearings, and the nine months that led up to them, were a Washington classic. It would be late in November before Koop got the job. But he had meanwhile made many connections inside and outside the Department of Health and Human

Services, including with two pediatricians on staff with the department, who advised and sustained him through the confirmation process, and became long-term friends—Samuel "Woodie" Kessel, and Edward Martin.[38]

Kessel first met Koop soon after his arrival at HHS. He was then serving as a special assistant to the assistant secretary for health, and introduced himself as a fellow pediatrician from Philadelphia. He rapidly became friends with "the godfather of pediatric surgery," as Kessel helped him through the confirmation process.[39] "We'd have breakfast virtually every day. And you know, he would fuss about food, and, he would make an omelet. If he said show up at 5:30 a.m., you better be there!" Sometimes they had dinner, with their wives. "Betty had this endearing warmth." Later on, they had fun together. Kessel recalls the august Surgeon General singing along with the comedy troupe Capitol Steps' satirical "Little Doc Koop." Once when they were traveling in uniform, a woman mistook them for redcaps and asked Koop to carry her bags. Koop replied "Of course, ma'am," and handed them to Kessel. Kessel duly carried them to her car—but felt obliged to decline the tip. She was no doubt even more confused when he added, "Delivered to you courtesy of the United States Surgeon General."[40]

Kessel recalled Koop's making negative public comments about video games. "And he came back to the office, and said, 'How'd you like that one?' I said, 'You're the Surgeon General of the United States. On what basis did you condemn those videos? You've got to show me the evidence and the papers.' He and I had the kind of relationship where I could talk to him like that, you know, we loved each other. When we were having breakfast in a hotel . . . it was a buffet. And I said to him, you know, Chick? I don't think you should eat all that bacon in public.'"[41]

Edward Martin was a top HHS official. Like Kessel, he was an officer in the Commissioned Corps, and had originally trained as a pediatrician. Like Kessel, he introduced himself early in Koop's confirmation process, and he later came to play an unorthodox but highly significant part in Koop's success.[42]

uot; per the *Boston Globe*.[45] "Dr. Kook," said
another editorialist, and this smart-aleck sobriquet stuck.[46]

Koop found the whole experience traumatic. "It was unbelievable. . . . Everything I had done in my life became a liability." But, in the
process, "I learned a lot about people." Koop was finally confirmed on
November 16. "Now, that's a long time from Valentine's Day."[47]

Meanwhile, Koop assured anyone who would listen that it was
not his intention to use the office of Surgeon General to campaign
on abortion. While many on both sides either hoped or feared this
was a mere ploy to aid confirmation—an "election day promise," in
Bowman's term—they would soon learn that he had actually meant

it.[48] In retrospect, it seems remarkable that he could say that, when the sole reason he had been selected for the job was his celebrated opposition to abortion. Had there been no actual discussion of how he would deploy that opposition in government? One insider admitted, "I know how the personnel system works . . . . It's very possible that he was not asked, What will you do about abortion as Surgeon General? They would have asked him about his background and his expertise and his managerial ability. And was he committed to President Reagan? And did he share President Reagan's views? All without saying, What will you say about abortion?"[49]

Meanwhile, Koop's friend Carl F. H. Henry, founding editor of *Christianity Today*, wrote with best wishes from a meeting of the Institute for Advanced Christian Studies, an evangelical academic network with which Koop had been associated. "We are proud and believe that our entire evangelical cause is honored and dignified by the choice."[50] Good wishes also arrived from a surprising source, Shepard Pollack. Pollack began by sharing his reluctance to come forward with congratulations, "because of the fear that in spite of the many years we have known each other as doctor and father of a patient, the activities you will be involved with and the name on this letterhead would appear to imply conflict." Pollack was the president of Philip Morris. He has changed his mind for two reasons. The recent *New York Times* editorial "attacked you and outraged me." And a friend had lately reminded him that "the highest morality lies in the support of one's heroes when they are under attack, and not in petty niceties." He added that his daughter Susan, who had been Koop's patient, has after more than one attempt finally made it to medical school. Three days later, Koop replied in the most cordial terms, asking that Susan keep in touch as she makes her way into medicine.[51]

He was also sustained by friendship with his two final trainees, who happened to have taken jobs in the Washington area, Martin Eichelberger and Victor Garcia. He describes them as "two surrogate sons."[52]

As the formal confirmation process progressed, the most virulent critique of Koop's suitability came from the American Public Health Association, whose executive director, William H. McBeath, gave oral testimony on behalf of their fifty thousand members on October 1, 1981, before the Senate Committee on Labor and Human Resources. It's an interesting speech, alternating between long dull recitals of detail, and punchy denunciations. McBeath backed it up by attaching copies of nine major newspapers' anti-Koop editorials.[53]

The core issue, he declared, is that of qualifications. "What public health qualifications does the USPHS Surgeon General need?" The office demands someone who is a "clearly qualified, specially trained, broadly experienced community health professional of demonstrated expertise and recognized ability." Koop is "clearly unqualified" for the job. Koop is indeed a distinguished surgeon. But "Koop is . . . *uniquely* unqualified. . . . Utterly lacking." The overkill continues. "It is ludicrous to treat the USPHS Surgeon General as an entry-level public health career position."

Just sixteen days later, McBeath's twenty-year-old daughter Angela was killed in the fiery crash of a small plane.[54] Word reached Koop through Woodie Kessel, who had drafted a note of sympathy. It's a comment on how offended Koop had been by McBeath's entirely predictable attack, and how thin-skinned he could be, that he refused to sign. But Kessel brought him round, and the letter was mailed. They have suffered "almost the same thing that Betty and I did 12 years ago. Betty and I were shocked to hear of the loss of your daughter . . . our hearts go out to you in a time of great distress."[55]

In his analysis of the confirmation process, Gregg Easterbrook highlights the significance of the religion factor. "Though Koop's views . . . were big factors in his confirmation struggle, what really unnerved opponents and some in the press was Koop's religiosity. It is common in Washington for public figures to make God-fearing noises at tactically advantageous moments. Actual religious fervor is another thing altogether. Thus the Washington establishment was uncomfortable with Jimmy Carter, who seemed genuinely worried about the ultimate disposition of his soul; Ronald Reagan did not generate a similar level of discomfort. . . . He rarely attended church, and his lifestyle gave scant indication that Christian teachings weighed heavily in his thinking."[56]

Meanwhile, back in Philadelphia, "Children's staff physicians, among them Koop's friend Dr. Anna Meadows, a *Roe* supporter, began calling reporters to speak in Koop's defense. But little of what they said filtered into the press's coverage of the confirmation fight. Gregg Easterbrook summarizes the situation:

> Shirley Bonnem, who had manipulated the national press corps so masterfully during the 1974 twins operation, was frustrated in her efforts to exercise spin control. "The *Washington Post* absolutely refused to listen to me because I was saying things they didn't want to hear," Bonnem says. "I begged the Post to send a reporter here and ask anyone they wanted what Dr. Koop was like. No one came. This was for a story they were putting on their front pages day after day. I begged them to call our doctors, nurses, or even patients who disagreed with Chick's views, and ask whether he was a man of principle. They would not."[57]

While the law required that the Surgeon General have public health experience, it's plain that the administration's lawyers reckoned they had enough wiggle room on this point. But they could not avoid the age requirement, that: "A commissioned officer of the [Public Health] Service shall be retired on the first day of the month following the month in which he attains the age of sixty-four years."[58] Since the law required the Surgeon General to be a commissioned officer, and since Koop had attained the aforementioned retirement age on November 1, 1980, following his sixty-fourth birthday on October 14, the law needed to be changed.

This led to a highly unusual situation in which the House of Representatives became embroiled in the process of confirming a presidential nominee, a responsibility assigned by the Constitution to the United States Senate. The House had to amend the Commissioned Corps regulations, such that "the President may appoint to office of Surgeon General an individual who is sixty-four years of age or older."[59] A trivial matter it might have seemed, not least as the Speaker of the House was actually almost four years older than Koop at the time. The only problem was that, unlike the Senate, the House was in the hands of the Democrats. Senator Jesse Helms, Koop's strong backer, attempted to bounce the required change through by attaching a suitable amendment to a bill on another topic—a standard procedure in minor matters. But the Democrats in the House were able to channel the issue through the Subcommittee on Health and the Environment, chaired by the redoubtable Henry Waxman, already on record as a vigorous opponent of the candidate. "Dr. Koop scares me. He is a man of tremendous intolerance," he had declared.[60] Waxman held a hearing, and invited Koop to participate, though his handlers in the administration told him to stay away. Months of horse-trading and procedural jockeying followed, before the House finally did approve the change.[61] The President then appointed Koop to the Commissioned Corps, as required, and on September 16, 1981, formally nominated him to be Surgeon General.[62]

In the event, the Senate voted a lopsided 68–24 in favor of Koop's appointment, with even a majority of Democrats who participated voting on his side. As the *New York Times* noted in its obituary, "Some senators who had been hesitant to support him said he had convinced them of his integrity."[63] Senator Edward Kennedy had been one of his most vocal critics, accusing him of holding "cruel, outdated and patronizing stereotypes" of women.[64] Koop recalled that when he had met with the senator, Kennedy was smoking a ten-inch cigar and blew the smoke into his face.[65] The day before the preliminary committee vote, Kennedy had a staffer call Koop—he reached him on a visit to France—to confirm, as a courtesy, that he would not be voting for him. Koop later described it as an "olive branch," but it can hardly have seemed that way at the time.[66] Kessel recalls how Washington worked back then, in somewhat more civilized times. Much of what took place was adversarial drama, "between nine and five." And then? "You play tennis and have dinner." Koop never quite grasped that. In Kessel's phrase, he "personalized the negative energy." After the full Senate vote, on November 16, Kennedy was "very gracious," and walked across to congratulate Betty. Then he turned to shake her husband's hand, but Koop turned away.[67]

The turnaround in Koop's relationship with Kennedy, after the AIDS report was published, was spectacular. Medical journalist Mona Khanna interned with Kennedy's office and told me what followed.

"So then HIV happened. And Koop came out the way he came out and shocked the hell out of all the progressives and the liberals." Since Kennedy was chairman of the relevant Senate committee, they began to work with each other. "They developed a great friendship, so much so that he and Ted—it's kind of bringing tears to my eyes. He and Ted Kennedy, once a week, would take an hour, usually at lunchtime, but sometimes in the afternoon, and walk across the Great Lawn in the White House, and just talk about HIV . . . and how they could further the cause." In his memoir Koop is much gentler about Kennedy's earlier opposition than he was at the time.[68]

Another Koop

As part of the administration's preparation for the confirmation process, they had drafted a memo listing Koop's professional efforts that could arguably fall under the category of "public health." This was the memo dismissed by McBeath as "dress[ing] up events in the nominee's clinical career which can hopefully be sold to this Committee and the Senate as 'significant experience' in public health." It was actually rather remarkable.

Here are some examples:

He worked hand in glove with his good friend Ray Knighton in developing what was first called the Medical Assistance Program, and later MAP International. At the time of his confirmation, MAP International was the largest international relief agency in the United States after the Red Cross.

While working with a committee of the American Academy of Pediatrics, Koop conducted a public relations campaign against the use of X-ray machines in shoe stores to determine whether children's shoes had a "scientific fit." The machines were high-dose models that likely harmed salespeople even more than children.[69]

Again working with the AAP, he led a critique of the sickly sweet scenting of corrosive cleaners, that encouraged children to regard them as candy and had led to a rise in burns of the mouth and the esophagus, a practice which was in due course banned.[70]

He made "substantial contributions to public health" during World War II, as "surgical consultant to an epidemiology team . . . assigned the task of investigating the incidence of hepatitis during the allied invasion of Italy. In the course of his work, he described the first transmission of the hepatitis virus across the placenta to affect the fetus without presenting any signs of the disease process in the mother."[71]

In 1960, he worked with the State Department to establish a medical school in Ghana, and then with the College of Physicians in Philadelphia to recruit its faculty."[72]

In 1965, he worked again with the State Department and other agencies to build a 180-bed hospital in Hong Kong.[73]

"At the request of the public health department of the Dominican Republic, he conducted an assessment of the needs stemming from a diarrhea epidemic . . . with an infant mortality rate between 50 and 70%. He planned and established nine hydration stations for administering intravenous fluids. He procured physicians and nurses for the stations, and arranged the necessary supplies. The epidemic was stopped as a direct result of Dr. Koop's administrative and clinical skills."[74]

Koop later reminisced: "I really did a lot to establish pediatric anesthesia, not only here but in many places around the world, and I had experience staffing a medical school in Ghana, working with the Rockefeller Foundation, so I had the benefit of that kind of prestige and money behind me and also working for the State Department. . . . I did a lot of things that I thought were public health, and that stood me in good stead for decisions I had to make. It wasn't nearly the leap that some people think . . . to go from being a surgeon of individual patients who had a surgical problem to 347 million people, which is the population when I went to Washington."[75]

"By the time the Senate finally confirms him in November, 1981," writes *US News and World Report*, "Koop has come to view his appointment as a moral mission to 'espouse the cause of those who lack justice.' And he finds injustice everywhere. In the case of Baby

Doe, an infant born with multiple defects whose parents deny the child life-prolonging medical care; in unknowing smokers, victimized by the 'reprehensible' tobacco companies; in AIDS patients, helpless and despised by their neighbors."[76] Bowman assesses him like this: "The sanctity of life he so jealously guarded for individual patients as a physician would now be protected for entire groups of people—smokers, Baby Does, AIDS victims, pregnant women, and more—as surgeon general."[77] Philip Yancey quotes one of Koop's closest aides: "What people didn't understand about Dr. Koop is that he is pro-life in the purest sense of the word: not *antideath*, but *pro-life*. I have seen him with thousands of people—malnourished children, Washington socialites, dying AIDS patients, abused wives, abortion-rights-activists—and he treats every one of them as if he truly believes, which he does, that they are created in the image of God. He'll interrupt his busy schedule to meet with some disturbed person who insists on talking to 'the top doc.' He truly does respect the value of all human life."[78]

Martin Eichelberger was in an unusual position to observe the confirmation process, as chief of trauma and burns at Children's National Health Center in Washington, DC. When the Koops arrived in Washington, he and his wife Nancy invited them to stay. Until, that is, "after about three weeks he realized he wasn't going to get appointed Surgeon General real fast," and the Koops moved into an apartment at 1111 30th Street in Georgetown.[79] Eichelberger's take on Koop's apparent reorientation is simple. Koop was a surgeon, and looked at his new situation in DC exactly as a surgeon would. He analyzed the situation, and focused on "what was the next step in what he had to do?"[80]

Since Schweiker's approach the previous summer, Koop had had many months to mull his situation.[81] As he moved on from pediatric surgery, he had decided that it was also time to end his briefer career as a pro-life crusader. He had plainly reflected on the political advantages of announcing right at the start that he was stepping out of what he somewhat dismissively referred to as "the pro-life circuit." If he lacked experience in the ways of Washington, he retained a healthy skepticism of government, as he had stated when he was first approached about the job: "I've always felt that the government and medicine didn't mix right."[82] And as his friend Harold O. J. Brown noted, Koop held a deep suspicion of ideology.[83] He had no plan to be co-opted into the ideological agenda of the social conservatives within the administration.

"Chick works with dispatch," his wife Betty would say. But it's hard to believe that he quite grasped the political significance of what he was doing—essentially walking away from the sole justification of his nomination. As one pro-life leader put it to me, with heavy understatement, "if you want the truth, we were disappointed."[84]

When it came to public pro-life events, Koop felt initially that he should be silent.[85] On June 5, 1981, he declined an invitation to speak at the annual Right to Life Dinner Dance, since "in my new role in the Government, I can't say the same things I did before."[86] Yet things soon loosened up. In September of 1982, he addressed a dinner for the benefit of pro-life Alpha Pregnancy Services in Philadelphia.[87] In January of 1984 Koop was guest speaker at the Rose Dinner, a major annual pro-life occasion held in association with the March for Life.[88] In 1985, he was keynote speaker at the National Right to Life Committee banquet.[89] In 1985 he spoke on euthanasia at a University of Notre Dame conference, an address that subsequently appeared under the coauthorship of Americans United for Life (AUL) executive director Edward Grant with the title "The 'small beginnings' of euthanasia: Examining the erosion in legal prohibitions against mercy-killing."[90]

All along, he maintained a particular commitment to AUL, a Chicago-based public interest law firm whose board he joined soon after its founding in 1971. He continued quietly fundraising for AUL while in office, in collaboration with development director, Guy M. Condon. For example, on August 14, 1985, he sought Cardinal Krol's aid in securing funding from the Catholic welfare agency the Knights of Columbus. On July 21, 1986, he wrote (on HHS letterhead) to major conservative funders he knew, confirming to Condon that "The letter has gone off to Joe and Holly Coors." This was not his only solicitation

for AUL. In October of 1988, Condon—by then executive director—
wrote to thank Koop for his personal contribution of $300, and also
for his introduction to "Mrs. De Moss," which had netted a somewhat
larger gift to AUL of $2.5 million.[91] Koop told Condon he would be
happy to rejoin the AUL board once he was out of office.[92]

Although the drawn-out confirmation process was a trial at the
time, Koop later reflected that these months helped him prepare.
"What I was able to do at that time was to make friends, study the situation," Koop recalled. "I'm probably the only, the first, surgeon general to step into the job with an agenda. I had seen, for nine months,
things that I thought were really bad. So I had some priorities."[93]

He was finally sworn in on November 17. Shortly after, Mike and
Sandy Roberts were surprised to see him turn up at the annual Surgeon General Dinner Dance—and in uniform! Mike was President
of the Commissioned Officers' Association, and Sandy of the USPHS
Wives' Club. The Roberts would get to know the Koops well. "Dr.
Koop loved a party," Sandy told me, "and always stayed until the
very end. He also loved Maraschino cherries . . . and was not opposed
to picking one or two from empty glasses around the room." Betty,
on the other hand, merely "tolerated" these social events, though
was an eager volunteer with a program Sandy directed to welcome
young scientists from overseas at the NIH's Fogarty Center. "She was
a quiet, gentle, kind, caring woman who made everyone around her
feel comfortable and welcome."[94]

Meanwhile, a crisis was brewing in the Commissioned Corps. As
Richard Kluger notes, "During the nine-month confirmation period
when Koop was nastily pilloried, the Reaganites had applied their
scalpels to the PHS's uniformed commissioned officers' corps, letting
go 1,600 physicians and public health workers, more than a quarter
of the total, and ordering nearly all the PHS hospitals closed. Finding morale understandably low in the corps as he took office, Koop
decided that it was fitting for the Surgeon General to don a uniform
and so routinely appeared in public in navy blues or dress whites
with a splash of gold braid. 'I was fighting for recognition of a service
that the Administration was trying to destroy,' he recounted. 'You

can rally people around a uniform.'"[95] As early as February 1982, we find him asking the editor of *Military Medicine* to make sure any photos they use in the future have him in uniform.[96]

The Beginnings of Celebrity

Meanwhile, he was meeting all kinds of people and revealing himself as a charming, thoughtful, friendly fellow; far from the anti-abortion "kook" they had read about. And in parallel, Koop was in the opening stages of becoming a political phenomenon far more significant than the diminished office of Surgeon General. The thunderous denunciations of a dozen major newspapers, and their eager reporting of every savage rebuke of his nomination, meant that with every day that passed for those long nine months he was better known right across America.

CHAPTER 8
Bully Pulpit

I have learned that, when an idea's time has come—and it is on your
watch—you must seize the moment.

—CEK, Glasgow speech

It would take C. Everett Koop, MD, ScD, just an hour, one very well-
prepared hour, to overturn nine months of obloquy and ridicule.[1]

In the process, he re-ordered the public face of the PHS, setting the
Surgeon General head and shoulders above his boss, the man sup-
posed to have the real power, assistant secretary for health, Edward
Newman Brandt, Jr., who months before had dismissed the Surgeon
General's office as an anachronism ripe for abolition.

In the process, Koop also shattered the easy assumption of Big
Tobacco that the favored nominee of smokers' patron saint Jesse
Helms, an old-time conservative, bearded, former pipe-smoker, would
prove a milquetoast.[2]

To the savvy, and the savaged, the morning editions of the *Times*
and the *Post* on February 23 made it unambiguously clear. The *Times*
devoted the top left-hand corner of its front page to a picture of the
man it had lately deemed "Dr. Unqualified," declaring smoking
"Society's chief cause of preventable death." (It's paragraph three
before we read a reference to "his superior, Dr. Edward Brandt Jr.")
The *Post* led with the announcement that smoking is now linked to
additional cancers. (In this case, Brandt would have to wait until
paragraph six before he found his name, after six consecutive references to the Surgeon General.[3])

As planned, Koop had stolen the show.[4] He ended by saying:
"Fifty-three million adults in this country still smoke cigarettes and
young people are still taking up the habit. On the evidence of the

report we submit to you today, this can only presage human tragedy in the years ahead and enormous economic loss to our country."[5]

"If you ever saw a press conference where someone really knew their shit, that was the press conference,"[6] said Donald Shopland, longtime US government tobacco control expert and author/editor of the document, on Koop's first presentation of the annual Surgeon General's report on smoking on February 22, 1982, just three months after his confirmation.[7]

Brandt got to open the event, and to introduce Koop to play what Mike Stobbe, historian of the Surgeon General's office, terms "his assigned bit part."[8] With his bulky presence and booming voice, Koop immediately dominated the proceedings. After nearly forty years of Surgeon General reports, this one was "the most serious."[9] And, he added, "Our choice of cancer as a subject of this report should not distract attention from the even larger costs of cigarette smoking, which become apparent when deaths from coronary heart disease, chronic lung disease and other diseases and conditions are taken into account." Smoking kills 340,000 Americans every year.

The Tobacco Institute, the industry mouthpiece, pushed back with its increasingly risible claim that "the question is still open," whether smoking causes cancer. Koop dismissed them out of hand. "The evidence is strong and scientific and we stand by it," according to the *Times*' frontpage account.[10]

In an hour, Koop had palpably altered the relationship between the US government and one of America's most important industries. "What had settled into a gentlemanly enmity was kicked into an all-out war," according to one observer.[11] "I never withheld any of the venom that I had for the cigarette companies."[12] Koop learned to despise the industry, and to convey his contempt whenever he addressed the issue. "The thing that impelled me," he later said, "was the sleaze with which the tobacco industry foisted their products upon an unsuspecting people with unfair advertising."[13]

Koop had been working for months on how to turn around the image the press had built of him during the anguished process of confirmation. He had come to the conclusion that the tobacco report provided him with that opportunity. "I think I saw smoking as the most visible thing my predecessors had done, and if I wanted to have some kind of platform from whence to jump to other things, I better do that one well."[14] It was a popular, "apple pie" issue, because tobacco consumption was already on the decline, and while the industry was powerful smokers were not a well-organized interest group. "This was a topic on which he could establish himself as a person to be reckoned with and to do—at least what others considered—the unexpected."[15]

February 22, 1982, would mark the turning point. "It was the beginning of a long and increasingly warm relationship between me and the press . . . their point of view was changed."[16]

To put it another way, just ninety-seven days after being sworn in as thirteenth US Surgeon General, Koop had his bully pulpit.

The Department of Health and Human Services

Koop now had a job, in an enormous and complex government department—with scores of bureaus and programs, scores of thousands of staff, and a budget for 1981 of $222,948,642,000.[17] His office held no responsibilities on the policy front, and therefore scant apparent opportunity to influence events. It had an appropriately tiny staff. The annual smoking report, his one specific assignment which had been requested by Congress of the Surgeon General since the 1960s, was as noted not actually produced by the Surgeon General at all, but the product of the separate (and much larger) Office on Smoking and Health, an office that reported to the assistant secretary for health. The Surgeon General's "bit part" was simply to sign it and introduce it.

Koop's approach, once he settled into his office in Washington's Humphrey Building, was exactly the same as it had been over the years at the Children's Hospital: to build a team—first by establishing strong relationships with his senior colleagues, and then by gathering able men and women around him to extend his reach and his resources.

As Stobbe notes, Koop "established rapport with key officials at the FDA, the CDC and elsewhere in the department," a process he had begun during his pre-confirmation time in the political wilderness.

"Out of those tough months I made a number of very important friends in HHS," Koop said. They would in due time lend him staff and help fund the workshops and reports that defined his time in office.[18]

During Koop's time at HHS, there were nearly a dozen top political appointees within the department who were key to his work, including three secretaries appointed by President Reagan (Schweiker, Heckler, and Bowen), and one by President Bush after the 1988 election (Sullivan).[19] Koop also had three immediate superiors (Brandt, Mason, and Windom), in the office of the assistant secretary for health.[20] We should also note the key roles played by two of the chiefs of staff to the secretary, C. McClain "Mac" Haddow and Thomas Burke, as well as that of Edward Martin, a senior administrator in the Bureau of Health Care Delivery and Assistance.

Koop had known Secretary Schweiker from his time as a US senator for Pennsylvania, though likely overestimated his support. "The men were on friendly terms," notes Stobbe in his history, "but by several accounts Schweiker and many PHS veterans were leery of giving Koop any power at HHS."[21] This may refer to the job description drafted for Koop in his holding role as deputy assistant secretary for health, which (unsurprisingly) excluded him from standing in for the assistant secretary. Stobbe remarks, "Koop was only dimly aware of the organization chart machinations going on at the time."[22]

Things changed for the worse when Schweiker stepped down in 1983, and former congresswoman Margaret Heckler was appointed to succeed him. Heckler formed a dislike for Koop and determined to keep him out of various efforts that she supervised, including Baby Doe and AIDS. But she hired a new chief of staff, Mac Haddow, who had long worked with Senator Orrin Hatch (their families were friends). Hatch was Koop's closest ally in the Senate, and Haddow and Koop would enjoy working together, not least to conspire against Heckler.

Soon after, in 1984, Brandt stood down, and James O. Mason, the director of the CDC, took over in an acting capacity as assistant secretary right through late 1986.[23] Mason, an officer of the Commissioned Corps and also a prominent Mormon, developed a cordial relationship with Koop. He freed him to speak about AIDS and added him to the AIDS task force from which Brandt had excluded him.[24] In 1986, a permanent replacement for Brandt was finally appointed, Robert Windom, who served until the end of the Reagan administration. "Bob Windom was very, very supportive" of Koop, Martin recalled. "They got along famously."[25]

At the end of 1985, after friction with colleagues elsewhere in the administration, Heckler was pushed into resigning, and made Ambassador to Ireland.[26] Her successor was Otis Bowen, the former governor of Indiana, who happened also to be a physician. Stobbe describes him as "an astute politician who recognized Koop had built tremendous credibility with the media. He was content to . . . give Koop a long leash."[27] Koop, in turn, later acknowledged that he owed much of his success to Bowen.[28] They developed a strong working relationship, and Koop also got on well with Tom Burke, Bowen's influential chief of staff.

His life was getting easier.

Eight years

Koop was strong-willed and opiniated. And he did surprise many people across the political spectrum with his positions and priorities. But the story of his nearly eight years as Surgeon General is not a simple one. We need to get under its skin.[29]

In fact, Koop has left us many clues as to just what *was* going on. Midway through his second term he gave a remarkably personal lecture on a visit to the Royal Children's Hospital in Glasgow, Scotland, starting out by facing head-on the fact that he had strong convictions. "Well, what happens when a person with strong, controversial, and publicly advertised ideas enters government? Must you deposit your religious beliefs in a blind trust? Should you donate your moral values to charity? Before you move to Washington, should you hide your ethics in an attic trunk? I say, No. . . . None of the above." He continued: "Since November 1981, when I was sworn into my position, I've had a number of opportunities to test my ability to apply to the public business the stuff of who and what I am. I will admit that

I was not always quick enough or sure enough to seize some of those opportunities as they went by. But with others I was more swift and more fortunate."[30]

While he later clashed with officials elsewhere in the administration over his approach to AIDS, Koop generally maintained cordial relations with the White House and cooperated with its political agenda. He later reflected on the many times he addressed visiting groups of Reagan political supporters, usually in the splendid Indian Treaty Room of the Old Executive Office Building. "I'd get a call in the morning that the president's entertaining some people this afternoon, he's going to speak to them from 1:00 to 1:05, could you take over until 2:00 o'clock? And so it would be on all sorts of things that had nothing to do with my job, really, and I had one big collection of talking points. And I used them many, many times, but never gave them a title. . . . And so my staff, to file it someplace had to give it a name, so they called it, 'A Really Good Sermon.'" And what was the sermon about? "It was [the President's] political social agenda. Really. It was his pro-life position, it was a conservative view of life in general."[31]

The version of this "sermon" on file is essentially a call for a revival of voluntarism within American society. Koop recalls "the president's first meeting with his task force on private sector initiatives," where "he said we need to rediscover America . . . the America beyond the Potomac river, the America whose initiative, ingenuity, and industry made our country the envy of the world, the America whose rich tradition of generosity began with simple acts of neighbor caring for neighbor."

Koop continues in distinctly Reagan-esque prose, calling for an "answer to weaning the country away from the support of the public treasury," calling it back to "a higher degree of self-sufficiency and self-reliance. It's there. It's always been there. We need to find it again. It was discovered in this rich and beautiful country three centuries ago. Now we need to rediscover that spirit of self-help, of community, of family strength, that spirit of independence that is fundamental to the human spirit in America. . . ." In sum, "I believe, as the President believes, that we have to return to a familiar, time-tested, American way of getting at many of our problems in health and social services."

Koop notes the high levels of Americans' charitable contributions, but brings things down to local level with a striking image.

> This is not a money issue, this is a caring issue, this is a compassion issue, this is an issue that illuminates the essential decency and humanity of our society. Not long ago, the Congress had to pass a law that allowed this country to have a debt in excess of one trillion dollars. That's a lot of money, even to people who can conceive of such a number. I can't, and so I've been told on good authority that one trillion dollars is a lot of money. But it is a few dollars short of the value of a visit by some young people each week to the apartment of an elderly person shut in by illness. One trillion dollars is not quite the price you ought to pay for an older man to spend a few hours each week with a young boy who may be fatherless, out of school, and out of work. A trillion dollars is less than half the value of a neighbor keeping tabs on how well a young woman is doing during her pregnancy, offering to do chores for a person recovering from an auto accident, preparing meals for a person at home and disabled by a deteriorating disease.
>
> These are the good works of the spirit. They are priceless. There is no county, state, or federal budget that will ever be big enough to buy the acts of goodness that Americans voluntarily perform.[32]

Koop often spoke of his involvement in the celebrated case of Katie Beckett as the first task he was allocated as Surgeon General.[33] Katie was a three-year-old who after contracting viral encephalitis at four months needed a ventilator to survive. Medicaid was paying for her treatment in the hospital but could not by law pay the much lower cost of her being treated at home with her family. Her mother caught the attention of her member of Congress, who spoke about the case with the vice president. President Reagan liked to get involved in sympathetic cases involving individuals, especially when as in this case they involved bureaucratic indifference and the waste of public funds. He promptly raised the story of "cold bureaucracy" at a press conference on November 10, 1981, and asked Secretary Schweiker at HHS to sort it out. Two days later, Schweiker issued a waiver, and

Katie was home in time for Christmas. A three-person "Katie Beck-ett Review Board" was established, in April of 1982, to handle further cases of this sort. It was chaired by Koop.[34]

Koop maintained a voluminous correspondence, some of it needed for the work of the Surgeon General, some not quite so much. Old friends kept in touch, and were not averse to asking for favors. Harold O. J. Brown was in Germany in 1982, but eager to get an appointment to a federal advisory panel. Koop pushed back. These appointments "usually go to big contributors or very special friends of the president."[35] To another friend: "they usually go to big contrib-utors or very special friends of the president. . . . Armand Hammer is chairman of the three-man advisory committee on cancer. Just to give you an idea of his wealth, his personal office plane is a 747."[36] These responses are somewhat disingenuous, and illustrate Koop's deep-seated unease about the use of his office for political ends, even to help out his friends.[37]

Arising from his role in the Indian Health Service, Koop wrote to the US Department of Agriculture asking if they could supply a green-house to a small tribe called the Picuris, who he says could make good use of one.[38] He sent Secretary Schweiker condolences on the pass-ing of his father, and would be making a gift to the Schwenkfelder Church in his memory.[39] He wrote more than once to Cardinal Krol, Archbishop of Philadelphia, seeking support for one John Amato, a prisoner he believed deserving of parole.[40] He lobbied the dean of a medical school, seeking to derail the appointment of a surgeon-in-chief he considered inferior to his preferred candidate. "I hope you will not think it presumptuous of me. . . ."[41] He pursued correspon-dence with friends in France who had to do with a memorial there to his son David. He had visited as an adjunct to his recent time at the World Health Assembly just over the border in Geneva, and one of his staff would like to visit as well.[42]

Meanwhile, Koop maintained his remarkable work discipline. In a later comment on the context of a speech he made on March 8 of 1982, he shared this story. "I had been awake for most of the night in an effort to pass my fourth or fifth ureteral stone with much pain and no apparent accomplishment.[i] I had taken morphine in the middle of the night that brought me some relief . . . but just as I was about to leave my home in Georgetown for Alexandria, the place of the meeting, the ureteral colic started again. I had two choices: cancel the meeting or take some more morphine and go." He chose the latter, warned the audience that he was under the influence of "heavy sedation," and was relieved when his presentation seemed to go all right.[43]

Koop was disturbed by news from the Children's Hospital that the distinctive ethical framework he had long set was already beginning to fray. One staff member, a "selfstyled ethicist," is an "undermining influence." In a recent case, Dr. Jean A. Cortner (1931–2005), physician-in-chief, had felt it necessary to issue a statement that it would not be the policy of the hospital "to let patients die because they were mongoloid." Koop shared this with former colleague and friend Al Bongiovanni (1921–1986), who had served as physician-in-chief of the hospital from 1963–1972 and written him a note of appreciation and alarm: "I overheard a remark that with Koop's departure from the clinical arena it should prove easier to 'pull the plug' on certain infants."[44]

Koop had actually entertained hopes of continuing to practice part-time while serving as Surgeon General, though he soon realized that, even with his work ethic, that would prove impossible.[45] But he still found time to aid his Czechoslovak friend Miroslav Kabelka, who is embarking on a conjoined twin separation. Koop inquired of various colleagues, and in his reply enclosed a letter from the top heart surgeon at NIH and a review of the patients' angiograms by another specialist. "Mirko, I think you have a very good chance of separating these children."[46]

As early as spring of 1982 efforts are in hand back at the Children's Hospital to establish the C. Everett Koop Chair of Pediatric Surgery. Koop wrote of his appreciation to board chair Richard D. Wood.[47]

---

i   Kidney stones can be extraordinarily painful, not least when they are passed through the urethra, in the case of men through the penis.

Colleagues and Friends

Just as he had at the Children's Hospital, and despite political Washington's very different culture, Koop sought to make friends of his colleagues, including the small staff of his office.

One Corps officer who worked closely with him lifted the lid in a candid interview on the Koop his little team got to know.[48] For his staff, it was "almost a family kind of relationship." She never saw anyone who did not get along with him, and the team proved extremely loyal. When they traveled to conferences and other events, Betty would often go along, and the Koops would take staff out to dinner as their guests. Toward the end of his time in office, at the annual Surgeon General's dinner, he surprised Betty by presenting her with the Surgeon General's Medallion![49]

The Koops also welcomed colleagues into their home. She remembered Koop as an enthusiastic cook; he would make "a wicked shrimp cocktail." She recalled Betty as "calm, stable, powerful." And she shared an amusing sidelight. Before a major speech, Koop would run through the jokes he was planning to use with Betty, to see if she thought any sounded inappropriate. If she flagged one of them, he would have the staff take a vote! He also needed his ego stroked.

Mac Haddow, who had served in various roles at HHS and was Secretary Heckler's chief of staff, shared a remarkable personal story. Mac and Rachel Haddow had a new baby, and he developed jaundice soon after they took him home; back in the hospital in Virginia he was diagnosed with a staph infection. But there was an ice storm, and confusion at the hospital. They turned up to collect him, but the hospital couldn't tell them where he was. They persisted, and finally discovered that he was in the NICU. Haddow, upset and angry, barged in. A nurse pushed him away, and after overbalancing he found himself on the floor. He "came up fighting." Someone called security. Meanwhile, Secretary Heckler has been looking for him, and (in pre-cellphone days) had called the hospital administrator. The administrator walked in on the rumpus in the NICU just in time, as security guards were about to escort Haddow off the premises. Haddow called his boss back and told her what was going on with his son. She told him simply: "Call Chick."

And he called him, and Koop replied, "I'm on my way, tell them we're airlifting him to Children's Hospital in DC." Koop arrived forty-five minutes later, and "he walks in and starts ordering people around." Then he bumped into another pediatrician, and it turned out they have worked together in the past. "And so Chick got very comfortable. They gave him permission to be a physician at that hospital to take care of our boy." Haddow reflects, "What he did was just amazing. Obviously, he didn't have to do any of this, he just jumped into the breach and took care of it. . . . And for a year and a half, two years later, he was calling me all the time, checking up on him. And that was the quality of who the guy was."[50]

The President and his Underlings

Since the reorganization of the 1960s, the position of Surgeon General had been low on the political totem pole. The Surgeon General reported to the assistant secretary, who reported to the secretary (through the deputy secretary), who reported to the President. Koop complained that it was difficult to connect with the President directly, as White House staff would prevent their meeting. This standard protocol to shield the President's time could also be used to keep him from opinions contrary to those of close advisers. Koop believed all along that as Surgeon General he should have the President's ear, and he lost no opportunity to seek it. From time to time he was successful. But his bosses faced exactly the same issue. Secretary Bowen later complained: "That was one of the problems that we had. In this job, you'd think that you'd have access to the President if you gave a good reason. Well, of course, we thought . . . that there were so many times I'd like to say, Mr. President, does this suit you? But the underlings at the White House had total control."[51]

Haddow recalls the time when AIDS first came onto the horizon in the early 1980s, and there were disagreements between the FDA and NIH as to how to proceed. He remains critical of Heckler. "She was a political animal completely. She looked at everything through the lens of politics. She and Chick clashed immediately on the issue. Chick came to me and said, 'You've got to help me get to the President.'"[52] And he did. "I worked out a deal where he got to see the President. And he wanted to have some political cover when that happened, because he knew the blowback that was going to come from Secretary Heckler, because his request was that President Reagan name him the AIDS czar." When she heard, Heckler "made Chick persona non grata with her for the rest of her time there, which was terribly unfortunate."

Despite that fact, "Chick talked to the President, not in a meeting, but he talked to the President relatively frequently about updates. He didn't go over to the White House because we knew the sensitivity."

Koop recalled exploring unorthodox channels of communication. "I had a secret way of communicating with the President." At the end of each day the director of the White House mailroom would pass the President a handful of letters to sign to representative individuals who had written to him. "She was my contact," and Koop somehow had this person pass on private notes.[ii] He gives a rather curious example. The President had said on television that he was concerned about liver transplants, because he had heard of a little girl in need of one. In his note, Koop explained some of the problems involved. The President replied with a call, and "we had a great talk about liver transplant on the telephone. But those were the kind of opportunities I used, and I think he appreciated the fact that I protected him and informed him about things like that. Which I would much rather prefer to do eyeball-to-eyeball, but his minions would not permit that."[53]

The Office of International Health

In May of 1982, Koop was appointed director of the HHS Office of International Health.[54] He was excited. "It gave me a whole new opportunity." He seized it with both hands.[55]

---

ii   Someone with knowledge of the mailroom procedures assures me that this was entirely possible.

Brandt had made the decision to add to the Surgeon General's portfolio for financial reasons. Budget cuts required that the office be reduced in size, as well as downgraded, with the loss of its own deputy assistant secretary. He had evidently been pleased to observe Koop at work in Geneva the year before.

Koop decided to launch a reorganization of the office, and in characteristic fashion raised the profile of the whole effort. On April 8, 1982, he circulated a memorandum to PHS Agency Heads (that is, the heads of CDC, NIH, FDA, and so on) and International Program Offices, attaching a staff paper and inviting these heads or their representatives to a meeting two weeks later. Koop announced that he was forming an "Advisory Committee on International Health to the Surgeon General," to consist of said agency heads (all of them, of course, more senior than the Surgeon General in the government hierarchy) or their designees.[56]

Koop greatly enjoyed his nine years of service with the World Health Assembly. During his final visit, on May 10, 1989, the Executive Board presented him with the Leon Bernard Award, for "outstanding service in the field of social medicine."[57] In response, "I spoke of the pride I had as a physician and as an American in the tireless selfless work the WHA did on behalf of the health of the human race in every corner of the world. . . . I made it clear that I knew that many in the audience often accomplished their task in the face of what seemed to be overwhelming adversities, whether natural, social, political, or economic."[58]

The Workshops: Koop's Agenda for Public Health

Koop often recalled how before his confirmation he had had time to mull an agenda for his time in office. He would address his concerns, one by one, through a series of workshops. "These workshops were really the backbone of the innovative and creative things that I accomplished as Surgeon General."[59]

In James Bowman's words: "With the goal of building a consensus around a problem, a planning committee would determine the workshop agenda. . . . Participants were selected from a broad range of organizations that could produce working papers and had access to large groups. The 3-day events were limited to approximately 100 participants, as the meetings were designed as work sessions with expert panels on specific topics."[60]

Though less newsworthy than the big controversies in which Koop engaged, throughout his tenure he leveraged resources from many places to develop these high-octane "Surgeon General's Workshops." These efforts well illustrate the freedom his office gave him, and his grasp of what in Washington is known as the "power to convene." You don't need to be in charge of something to be able to get people together to talk about it—on your terms. Each of the workshops was run on similar lines, bringing together both private sector and federal players on a succession of crunch points in public health, from domestic violence to the challenges faced by the families of handicapped children to "self-help" healthcare groups.[61] One workshop was convened in response to the President's interest in organ transplantation, another in connection with Attorney General Meese's report on pornography.

The usual format was this. On the evening of the first day (or in the morning, if that's when the workshop began) Koop would give a short keynote, the "charge" to the group. Other speeches might follow from senior colleagues at HHS, before expert presentations and then breakout sessions on the second day. On the third day, the first half of the morning consisted of reports from the breakout groups on their assigned topics, and the second half was the Surgeon General's response. It was "obviously not prepared in advance, was tricky to give because it represented a statement by government about a health problem and I had to be careful that I wasn't committing the government to something that it could not do either politically or financially."[62] But Koop never had any trouble thinking on his feet.

The agenda he had devised was broad, and he pulled into a "public health" framing issues that might not normally be seen there.

Koop began the series with a topic on his home turf, responsive to the President's interest in the Katie Beckett case, on December 13

and 14 of 1982; and he held it back at the Children's Hospital of Philadelphia.[63] The goal was "to lessen the handicaps imposed on disabled
children and to promote child and family self-sufficiency and auton-
omy."[64] This was a bigger event than those that followed—there were
more than one hundred fifty invited participants, including handicapped persons and their families, and a further hundred attended
part of the time. Participants paid their own way, except for patients
and families. "Those attending the workshop concentrated on the
severe, specific problems of the ventilator-dependent child"—such
as Katie Beckett—"and the findings for this prototype were extrapo-
lated for their implications for all handicapped children."

Koop achieved a remarkable co-mingling of the many stakehold-
ers. "Parents met insurance people, government executives saw and
talked with handicapped patients who were in wheelchairs and on
ventilators, executives of service organizations walked the acute and
intermediate wards of the hospital and interacted with children who
have lived there all their lives, 3 or 4 years; legislative aides participated with physicians and hospital administrators. During this brief
time a mechanism evolved which cut through the intermediaries of
typed letters, impersonal phone calls and layers of formalization."

More workshops were to follow: on Solid Organ Procurement for
Transplantation,[65] Breast-feeding and Human Lactation,[66] Violence
and Public Health,[67] Pornography and Public Health,[68] Self-Help and
Public Health,[69] Children with HIV Infection and Their Families,[70]
and Health Promotion and Aging.[71]

A 2008 essay on reducing global violence takes the Surgeon General workshop as its point of departure. Under the title, "Reducing
Armed Violence: The Public Health Approach," Jennifer M. Hazen
draws attention to Koop's pioneering role in the development of a
public health approach to violence. "In 1985 the US Surgeon General,
C. Everett Koop, convened a landmark workshop on violence and
public health. . . . This conference 'signaled public health's entry into
the field of violence prevention,' and set the stage for a proliferation
of research and action. . . . In 2002 the World Health Organization
(WHO) released its World Report on Violence and Health, bringing

the issue of violence, its effects on population health, and the role of the public health community in prevention efforts to the attention of the international community."[72]

As ever, Koop was thinking big. The original plan had been to launch the recommendations of the workshop at a press conference in Washington on Wednesday, the day after it concluded. Instead, he and six other presenters testified at Senate committee hearing.

Koop later reflected: "I consider one of the contributions I made to the American scene was lifting personal violence, with its sub-headings of child abuse, child sexual abuse, spousal abuse, abuse of the elderly, out of the exclusive fields of law, and jurisprudence, and putting it where I think and more properly belongs, and that is in the field of public health."[73]

The *New York Times* reported on April 7, 1987, that Koop had warned that AIDS is "a growing menace to the nation's children," and "reiterated his call for early sex education as part of the general effort to halt its spread." Since this workshop was on AIDS, hard on the heels of his October 1986, report, Koop had decided to depart from the usually semi-private nature of these events and began the AIDS and Kids workshop with a press conference. Provocatively, he announced that "sex education should start in kindergarten. . . . You have to tell them about AIDS and that requires sex education." He added: "If parents don't do it, they've abrogated their responsibility and somebody else has to do it."

He was again back at the Children's Hospital. "Dr. Koop said the problem of AIDS and children had been widely overlooked but was spreading. . . . The Public Health Service estimates that at least 3,000 children will have the disease by 1991 and that 'virtually all will die.'" Following up on Reagan's Philadelphia speech the previous week, in which he had endorsed sex education within a moral framework and urged young people to abstain from sexual relations to avoid AIDS, Koop stated that as "a health man" he must focus on protecting kids' health.[74]

In May of 1988 twenty-four children and three adults died in a fiery crash that was called "the worst drunk driving crash in American history," when a thirty-four-year-old Kentucky man with more than twice the legal limit of alcohol in his blood drove the wrong way down an interstate and hit a school bus full of kids returning from a church trip to a Cincinnati amusement park. "The image of children vainly scrambling to escape the flames made the story even more heart-wrenching." As physician and historian Barron Lerner reported, the issue was forced upon him. In an extraordinary display of Koop's political profile, the House voted unanimously and the Senate 99–1 to call on him to declare drunk driving a national emergency.[75] In an equal display of stubbornness, Koop resisted pulling drink-driving into his public health agenda.

A reporter named Ross published the address of the Koop house on the NIH campus and urged his readers to mail the Surgeon General direct. Former trainee Howard Filston shared with me the conversation he and his wife had with Koop. They were urging him to address the subject, while Koop was fretting about the mail. So much mail was arriving, as a result of Ross's campaign, that one day the door jammed and they could not get into their home. "And I said," Filston told me, "you know, you're talking to someone whose kid was killed by a drunk driver, so I've not got a lot of sympathy for your mail-slot problem."[76]

CHAPTER 9
Saving Baby Doe

Baby Doe . . . starved to death because he had Down's Syndrome and
some people didn't think his life would be worth living.

— RONALD REAGAN

I don't think parents should have the discretion to kill their children.

— CEK, quoted in his *Bloomberg* obituary

Six days of life in Bloomington, Indiana

Koop had argued in his 1976 Ladd Medal speech to the AAP
that judging a human life with congenital handicaps to be
"not worth living" is both terribly wrong and terribly dangerous. "If
indeed we decide that a child with a chronic cardiopulmonary disease or a short bowel syndrome or various manifestations of brain
damage should be permitted to die by lack of feeding, what is to prevent the next step which takes the adult with chronic cardiopulmonary disease who may be much more of a burden to his family than
that child is, or the individual who may not have a short bowel syndrome but who has ulcerative colitis and in addition to his physical
manifestations has many psychiatric problems as well or the individual who has brain damage—do we kill all people with neurological
deficit after an automotive accident?"[1] It will put us on "The Slide to
Auschwitz."

Six quick years later he found himself at the center of a nationwide
firestorm over just this matter. The storm would rage over the greater
part of the decade, and across all three branches of the federal government. Curiously, it did not at first involve Koop at all. But soon
it did, and the man who had retired from pediatric surgery, and forsworn campaigning for the sanctity of life, suddenly found himself

as the nation's leading public health official—with all three roles in alignment.

A little boy had been born, weighing 6 lb., in Bloomington Hospital, in the town of Bloomington, in south central Indiana, at 8:19 p.m. on Good Friday, April 9, 1982. No one knows his given name except those who were closest to him.[2]

This newborn son had Down Syndrome,[i] and in addition a blockage in his digestive system. As with the cases at the Yale-New Haven Hospital described by Duff and Campbell in their celebrated article, a decision was soon taken to bring about a death "related to withholding treatment"—the needed treatment in this case being surgery to correct the digestive problem.[3] Dr. Walter Owens, the obstetrician who delivered the baby, told the parents, in the traumatic aftermath of the delivery, that even if corrective surgery for the blockage was successful, their son would end up a "blob." In any case, such surgery had only a 50 percent chance of success, he assured them. So they came to an agreement. There would be no surgery. As a result, that Good Friday evening, the little newborn baby was left untreated for his medical conditions, as well as his hunger, and his thirst.

This decision provoked a great deal of dissension in the hospital.

As nurse Linda McCabe later recalled, when "the orders came to give the baby nothing by mouth and no intravenous feeding," she and her colleagues in special care "told the hospital administration we would not help starve that child." So the baby was moved, to starve and dehydrate in a room elsewhere in the building, and the parents were forced to hire private nurses to supervise the process. "By the fourth day it got so bad, thinking about that baby just lying there, crying, that some of us nurses started checking in law books to see if we could find some legal arguments to stop the killing of that baby."[4]

---

i   Down, or Down's, syndrome, named for the 19th-century English physician who first fully described it, used often to be called "mongolism." It is a chromosomal abnormality formally known as Trisomy 21, with a wide range of outcomes. Some Down syndrome kids attend normal schools; some have married. Others are affected more profoundly. They are characteristically happy people. Current US usage is Down, not Down's, syndrome, though as our quotations from Reagan and others show, in the 1980s Down's was still widely employed.

The nurses had not been alone in their concerns. Doctors other than Dr. Owens were alarmed by the course that events were taking. The baby's parents themselves had two further physicians, Dr. James Schaeffer, their pediatrician, and Dr. Paul Wenzler, their family doctor; neither of whom agreed with Owens.[5] There was evidently a fair amount of discussion between them all. Dr. James Laughlin, described as a "consulting physician in the case," said he had recommended the baby be transferred to Riley Hospital for Children in Indianapolis, which would have been necessary for surgery, but he lost the argument.[6]

As a result, the hospital's attorney decided to seek an urgent opinion from a judge. So, next day, on the evening of Saturday, April 10, at 10:39 p.m., in somewhat dramatic circumstances, Monroe County Superior Court Judge John D. Baker opened his emergency court in a room on the sixth floor of the hospital.[7]

The court was presented with the narrative of the previous twenty-four hours. Owens, Schaffer, and Wenzler had consulted. Wenzler and Schaffer indicated that the proper treatment was immediate transfer to Riley Hospital for corrective surgery. Owens, representing the concurring opinions of himself and his colleagues Anderson and Ludlow, recommended that the child remain at Bloomington Hospital with full knowledge that surgery to correct "trachioesophageal" [*sic*] fistula was not possible there, and that "within a short period of time the child would succumb due to inability to receive nutriment and/or pneumonia."

Owens went on to explain what he had previously told Mr. and Mrs. Doe, that "even if surgery were successful, the possibility of a minimally adequate quality of life was non-existent due to the child's severe and irreversible mental retardation."[ii] He had presented them with a choice of two alternate "courses of treatment." The debate went back and forth, with Wenzler sharing that he knew at least three

ii   The term "retarded" and cognates were in general use in the 1980s but are now regarded as prejudicial. In 2010 the federal government started to require the use of the term "intellectual disability" in place of "retardation." "Why you shouldn't use the R-word," *Washington Post*, June 27, 2011.

instances of Down syndrome children who had a "reasonable quality of life," though he was unsure how the fistula would affect the baby's health. Mr. Doe then spoke up, explaining that he had spent seven years teaching public school, and had on occasion worked with children with Down syndrome. "He and his wife felt that a minimally acceptable quality of life was never present for a child suffering from such a condition. Mr. Doe was lucid and able to make an intelligent, informed decision." After speaking with the various doctors, he and his wife had determined that "it is in the best interest of the Infant Doe and the two children who are at home and their family entity as a whole, that the course of treatment prescribed by Doctor Owens should be followed." They had signed a statement to this effect in front of witnesses at 2:45 p.m. that afternoon.

The court recessed, and subsequently Judge Baker took several decisions.[iii] He first announced that he had concluded that the hearing had been able to proceed without the need to appoint a guardian *ad litem*. He then directed the hospital to carry out the regime prescribed by Dr. Owens, since "it is the opinion of this Court that Mr. and Mrs. Doe . . . have the right to choose a medically recommended course of treatment for their child in the present circumstances." Finally, he returned to the question of a guardian *ad litem* and appointed the Monroe County Department of Public Welfare to serve in this role, "to determine whether the judgment of this Court should be appealed."

Owens would later testify at length to the U.S. Commission on Human Rights about his role in the Doe case, and his views of the appropriate way to manage newborns with Down syndrome and other serious handicaps. He produced a letter from a satisfied former patient thanking him years later for helping her decide to ensure the death of her spina bifida newborn. He railed against people with Down syndrome as a huge cost on the public purse. And when offered, as a courtesy, a draft of the commission's report for his review, he responded unapologetically in a letter dated September 16,

---

iii   The written judgment is dated April 12.

1988: "Baby Doe died with little suffering after a few days. A family which probably would have been destroyed by the situation has not only been preserved, but they have had another very healthy child, which almost certainly would never have been born, had the pediatricians been able to enforce treatment to preserve Baby Doe's life." He signed off: "Meanwhile, I hope that you and the commission members may have the privilege of living in blissful isolation from the hard decisions of real life." The commission decided to include the letter as an appendix to their report.[8]

It's evident from the *Indianapolis Star* of April 16 that the Monroe County Prosecutor's Office had been working round the clock to try and save the baby. The county's deputy prosecutor, Lawrence Brodeur, had been appointed the baby's guardian. But Judge Baker ruled again that the parents remained free to choose which doctor's advice they wished to follow. On Monday April 12, other attorneys sought to apply Indiana's child neglect law to the baby; but another judge turned them down. One of the lawyers sought an order to require intravenous fluids for the baby, to keep him alive while the legal process continued, but this too was turned down. According to the *Times*, ten separate couples had expressed interest in adopting the baby. On Tuesday April 13, an attorney for Shirley and Bobby Wright of Evansville, Indiana, the parents of a three-year-old girl with Down Syndrome, petitioned the court for legal guardianship; but he was refused.[9] Meanwhile, the child neglect case was appealed, and the appeal was refused. On Thursday 15, four things happened. First, describing the baby's state as "grim," deputy prosecutor Brodeur and Patrick Baude, a professor from the Indiana University law school, flew to Washington, and were due to appear before Justice John Paul Stevens of the US Supreme Court the following morning. Second, in case the Court declined to issue an order, prosecutor Barry Brown was set to try again at the state Supreme Court in Terre Haute. Third, at the hospital, the chief of staff ordered Dr. Schaeffer to give the baby intravenous fluids but was blocked by Dr. Owens.[10] And fourth, at 10:03 p.m. that night, after a priest had been summoned and the child had been baptized and named and given his last rites, Baby Doe died.[11]

By the following morning, he was in the *Washington Post*. The hospital had referred to him on the telephone as "Infant Doe," and the name stuck.[12] The following day, April 17, he was in the *Post* again, this time on the front page, and he made his first appearance in the *New York Times*.[13] The *Post*'s conflicted use of language is interesting. The headline tells of the "demise" of the baby. The sub-head and the headline on the inner page speak of the "permitted death" of the baby. The opening sentence of the article comes closer to the point. The baby's death marks a new chapter in the debate over "the right to end someone else's life."

On Monday, April 19, Monroe County Coroner Dr. John E. Pless ruled that the baby had died of "natural causes." So the parents, who have two other children, "will not face criminal charges for withholding life-saving treatment from their son," as the *Star* put it.[14]

Since both the *Washington Post* and the *New York Times* were writing prominently about Baby Doe, the story spread fast and attracted immediate political attention. The *Post* would run fifteen Baby Doe stories in 1982, and nearly eighty in 1983.

Ten days later, the *New York Times* followed up its initial reporting with an editorial that strongly criticized the courts for their failure to intervene. "Had that baby been normal, his death by starvation would have been a public concern. But because he had been inadvertently robbed of perfection, he was deliberately robbed of life. His flaws somehow canceled out his rights. Two county courts and the Indiana State Supreme Court appear to have agreed: they declined to force his parents to feed 'Infant Doe.' But if children have a chance to live, shouldn't they get it, whether or not their parents are willing?"[15] That question was starting to preoccupy many Americans, from the President down. As Koop would later summarize the situation: "If baby doe had only had Down Syndrome, he would have been nourished and cared for, if he had only had esophageal atresia, he would have been operated on and cured."[16]

Before the month was at an end, President Reagan had sent a memo to HHS Secretary Schweiker and Attorney General William French Smith, "making it clear that he considers withholding treatment from such infants illegal." According to the *Washington Post*, he asked Schweiker to remind health care providers that "if they receive federal funds they must abide by that law." And he told Smith to notify him of "federal and constitutional remedies" that could be employed against those who break the law.[17]

Schweiker responded promptly with a two-page letter to nearly seven thousand hospitals from the HHS Office of Civil Rights, that included what the *Post* properly described as a "novel application" of the federal law prohibiting discrimination against the handicapped, Section 504 of the Rehabilitation Act of 1973. In what would be the first of several efforts to capture the need for appropriate medical treatment for handicapped newborns in just a few words, the note said that it was "unlawful" for hospitals to withhold food or medical or surgical treatment "required to correct a life-threatening condition"—if the handicap "does not render the treatment or nutritional sustenance medically contraindicated." It goes on to state that hospitals should not aid in such decisions by parents and would be held responsible for the "conduct of physicians" in such cases.

There was immediate, and predictable, pushback from the American Hospitals Association.

On October 11, 1983, the flames of debate were fanned when "Baby Jane Doe" was born on Long Island, with spina bifida[iv]—by chance, in the same hospital where Koop had spent his summers when he was in high school and college, and where he had performed his first amputation.[18]

Once again, the baby's parents had been offered a bleak assessment of her prospects by physicians, and encouraged to refuse treatment for what was generally recognized as a treatable condition. "Based on doctors [*sic*] reports that Keri-Lynn would live a life of pain even after surgery, her parents, Dan, 31, and Linda, 24, who ask their last name not be publicized, decided against operations to close the opening on Keri-Lynn's spine and to implant a shunt to drain fluid from her skull."[19] They did not, however, require that she be starved. Five

---

iv   A birth defect in which part of the spine does not form properly, leaving a section exposed through an opening in the back.

months later they finally did approve a surgical intervention, though by then her spine had closed naturally, and the delay had led to infection and brain damage.[20] Nonetheless, when reporter Lee Comegys joined her first birthday party, she found a "smiling, playful little girl." Keri-Lynn would go on to celebrate her thirtieth birthday in 2013, "happy, joking, learning," a "talkative and smiling young woman," according to reporter Nicole Fuller, leading a semi-independent life in a group home and spending weekends with her parents.[21]

Koop remained excluded from the Baby Doe decision-making, and found this situation increasingly intolerable. He recounts how when he was flying from Cairo to New York City with Secretary Heckler, he knelt down in the aisle beside her seat to try and persuade her to hand him the file so he could sort things out—not least, as he was taking the blame anyway.[22] He later summed up the situation like this: "President Reagan said he never wanted to see that happen again on his watch. And machinery was put into place that was improper. There were signs put up in hospitals that made parents suspicious of doctors and nurses. . . . They were getting ready to do the third set of rules and regulations, when I went to Margaret Heckler, who was the Secretary of HHS, and said, If you expect me to be the expert witness to defend the government, I want to write the rules and regulations."[23]

Heckler's chief of staff, Mac Haddow, recalls, "I know that conversation took place, because I had to go in and see if I could validate her willingness to allow him. She said, No. She didn't trust him. She had her litany of complaints. But there were a couple of other people who were very close to her who persuaded her to let that happen. She was dragged, kicking and screaming into it."[24]

Bowman briefly summarizes the course of events. "President Reagan ordered HHS to prevent such actions. It issued regulations in 1983 to set up hotlines for reporting these events, designated federal personnel to investigate tips, and threatened to hold hospitals in violation of civil rights and rehabilitation laws if they withheld treatment. Health care groups filed suits, and a federal judge declared the rules invalid on a technicality. The government published revised regulations that were again challenged. While the legal contest was under way, the department began work on a third set of regulations."[25] Meanwhile, Koop had been coming under increasing criticism, even receiving a letter of complaint signed by scores of house staff at the Children's Hospital of Philadelphia, who assumed this was all his doing.

When the latest regulations were struck down by the Supreme Court, and Koop was finally freed to take the lead, he took a different tack, meeting with the AAP and other groups, to develop a compromise "based on local hospital patient-care review committees and medical standards that required treatment when it would be clearly beneficial," which aided Congress in amending the Child Abuse Prevention and Treatment Act of 1974.[26] Koop's comment: "We sat around a table . . . and people who were enemies began to work together. . . . We wrote something called the patient's bill of rights for newborn infants." He continued: "It was one of the best times of my life, to see how you could bring people together. We were still sued, and we still lost the case, but in the meantime Ted Kennedy . . . lifted the whole problem of Baby Doe out of the problems of handicapped children and put it in the child abuse situation."[27]

Koop's efforts at compromise were heavily criticized by some conservatives. He later reflected that "the Baby Doe controversy made me see the self-defeating quality of some pro-lifers' absolutist frame of mind—their all-or-nothing mentality." He was denounced for writing regulations that would offer protection to 97 percent. "Certain pro-life leaders wanted 100%. . . . I thought 97% was better than risking getting nothing."[28]

Kennedy's amendment "defined refusal to treat handicapped newborns as child abuse and permitted the federal government to withhold money from states that lacked procedures for guaranteeing the rights of disabled infants."[29] As a result, "if a case involves parents or their doctors choosing to withhold treatment, the review boards are obligated to report the case to child services as an instance of medical neglect. Under the rules, withholding treatment is only permissible if the newborn is irreversibly comatose, if treatment would only prolong its death, or if treatment would be inhumane. Furthermore, the law also holds that a physician's decision for neonatal care cannot be based on quality of life, or other abstract concepts."[30] The debates in Congress brought together members who disagreed about abortion. Pro-life leader Henry Hyde spoke for many pro-choice advocates also when he declared, "The Constitution ought to protect that child. . . . Because they are handicapped, they are not to be treated differently than if they were women or Hispanics or American Indians or black. [Their handicap] is a mental condition or a physical condition; but by God, they are human, and nobody has the right to kill them by passive starvation or anything else."[31]

Stanford's Alyssa Burgart, who trained first in bioethics, reflects on the difference that the Baby Doe case made. "I work as a pediatric anesthesiologist. We're operating on kids with Trisomy 21 all the time. Like this is Tuesday, just a regular day." She added, "The idea of declining treatment solely due to potential intellectual disability is unheard of now. . . . The kinds of issues Koop faced with Trisomy 21, we face those now with different complex and sometimes unnamed conditions. Koop's a fascinating person. I think we would have a lot of interests in common. The intersection of ableism, disability rights, and pediatric critical illness really all come together in his story."[32]

In his remarkably candid Glasgow speech, on September 30, 1987, Koop looked back on the early days of the controversy—under the title, "Private Thoughts on Public Issues." "In my pediatric surgical practice," he stated, "I had come upon variations of this kind of situation . . . often . . . enough so that the experience was engraved in my mind forever: A tragically disabled child . . . parents who are confused, angry, grieving . . . a divided medical staff. What then? My considered judgment—worked out over some years—tells me that we have a clear legal and a crystal-clear moral responsibility toward these patients and their families: We ought to do those things that will give a person all the life to which he or she is entitled, but not do anything that would vainly extend that person's act of dying."[33]

Koop was in reflective mood as he shared his public private thoughts:

The Baby Doe experience was a hard lesson for me. It taught me once again that contemporary society, with all its technology and sophistication, is still slowly working out its responses to the most basic questions of ethics and morality. Hence, if you are committed to saving lives that are put at risk because of ethical conflicts, you have to be prepared to negotiate hard and fight hard for each life, and that battle is very difficult. Because your adversaries are not monsters. . . . They are just as human as you are.[34]

CHAPTER 10
Smoke-free Society?

Smoking was once a ubiquitous public practice; it is now a shameful private vice.

—SARAH MILOV, *The Cigarette*

For smokers, chewers and snuffers who find his approach too heavy-handed, Dr. Koop offered in his latest report examples of how other government officials down through the years have opposed tobacco. Many, it seems, have made the use of the substance doubly dangerous to one's health. . . . In 1633, the Sultan Murad IV of Turkey, maintaining that tobacco caused infertility and reduced the fighting abilities of his soldiers, ordered tobacco users hanged, beheaded or starved.

—IRVIN MOLOTSKY, "From our Mild-Mannered Surgeon General," *New York Times*

May of 1984 found Koop once again in Geneva, leading the US delegation to the annual World Health Assembly. But his mind wasn't focused on the elaborate diplomatic dances. It was on a speech that he would deliver almost immediately on his return stateside, a speech he had been preparing with particular care. Years later, he reflected that he had never before put so much effort into a speech.[1] Forewarned by Washington colleague Ted Cron of likely opposition from Secretary Heckler, and figures in the White House, Koop decided to go one further than his occasional tactic of side-stepping the formal vetting process for public statements. He avoided even his own staff and arranged for the speech to be typed and printed, under conditions of strict secrecy, in the offices of the American Lung Association. Only one typist and one official would know of its existence.[2]

It proved his most influential speech on tobacco; likely the single most influential speech of the century-long American struggle for tobacco control.

The Julia M. Jones Memorial Lecture for 1984 was delivered in Miami Beach, Florida, at the annual meeting of the American Lung Association, held in conjunction with the American Thoracic Society.[3]

Koop kicked off by noting that 1984 was the twentieth anniversary of Luther L. Terry's famous Surgeon General's report, in which the risk of smoking for health was for the first time laid out by a federal official with unambiguous clarity. The most prominent Surgeon General before Koop, Terry had been appointed by President Kennedy in 1961. His landmark 1964 report laid out in grim detail the evidence that smoking can cause both lung cancer and chronic bronchitis, and it led directly to the Federal Trade Commission's health warning requirement and the congressional mandate of an annual report.[4]

In the twenty years since then, Koop observed, there had been fifteen more such reports, each deepening the evidence and underlining the risks. The next in the series was due out the following week. But, he asked, what is going on, as research is done, reports are published, and warnings issued? It's been thoroughly established that "smoking was—and still is—a grave threat to individual and family health."[5] He reviewed the numbers. His 1982 report implicated smoking in 129,000 annual US deaths from cancer. His 1983 report showed the close relationship between smoking and cardiovascular disease. "We estimated that cigarette smoking was directly related to 170,000 coronary disease deaths each year." But people were still smoking.

He noted how American society had responded to other high-profile cancer threats of the day. The most striking was Agent Orange. Despite weaker evidence, and much smaller numbers, everyone seemed to have agreed on the problem and the need for a solution. Then there was the case of ethylene dibromide (EDB), a pesticide that had been labeled carcinogenic. It was in process of being banned, despite the lack of any direct evidence of its causing cancer in any one individual.

In both these cases, the argument had been made that people affected by these agents have had no choice. "That, of course, is a vital difference between the tolerance of those cancer-causing agents and cigarettes. The act of smoking is not mandated by law. It's a voluntary act: you don't have to smoke if you don't want to."[6]

In fact, smoking numbers at that point were already in gradual decline. Koop asked why.

He offered three reasons, the third of which developed into the core of his speech. First, the health arguments were slowly getting through. Second, economic factors were at work. But the third factor was "the new militancy of the non-smoking consumer, voter, and tax-payer."

Starting with Arizona in 1973, more than thirty states and hundreds of communities had prohibited or restricted smoking in "places like restaurants, government offices, theaters, indoor sports arenas, bus station waiting rooms, clinics, retail stores, and so on." One of the toughest was Minnesota, where the Clean Indoor Act banned "the smoking of tobacco in any public place unless a sign is posted saying you may."[7]

The key point was that smoking was "becoming socially unacceptable." And in this process lay the key to the future. Yet the piecemeal publication of reports and enactment of ordinances required a context. "Toward what goal are we moving? . . . I believe our ultimate goal should be . . . a Smoke-free Society by the year 2000. . . . It is as if we suspected all along—and somehow silently agreed among ourselves—that the number 1 health goal for this country was, after all, a smoke-free society by the end of this century."[8]

The brilliance of Koop's approach was to set an over-arching national goal, and re-frame the conversation, by building on the myriad efforts of health promotion and grassroots anti-smoker advocacy across the nation. And to do so not only without any governmental authority, but deploying this lack of authority as a virtue!

As Sarah Milov writes, in her definitive history of the tobacco wars, "The speech demonstrated Koop's genius for spinning the dross of federal lassitude into the gold of vigorous state, local, and private activity. It was hard for even pro-tobacco forces within the administration to argue with Koop as he stood in his white, starched navy uniform, disavowing the heavy hand of the federal government while praising the thousands of cost-conscious decisions made by the private sector."

"Let me emphasize one important point," he stated, "before there is any misunderstanding. I think this ought to be the accepted goal for all Americans, *not* a goal set by the Surgeon General or the US Public Health Service. In fact, I will go further than that and say that the achievement of such a goal ought to be the triumph *primarily of private citizens and of the private sector,* and *not* of the government."

Koop's rhetoric, crafted in Swiss secrecy and typed up in the security of the offices of the American Lung Association, then took flight in a series of remarkable paragraphs.

> I believe it is my duty, as Surgeon General, when I see the need and the opportunity for a far-reaching public health initiative, to come before the public and suggest it. And that's what I'm doing now. I am calling upon not only the American Lung Association and the American Thoracic Society, but I'm calling on the individual agencies that comprise the National Interagency Council on Smoking or Health to join this march toward a smoke-free society by the year 2000.
>
> The drive for a smoke-free society ought not to depend on government grants or contracts. Rather, it must begin and end as the entire anti-smoking campaign has done so far: with self-motivated individuals . . . with free institutions . . . and with independent communities, both social and political."[9]

He concluded: "I call upon the Coalition on Smoking or Health . . . . Bend your efforts over the next 16 years so that we can have a senior high school class graduate that would be the *first* smoke-free generation to enter the adult world of family life and work. You can do it . . . and I pledge to you the full moral suasion of my office to help in any way possible."[10]

In this call to action to the coalition of anti-smoking groups Koop was not simply piling on the rhetoric. He had been meeting with them in private, sounding them out, "arguing that the country was ready to make such a commitment and that as surgeon general he had the forum to take a dramatic step. However, because he was not proposing a government program (and hence there was no need to clear the initiative through bureaucratic channels), a genuine commitment was needed from health groups. They accepted the challenge, and he participated in their follow-up planning and implementation sessions."[11] In an emollient remark after Koop stepped down, Gary Bauer, who had been one of his fiercest critics from inside the administration on the AIDS front, offered this assessment: "Dr. Koop was perceived as doing, I think, what a Surgeon General should do. What he was not perceived as was an individual who had the final say on what Administration policy would be."[12]

His speech "changed the course of how we thought about tobacco."[13]

Jack Henningfield had worked closely with Koop on tobacco policy. Shortly after Koop was appointed, he had asked for a briefing on smoking. All Henningfield knew about him at the time was what he had read in the *Washington Post*, that he had got the job because he was anti-abortion. The Office on Smoking and Health (then a part of HHS) "sent me to do an interview with him, because he wanted to take on tobacco. And he did a free ranging interview, and said that he wants to make sure that everything, anything we use is scientifically sound. That's what he wanted." So Henningfield was designated Koop's point person on tobacco issues and helped draft his first tobacco testimony to Congress.

The Office of Management and Budget reviewed the testimony and refused to permit Koop to use the word "addiction." The next time he was asked to testify, the administration denied him permission to do so at all.

"So what did Koop do?" In an act that symbolized his approach to political orders that conflicted with his convictions, Henningfield told me, "he shows up at the hearing. And the Chair Henry Waxman says, Dr. Koop, you are here to testify. And Koop says, Yes, but I have not been authorized to speak. "That was his statement!" Soon after, Koop spoke to the press. Nicotine, he said, was eight times more addictive than heroin. And the press went to HHS, and Henningfield was put on the spot and sought to defend Koop by speaking of the addictive character of smoking itself, and its social context, while all along knowing that while it "meets all the criteria as an addictive drug . . . logically speaking, it's not 'more' addictive."

In 1986 Koop went well beyond moral suasion, when for the first time a Surgeon General's report devoted "an entire edition" to "the health consequences of involuntary smoking."[14] That was red meat to the anti-smoking social activists, and also the lower levels of government—state and city—that the tobacco lobbyists found harder to control than they did the US Congress. As the 1970s ended, Milov notes, more than three-quarters of American workplaces still permitted unrestricted smoking. "Finding that appeals to the bottom line were more persuasive to their employers than simply registering their distress and discomfort, nonsmokers embraced the business case for smoking restrictions at work. Smokers . . . were bad employees; they had higher rates of absenteeism . . . they were less productive, took frequent breaks, cost more to insure, dirtied equipment, and caused accidents."[15]

Businesses had begun to make their own decisions. Beginning with the State Mutual Life Assurance Company of America in 1964, by 1987 eighty percent of insurance companies were offering discounts to nonsmokers.[16] While actuarial complexity delayed any such offering to consumers of health insurance, the trade associations of both life and health insurance companies had joined together by 1980 to encourage their members to adopt smoke-free workplace policies, and by 1984 were lobbying for legislation to reduce tobacco use.[17] By 1982, television characters were already smoking an astonishing nine times fewer cigarettes than they had been two decades earlier.[18]

The tide had begun to turn against tobacco. America was moving on from the old days when, just a decade before, the Children's Hospital of Philadelphia had—astonishingly—congratulated its surgeon-in-chief, one Dr. C. Everett Koop, on twenty-five years' service, with the presentation of an engraved silver cigarette box.[19]

While Koop was not kicking at an open door, it was loose on its hinges. His timing was exquisite, and he knew exactly where to land his blows.

"Dr. Koop Has Had an Impact."

Corporate consultants Bloomberg Industry Group[i] informed their clients in a special 1987 report that, in the three years following Koop's speech, a full 45 percent of US businesses had adopted workplace smoking restrictions for the first time.[20]

"Smoking in the workplace: For decades, it was a non-issue. Smoking and non-smoking employees worked side-by-side, without evident hostility, health fears, or argument. Where fire hazards or sanitation were not obvious concerns, smoking restrictions were almost unknown. The popular image of workers was often interwoven with smoking: Executives smoked cigars, professors smoked pipes, and hard workers everywhere smoked cigarettes. That is no longer the case."[21]

The report's core conclusion was stunning. In just one year, since its last edition in 1986, "The nature of the smoking issue has changed. . . . No longer is the primary question facing most employers whether smoking should or should not be restricted. Increasingly, the core question is: How should smoking be restricted in the workplace?" As Pete Lunnie of the National Association of Manufacturers would laconically observe, "Dr. Koop has had an impact."[22] Now, "smoking is under siege in the workplace. That is the central finding of this Special Report." And it is the evident impact of Koop's 1986 report on "involuntary smoking," which argued that—just like Agent Orange and the pesticide EDB—smoking is in fact *not voluntary at all* for millions of Americans.

Bloomberg also noted the impact of the 1985 Surgeon General's Report, with its focus on the interaction of smoking and various occupational exposures that are already hazardous but become much worse for smokers. The "most dramatic interaction" is that of asbestos exposure—ten times worse for smokers.[23]

Then there were cost considerations. "Marvin M. Kristein, professor of economics at the City University of New York, told BNA that

---

i   This is the current name of the business consulting firm, founded in 1929; in the 1980s it was still known by the curious and potentially misleading title the Bureau of National Affairs (BNA).

smokers use $500 to $600 more medical care each year than non-smokers, and that they are absent from work two days more each year than non-smokers."[24] As a result, the core issue for corporate America was whether smoking should be banned in areas shared by nonsmokers.

Bloomberg reviewed assorted counterarguments. A ban could actually increase health risks, according to some labor union officials, by removing the most obvious evidence of bad air quality. It could lead to legal action by "addicted" smokers on handicap grounds, or on grounds of racial discrimination by black males, since they are more likely to smoke.[25]

Meanwhile, Bloomberg noted, action at the state and city level continued. Fourteen states had restricted smoking in private businesses, together with some two hundred local entities. And, at the federal level, the General Services Administration, which manages the government's real estate, in February of 1987 had limited smoking to designated areas in the nearly seven thousand buildings it controls, a ruling affecting 890,000 federal employees.[26]

Detailed results from the private sector, focusing on shifts between 1986 and 1987, are remarkable. The number of firms with smoking policies of some sort in place had jumped by 50 percent (to 54 percent of all companies). The proportion of companies with no policy and none under consideration had halved to 22 percent. Three out of four policies ban smoking in meeting and conference rooms, an increase of one sixth over the year. Meanwhile, the number of companies banning smoking from all company premises had doubled, from 6 to 12 percent. The names of these companies read "like a who's who of U.S. business."[27] There is even a small list of companies and public bodies who will hire only nonsmokers.[28]

Meanwhile, labor unions pushed back hard. Ray Scannel of the Bakery Workers, whose membership included seventeen thousand tobacco workers, dismissed Koop as an "anti-smoking zealot." But the pushback was broader. The 1985 report "was roundly criticized by the AFL-CIO Executive Council."[29] Five AFL-CIO union presidents issued a joint statement attacking the 1986 report, and calling instead for improved ventilation systems, which "will also serve the more important goal of removing many of the other contaminants of the air quality to create a safe and healthy work environment."[30]

Laying the Foundations: Burney and Terry

Needless to say, concern over the health effects of tobacco was nothing new; studies in the 1930s and 1940s had already linked lung cancer to smoking, and an influential article was reprinted in the *Reader's Digest* as far back as December 1952 under the subtle title "Cancer by the Carton." A CDC historical review included in the Surgeon General's report for 2000 noted that the immediate decline in smoking precipitated by this piece prompted fresh attention by the industry to the novel filter tip, being introduced initially as a means of offering a milder smoking experience to new users. Now it offered a fresh marketing opportunity, even if it tacitly acknowledged the possibility of a risk to health. The market share for filter brands "increased from less than 1 percent in 1952 to 73 percent in 1968."

Public debate had ebbed and flowed in the 1950s. The monthly magazine *Consumer Reports*, for example, had noted "suggestive" reports about a connection between smoking and lung cancer, and recommended that until further research clarified the situation "those who can" should reduce their smoking to a "moderate" level—defined as not more than one pack a day. At the same time, smoking's health benefits were also touted, specifically that it could reduce stress in a way that was less harmful than alcohol or overeating.[31]

At another social level, smoking was one of the standard examples discussed by Leon Festinger in his classic study, *A Theory of Cognitive Dissonance*, first published in 1957. Among university faculty, who were as informed as anyone about the research and its direction, smoking remained extremely popular—together with various forms of intellectual justification, typically focused on comparisons with other examples of risk that were readily accepted, such as travel by (pre-seatbelt) automobile.[32]

Meanwhile, in that same year, 1957, 8th Surgeon General Leroy E. Burney (1906–98, in office 1956–61) weighed in with the first formal statement from the federal government on lung cancer and smoking.[33] "It is clear that there is an increasing and consistent body of evidence that excessive cigarette smoking is one of the causative factors in lung cancer."[34] Burney's role in the history of anti-smoking efforts should be better known, since he paved the way for his immediate successor, who is generally credited with initiating the federal critique of tobacco.

Luther L. Terry (1911–85), a "soft-spoken, Alabama-born physician," had, like Burney, worked his way up through the Public Health Service, including years of cancer research service at NIH, before President Kennedy picked him to be Surgeon General. Three months after Terry's confirmation on March 2, 1961, the Presidents of the American Public Health Association and several other medical groups appealed to the President to establish a commission on the health consequences of smoking. Early the following year, Terry secured approval from his boss, Secretary of Health, Education, and Welfare,[ii] to do so.

Terry took a somewhat political approach to his task.[35] As Allan M. Brandt tells the tale in his history of *The Cigarette Century*, his staff first assembled a list of some one hundred fifty experts as potential members of the committee who would write the report. They deleted the names of any who had already published on the issue and taken sides (thereby oddly excluding all actual experts!), and circulated the remainder to all relevant organizations, from the American Cancer Society to the Tobacco Institute, the cigarette industry's lobbying and public relations arm, with an invitation to remove any names they wished—an invitation of which the Institute took full advantage, in one case of an academic who was known at some time in the past to have decided to stop smoking. From those that remained, Terry selected ten: five smokers and five nonsmokers. It would be part advisory group, part drafting committee, and part jury.[36] Terry was scrupulous in his determination that the industry should not be able to undermine the work of the committee by suggesting that

---

ii   The department was re-organized, with education spun off, and renamed HHS in 1980.

its members were biased. "Photos of the committee meeting at the National Library of Medicine show a smoke-filled room with a conference table littered with ashtrays."[37]

The 1964 report that resulted was unequivocal, concluding that "there was no question as to the role of cigarette smoking in causing lung cancer." It was a matter of "national concern." The death rate from cancer was "almost 1,000 percent higher in men who smoked cigarettes than it was in nonsmokers." What's more, it played a key role in a string of other diseases, from chronic bronchitis and emphysema to coronary artery disease.[38] Or, in the summary with which Sarah Milov opens her history of the tobacco wars, "The nearly-400 page report concluded that cigarettes caused death." There was such concern in official circles about the potential significance of the report for cigarette consumption, and therefore for the tobacco industry, that it was released on a Saturday, to cushion its impact on the stock market.[39]

Legislation followed in Congress: the Federal Cigarette Labeling and Advertising Act of 1965. But as the 2000 Surgeon General's report observes, the Act "undermined much of the original proposal's strength by requiring a more weakly worded label than the FTC had proposed," and went on to preempt the FTC and any other government entity, federal, state, or local, from further tobacco restriction until the 1969 expiration of the law. Terry himself later referred to the law as a "hoax on the American people."[40] But federal health officials didn't make it too hard. In a 1969 hearing, for example, then Surgeon General Stewart (1921–2008) and three other top health officials all testified in favor of stronger warnings. A member of Congress pointed out that all four of them, including the director of the National Cancer Institute, were smokers![41]

The Reports

Koop signed the reports.[42] Then he went around making speeches about them and took the heat of the anti-anti-smoking lobby to such a degree that the FBI had to deal with death threats to the Surgeon General.[43] As Donald Shopland, who worked on the reports, explained to me, Koop actually had little to do with preparing them.

The Office of Smoking and Health strategy in the 1980s was two-fold. First, to follow up the 1982 cancer report with focused documents on two further major harms: cardiopulmonary disease in 1983, and chronic obstructive lung disease in 1984. Thus, in three successive years, the latest research on these three disease outcomes was summarized and employed as the basis for Koop's continued assaults on tobacco use and the tobacco industry itself.

Second, the theme of the annual reports then turned to fresh ways of making the case. As Koop had noted in the 1984 Julia Jones speech, the risk of tobacco use was seen as different from the risks of exposure to Agent Orange or toxic pesticide because it was a risk voluntarily undertaken by smokers. The three reports that followed undercut this argument by focusing intensively on aspects of non-voluntary smoking risk. First, its effect on disease in the workplace (1985), where smoking risk would intersect with other environmental toxic risks such as asbestos, with results that were worse all around. Second, the explosive matter of involuntary, or secondhand, or "sidestream," smoking, to use the technical term, smoking that is no more voluntary than Agent Orange exposure for the US forces in Vietnam (1986). And third, nicotine addiction (1988).[44] This succession of reports demonstrated that the idea of smoking as a purely personal and voluntary activity was false. In the workplace, other environmental risks made smoking more dangerous. Secondhand smoking was the very oppositive of voluntary. And the highly addictive character of nicotine suggested that the industry was locking smokers into a dangerous pastime that they would find hard to escape even if they so wished.

The industry was alert to the potentially devastating threat posed, especially by the report on secondhand smoke. Allan Brandt, in *The Cigarette Century*, shares notes from a war-room meeting planning their response.

> [S]econdhand smoke posed a potentially life-threatening risk—to the industry. As John Rupp, a lawyer at Covington & Burling working on tobacco accounts, put it, "we are in deep shit." Rupp was speaking at a 1987 conference for Philip Morris's Project Down Under, organized to devise new strategies to address the threat. Attendees continued to

hope for ways to upend the research implicating secondhand smoke as a serious health risk.

Minutes from the meeting reported, "A scientific battle was lost with the Surgeon General's '86 Report. Is there any way of showing the Surgeon General is wrong?" Even as the gathered executives recognized that they were losing the battle of public perceptions, they understood that they still had considerable advantages in resources and power. One theme discussed at the conference was "Make It Hurt." "Let pols know down side of anti activity," noted the conference minutes. "To do this, we take on vulnerable candidate, beat him/her, let people know we did it." At a brainstorming session, the Philip Morris executives came up with more than one hundred 'solutions to the problem.' These ranged from "create a bigger monster (AIDS)" to "undermine Koop et al."[45]

Koop's energetic prosecution of the Smoke-free Society campaign led to many initiatives. Actor Yul Brynner wanted to help. Koop reached out to Stan and Jan Berenstain, authors of the wildly popular children's Berenstain Bears series, and they responded enthusiastically.[46] He introduced an institute on occupational smoking to former Secretary Schweiker, who in 1985 was president of the American Council of Life Insurance.[47] He responded to an unusual letter from a physician seeking his help to persuade his wife, herself a pulmonary physician, to stop smoking. His daughters have bought her Nicorette gum, but she says she needs more motivation. Perhaps a personal letter from the Surgeon General would do the trick? Koop has printed up buttons saying, "the Surgeon General personally asked me to quit," and "I quit because he asked me." So he wrote to the smoking pulmonary physician: "Your husband . . . is very distressed about your smoking and thought that a word from me might do the trick. . . . I am enclosing two buttons, one to encourage you and one to brag about when you have been successful." Two months later he wrote a second time, with two more buttons.[48]

Koop later reminisced about something he had found particularly satisfying—stopping smoking on airplanes, for which he took personal credit. He worked with Air Canada, since he could not find a US airline prepared to cooperate, to research the impact of smoking on transcontinental flights. "We showed it didn't matter where you sat in an airplane, you got the same amount of noxious inhalations . . .

a nonsmoking flight attendant on the flight from Montreal to Vancouver would smoke three cigarettes, whether she wanted to or not, just from sidestream smoking. And we found that nonsmokers held onto the toxins in their bodies for a lot longer period of time than did regular smokers because they [smokers] apparently had learned . . . to get rid of these things that were killing them faster than the nonsmoker did. And from the day we started till the day we had the information we needed, it took two weeks."

Koop took the research to Senator Frank Lautenberg of New Jersey, "because I had worked with him on other smoking things, and it took him a year to get it through Congress." He reflected: "If you look back at it, I think, having cracked the airlines is what made it easy to crack everything else, from bars to baseball fields."[49]

In 1986, the National Academies had issued a report on the risks involved in airplane smoking and recommended a ban on all US commercial flights. Congressman Richard Durbin's bill only just passed the House, 198–183, after lobbying from both tobacco companies and the airlines. The Senate vote, where Senator Lautenberg took the lead, was 84–10, against entrenched opposition from Helms and other tobacco state senators that whittled the ban down to flights of ninety minutes or less, and for a period of two years only.[50] "People choose to smoke, but there is no choice about breathing," said Republican Senator Orrin Hatch. The ban went into force in 1988. Northwest Airlines took the opportunity to announce a ban on all smoking on its flights, and "heavily advertised" the new policy, which proved popular, and the other airlines dropped their opposition.[51] In 1989, Senator Lautenberg took the initiative in extending the ban from 1990 to all flights under six hours.[52]

Koop's Impact

"He was single-handedly responsible for reinvigorating the anti-smoking movement," said Guy L. Smith IV, then Philip Morris's vice president for corporate affairs.[53] Per the *New York Times*: He "played a crucial role in changing public attitudes about smoking."[54]

Smoking was trending down when Koop came into office, but it's striking to compare the raw numbers, decade by decade. During the

1970s, according to the American Lung Association, smoking fell a total of 4.2 percent: 6.5 percent among men, 2.2 percent among women. In the 1990s those figures were, respectively, 2.2, 2.8, and 1.8 percent. The 1980s contrast is stunning. 9.2 percent of American men quit smoking in that decade, 6.5 percent of American women, a total of 7.7 percent of the population.[55] Per Gallup, smokers in June 1981 were 35 percent; May 1989, 27 percent, an 8 percent drop during Koop's eight years in office—which is actually a drop of almost one-quarter in the number of smokers.[56] "It was during the 1980s," notes Michael J. Bowman, "that smoking became an antisocial activity.[57]

Looking back from the end of his tenure, the *Los Angeles Times* reflected on his impact. "In 1982, Koop wrote his rigid indictment of cigarette smoking, focusing exclusively on its connection with a dozen cancers . . . and was vilified by cigarette companies, their lobbies, their legislators and the governor of North Carolina.

"Today, the cigarette habit continues to decline and Koop thinks his smoke-free society may not be a pipe dream. Looking back, he presumes the crusade will be considered among the highest triumphs of public health." Looking ahead, "he would often say that he wants to create a world where it's as easy to get help in overcoming tobacco dependence as it is to go down to the corner and buy a pack of cigarettes."[58]

Yet just a few days before he died, Koop was visited by friend and Dartmouth colleague Joseph O'Donnell. "And, you know, he was fading," O'Donnell told me. "He basically said, Joe, I wanted to rid the world of tobacco. You got to be able to finish the job."[59] [iii]

[iii] US smoking rates were continuing to fall, if more gradually than during the 1980s. When Koop left office, the rate was 27 percent. In "Smoke-free Society" year 2000, it stood at 17.8 percent. As of this writing in 2024, the latest figure per CDC is 11 percent. Among those with graduate school degrees, it is below 3 percent.

CHAPTER 11

Confronting AIDS

I think what he did was extraordinary.
—MICHAEL GOTTLIEB, who first identified the HIV virus, interview

He was hailed as a kind of Paul Revere.
                                            —CEK adviser, interview

The recent material you sent on AIDS is the same rubbish that you
have been sending me in the past. I think you'd improve your peace of
mind if you didn't read it. Think of it this way, if you could get AIDS
the way these people say you can, we'd all have it.
                                            —CEK, to an old friend

June, 1989, and a remarkable scene is unfolding. A beautiful day
on Boston Common, temperature in the mid-70s. Eighteen thousand young men, gay activists, fundraising against a plague that has
already killed five times as many of their friends. And another man.
Oddly bearded, deeply religious, somewhat surly, an aging social conservative physician. Who had freely called gay sex sodomy, and once
actually made a movie standing on the site of Sodom as the embodiment of evil. The burly figure of Presbyterian elder Charles Everett
Koop could be seen stepping out in front of the crowd. As he slowly
walked toward the platform, in his curious navy-style uniform hat
and short-sleeve whites, and up the steps, and across the podium,
all you can hear, right across the Common, is the chanting. Koop!
Koop! Koop! He's at the mic, and they won't stop. KOOP! KOOP!
KOOP![1]

How on earth has this happened?

"AIDS entered the consciousness of the Public Health Service quietly, gradually, and without fanfare. I was at a staff meeting in June of

1981, as the Surgeon General designate, when the Centers for Disease Control published a report . . . concerning five previously healthy homosexuals, who had been admitted to Los Angeles hospitals with pneumonia caused by a very rare organism, pneumocystis carinii."[2] That's how it all began.

A few miles north, Anthony Fauci was sitting in his office at the NIH reading the same report.

> My life actually changed in the summer of 1981. I was sitting at my desk at the Clinical Center, Building 10 . . . and a publication from the Centers for Disease Control and Prevention called MMWR, for Morbidity and Mortality Weekly Report, landed on my desk a couple of days after its published date of June 5th, 1981, reporting five men from Los Angeles who developed a very unusual infection called pneumocystis pneumonia that you would never see in someone with a normal immune system. Curiously, they were all gay men. And I had no idea what was going on. I put it aside. I thought it was a fluke. I thought that, well, maybe they took a toxic drug or something that suppressed their immune system. But I was a little bit interested in it because they were immunosuppressed and I was an immunologist. I didn't make much of it. One month later, on July 4th, 1981, another MMWR appeared on my desk, this time reporting twenty-six men now, not only from Los Angeles but from New York and San Francisco. Again, complete puzzle, presenting otherwise well with a variety of infections, pneumocystis, cytomegalovirus, and also Kaposi's sarcoma, which is, again, a rare cancer found in people who are immunosuppressed, usually transplantation patients. Curiously, all of them were gay. And I remember sitting there in my office saying, Oh, my goodness, this is a brand-new disease.[3]

Like Fauci, Koop knew all about pneumocystis pneumonia; in fact, he was the only person at that HHS staff meeting who had actually seen cases with his own eyes: patients immunosuppressed by chemotherapy.

Two months later, CDC reported that cases were up to one hundred eight, with forty-three deaths. Koop recalls his "first real confrontation with the other members of the Public Health Service," when he told them: "If this is a homosexual disease, one of the things we will have to come to grips with, early on . . . is the forced sodomy which takes place in prisons and would be a source of rapid spread of the disease. No-one at the staff meeting agreed with me, and it was years before anyone, especially the Centers for Disease Control were talking about AIDS among prisoners."[4] This early "real confrontation" with PHS colleagues may have played its part in the decision taken by Koop's superior, Edward Brandt, the assistant secretary for health, to keep him right out of the AIDS loop—and, specifically, off the high-level AIDS task force he was putting together. Brandt wanted to avoid the "politicization" of the disease, as he saw it, preferring to leave it to sober science in the hands of sober scientists. He judged his firebrand social conservative Surgeon General to be quite the opposite.[5]

Meanwhile, Koop and Fauci were talking, and Koop was learning a lot about what would soon be known as HIV/AIDS.[6] As Fauci told me, "The Surgeon General by tradition lives on the NIH campus . . . there are houses originally meant for the directors of the Institute. So every night, when Chick Koop would come home from work, which was downtown in the Humphrey Building. His home was, literally, I can see it as I'm talking to you, I'm looking out of the window. So since we were friends, Chick was a gregarious guy who would often on his way home stop in my office. I've always worked until eight or nine o'clock, being somewhat of a workaholic." Then, "one night he said, You know, I really want to learn a bit about this disease, this HIV/AIDS disease, and we'd talk about it. And he'd spend literally hours of the evening, until he became so interested in it that he decided he was going to make it his thing."

Fauci went on: "And once we educated him about HIV, you know, I could see his mind working. You know, I'm sitting in my office, and I'm in the same office as I was back then. And I'm looking at the chair and the couch, where he sat for hours of the evening talking about it, and you could see him gradually getting transformed into saying, you know, there is a problem with the entity which is the virus, the entity is not the people." And Koop started to say, "We've got to be completely open-minded about trying to help them. There should not be any stigma associated with HIV. And then once he got that going, then that was it. I mean, he was off to the races. And that was pretty extraordinary back then. I mean given how social attitudes have shifted since."[7]

When Margaret Heckler succeeded Richard Schweiker as HHS secretary in March, 1983, she had never even heard of AIDS.[8] Heckler, a former congresswoman, loved the public eye, and was keenly aware of her image.[9] Not only did she support Brandt's decision to keep the Surgeon General away from AIDS, she immediately "injected herself into the AIDS issue."[10] Koop observed that, "Under ordinary circumstances, a non-medical person in that position would defer to the Assistant Secretary for Health for annunciation of scientific breakthroughs, dilemmas, and uncertainties. Not so, Madam Heckler. She . . . wanted the spotlight associated with AIDS and made major announcements and held press conferences." She wanted to speak in scientific terms and advised her speech writers accordingly. "When it was amply demonstrated that she faltered with the scientific language and she was advised to remove it, she settled for phonetic spelling which she also butchered." Koop recalled: "It was sad that people were actually giggling on one occasion at an Atlanta meeting where her mispronunciations provided the only levity for the occasion."[11]

While it was February of 1986 before President Reagan tasked Koop with writing the report on AIDS, Koop's claim that he was "completely cut off from AIDS" for "an astonishing five and a half years" is misleading.[12] As we have noted, everything changed when Brandt stood down and was succeeded as assistant secretary by James O. Mason. Mason was greatly esteemed as a public administrator. He had earlier run the Mormon hospital system, and combined that with longtime service in the Commissioned Corps.[i]

"It is difficult to comprehend the hysteria that surrounded HIV/AIDS in the United States in the first decade of the epidemic," the *British Medical Journal* later recalled. "When homosexuality was

---

i   Mason served as acting assistant secretary for health from Brandt's departure in 1984 until the end of 1985, doubling up as he continued to be director of CDC. He was later appointed by George H. W. Bush to be assistant secretary from 1989 to 1993. In that capacity he also took over as acting Surgeon General when Koop stood down.

still deemed taboo. When there was no effective treatment for AIDS, and when healthy young men would turn into shuffling cadavers in a matter of weeks, and then disappear." And, when "a firebomb drove the Ray family from their home in Arcadia, Florida, because the parents sought to enroll their boys—aged 8, 9, and 10—in school. The children had contracted HIV through blood products used to treat their haemophilia."[13] In 1986, conservative commentator William F. Buckley, Jr. called for the tattooing of gay men and drug users: "Everyone detected with AIDS should be tattooed in the upper forearm, to protect common-needle users, and on the buttocks, to prevent the victimization of other homosexuals."[14] Meanwhile, "Other conservative Republicans talked about quarantining HIV-positive people and 'rounding up' all gay men."[15]

The Reagan White House

President Reagan has been widely blamed for failing to address AIDS earlier. The President did not utter the word in public until 1986. New evidence has come to light that suggests this criticism may be ungrounded. In a later interview, Edward Brandt, who as assistant secretary for health from 1981–84 was in charge of the PHS, including the Surgeon General, NIH, and CDC, and therefore all aspects of AIDS policy, made the startling statement that this was actually his doing. With the agreement of the secretaries under whom he served—Schweiker and then Heckler—he had taken it upon himself to "ask[ed] the White House to stay out of the whole thing and for a whole lot of reasons."

Brandt continued: "And so I knew that White Houses are by their very nature political. . . . I was trying to . . . keep it as a basically scientific issue." So Brandt was prepared to take responsibility for something for which "the President got heavily criticized." He was asked to review various draft speeches that Reagan was going to make "in which they had put something in there about AIDS. And I asked them at the White House to take it out; and they did. So I think he was unfairly criticized."[16] A White House staffer at the time told me:

"the White House was a house divided. We had the Meese side of the White House, the conservative side of the White House, and we had the Baker side of the White House, which was the pragmatic. . . . We could probably come up with half a dozen names of people . . . wanting the President out front on this, wanting him to be sympathetic to the community that was primarily affected."[17]

Brandt followed up this confession by explaining why no one had heard it before. "I know of thirteen histories that have been written during that period of time. Only one author has ever talked to me."[18]

As for Reagan himself, biographer Edmund Morris noted the significance of his friend Rock Hudson's death on October 2, 1985. He and Nancy had called Hudson, then in hospital in Europe under cover of another ailment. Just two months before his death they invited him to the White House. Until then, says Morris, Reagan was "unconcerned" about AIDS. He began to ask one of his doctors "a few shyly clumsy questions: 'It's a virus, like measles? But it doesn't go away?' My research cards," continued Morris, "have him finding it a fit subject for humor as late as December 1986, and five months after that waxing biblical in his opinion that 'maybe the Lord brought down this plague' because 'illicit sex is against the Ten Commandments.'"[19]

Koop continued to take what opportunities came his way to engage with the President. On one occasion, he joined him visiting sick children at the National Cancer Institute, when a bomb scare led the Secret Service to thrust the two of them into a broom closet! "We were walking side-by-side and we were surrounded by Secret Service. . . . So it was just he and I in the broom closet, and I said with a smile on my face, 'We have very little time, Mr. President, but I have a few things to say about AIDS.'"[20]

Writing the AIDS Report

As 1985 drew to a close, there was something in the air.

First, a remarkable formal proposal was made by the White House to give the Surgeon General's office authority over all AIDS research and other activities across HHS, including the various efforts at NIH and CDC; in other words, to make Koop the AIDS Czar. "The Office of Management and Budget has proposed consolidating all federal AIDS programs in the surgeon general's office," reported Marlene Cimons in the *Los Angeles Times* for December 24, 1985.[21] In her deeply researched 1988 book *The AIDS Bureaucracy*, Sandra Panem suggests this proposal may have originated with James Mason, then acting assistant secretary for health. Mason stepped down from the role at the end of the year, and would therefore have been in no position to shepherd it through.[22] The proposal went nowhere.

Two more key actions were taken by the White House around the turn of the year. On December 17, the press office requested talking points on AIDS from the assistant secretary for public affairs at HHS, since a presidential press conference was planned for the new year.[23] Second, a paragraph was drafted for inclusion in the State of the Union, which in early January was passed to HHS for approval by the secretary.[24]

As it happened, on January 28, 1986, the day of the State of the Union, at 11:39 a.m. eastern standard time, the space shuttle Challenger exploded. At five o'clock in the afternoon the president made an emotional broadcast to the nation from the Oval Office, closing with the words of war poet John Gillespie Magee: "We will never forget them . . . as they prepared for their journey and waved goodbye and 'slipped the surly bonds of earth' to 'touch the face of God.'"[25]

The State of the Union speech was delayed by one week until February 4, and it opened with a further memorial to the crew. "We pause together to mourn and honor the valor of our seven Challenger heroes." That explains why reference to AIDS was taken out. And why it became the subject of another unusual move by the President, his visit the very next morning to the Hubert Humphrey Building, the HHS headquarters, to make a speech in the atrium.

Toward the end of his mostly humorous remarks, Reagan slipped in the statement cut from the previous day's speech: "One of our highest public health priorities is going to continue to be finding a cure for AIDS. We're going to continue to try to develop and test vaccines, and we're going to focus also on prevention. In this regard, I'm asking the Surgeon General to prepare a major report to the American people on AIDS."[26]

There had evidently been discussion in the White House about whether Koop or Secretary Bowen (himself a physician) should be asked to take the lead and write the report, and there was concern that the secretary might be displeased if it went to Koop. "We viewed him [Bowen]," a White House staffer told me, "as someone who didn't necessarily have the President's values." So, "the decision was made—Koop did get the nod."[27] According to James Bowman and Brent Wall, the secretary was not unhappy with this situation. His chief of staff, Koop ally Thomas Burke, said, "Let Koop be Koop."[28]

Koop wryly remarked later, "It's good that I was listening carefully, because that's the only directive I had from anyone about that report." One result of this lack of documentation was that no particular requirements were laid down, so Koop was free to shape his message any way he chose. He might have opted for the tobacco report model, which can run to six hundred pages of tightly packed text from a slew of experts. Instead, he chose to speak to the people in language they would understand, and to write the report himself at a standing desk in his basement.

While the report remained secret until published, Koop was not shy about his basic approach, telling the *Los Angeles Times* on September 14 that populations at risk of AIDS had no need to feel nervous about what was coming. "It doesn't matter how I feel about homosexuality. . . . That's not my job as a health officer. When I was a surgeon it didn't matter if I was treating the gunshot victim or the perpetrator caught by the police—they were both people." And, he added: "It will have the imprimatur of a name the public has come to rely on."[29]

Koop's approach was a model of inclusivity, as he sought both to understand people's perspectives and at the same time to build confidence in his work. He set out to engage the widest range of interested parties from across America; at one place he lists a total of twenty-seven such groups. He made clear that he was willing to meet with anyone who wished to meet with him—from major medical organizations to AIDS activists.

Jeffrey Levi, now a professor at George Washington University, was then leading government relations for the National Gay and Lesbian Task Force. "We were all scared out of our mind what he was going to report," he told me. Then they sat down with Koop and talked, at length. "We're initially incredibly skeptical. OK, so he's pretending to be objective and scientific and wanting to learn." But it became clear that he was for real. "He turned out to be this incredibly engaging person as well, who, despite sort of his gruff manner was very sensitive. There were just so many incredible ironies." And in the end, "He became, you know, to all of us a major figure that made a difference."[30]

Koop could be wily, and he became practiced at heading off challenges from within the government when he wanted to say something that others did not want him to. We have seen his Smoke-free Society speech typed up secretly by the American Lung Association. So once he was done, instead of sending the White House a draft to be scribbled on, Koop began by printing a thousand copies of the report on "expensive paper with a royal blue cover emblazoned with the silver PHS seal." He took a pile of them with him, numbered them, and explained that he would have to collect them after the meeting "for security reasons" lest they leak to the press. He evidently got away with it.

AIDS and the White House

Yet when the contents of the report had been absorbed, as one White House staffer told me, they were shocked. "I am sure that many people who were big Koop advocates on the front end of his joining the government were appalled." They had just assumed that "the number one recommendation would be abstinence."[31]

Yet as historian Jennifer Brier makes plain in her analysis, it is a mistake to assume that the approach of religious conservatives within the administration was homogeneous, with Koop as an outlier.[32]

The issue for Brier is not simply AIDS policy, but the politics and the players. "Putting AIDS at the center of a historical analysis of

Reagan's presidency unsettles our understanding of modern conservatism." There was actually a range of responses among the "family-values" types. While "Gary Bauer, William Bennett, and Carl Anderson, steered the administration toward a morality-based[ii] AIDS initiative that shunned homosexuality and hailed abstinence and heterosexual marriage as the only forms of AIDS prevention," Koop and Admiral James Watkins, who would go on to lead the Presidential Commission on HIV, "fundamentally disagreed" with them. In a welcome departure from the naive if conventional idea that Koop set his religious beliefs aside to address the AIDS crisis, Brier captures his approach precisely when she states that he maintained that "to address AIDS required a commitment to rational science and Christianity as well as explicit discussions of sexual practice, drug use, and condom distribution."[33]

Soon after, AIDS finally did make it into the (1987) State of the Union, with the Koop report center-stage—the final sentence giving evidence that the push in the White House to frame educational efforts more clearly in family-values terms has met with modest success:

> My Administration will also continue to invest in research to cure heart disease, cancer, and other life-threatening diseases. In particular, we will continue our work to find a cure for acquired immune deficiency syndrome, or AIDS. We are also increasing basic research to better understand the causes of AIDS and to find a cure for AIDS or a vaccine to prevent it. Last year the Surgeon General issued a report that was a landmark in public education about AIDS. We will expand that education effort this year, stressing that education about AIDS to schoolchildren must be grounded in the moral and cultural values of parents and communities.[34]

The White House Domestic Policy Council (DPC) had initiated three successive wide-scale efforts to shape the administration's response to AIDS. The first was the 1986 report to the nation, that Koop was asked to write. The second was the work of the presidential commission,

ii   This use of "morality-based" to characterize the approach of Bauer and others is less than helpful, since what's in review are two competing construals of morality, indeed, of conservative Christian morality, to shape AIDS policy.

soon to be known as the Watkins Commission, established in 1987. The third was the 1988 mass mailing, to one hundred seven million households. It is fair to observe that none of these initiatives turned out as more conservative/"religious right" voices in the administration had intended; they essentially lost control of all of them. The Koop report was the first—and, from their point of view, plainly, the worst, since it set a context for the commission, and the mailing that followed.[35]

AIDS discussion within the DPC had its origins in early outreach efforts in the developing crisis. In the summer of 1983, two meetings had been held under the auspices of the White House Office of Public Liaison (OPL). The first brought together representatives from HHS and two "gay activists"—Virginia Apuzzo, who noted that it was "the first meeting between the gay/lesbian community and the Reagan administration," and Jeffrey Levi, who as we have seen would later be a key Koop informant in his consultation process. Unusually, OPL chose to host this meeting at HHS.[36] It was followed by a second meeting later in the summer in which OPL responded to a request from representatives of the Moral Majority and the Conservative Caucus. It's interesting to note that these grassroots conservatives had been equally critical of the failure of the White House to do more early on in response to an issue of "overwhelming public concern." Brier reports that from her review of the records these were the only formal OPL AIDS-related outreach meetings until 1985.[37]

Meanwhile, various HHS efforts had been underway. In September of 1985, an interagency health policy working group laid out a proposed course of action to handle the AIDS epidemic, entitled "What should the federal government do to deal with the problem of AIDS?" Once it was passed to the White House, Carl Anderson, then special assistant in the OPL, amended the memo to add the need for a "special report on AIDS."[38]

Then, on December 19, the DPC reviewed the interagency working group memo, during a meeting somewhat unusually attended in person by the President.[39] The President is quoted in the minutes as saying that "AIDS must be dealt with as a major *public* health problem," seemingly weighing in at one end of the public health-civil rights axis, though minuting can of course be selective. The meeting recommended that the President sign the revised memo, and three days later, on December 22, he did.[40] The irony of Carl Anderson's role in all this stands out. As one of those who had been key to the original push to have Koop as Surgeon General back in 1980, when he was working for Senator Helms, he is now advocating for a special report on AIDS that Koop will be asked to write, but that in the event will much displease him. Yet, in Brier's understated prose, "in the minds of the upper-administration officials, Koop's beliefs made him the perfect candidate to write a special report on AIDS that would emphasize morality, defined as a commitment to heterosexual marriage as the key institution of the American family and nation, rather than condoms and sex education."[41]

Meanwhile, CDC director James O. Mason, three months after the Koop report was issued, had pulled together a sixty-page "information/education plan" to "prevent and control AIDS," with as its centerpiece "an immediate one-time direct mailing of AIDS facts to every household in the United States," in tandem with an "extensive media campaign" to encourage people to read their mail. The plan went up the chain to the White House, where it was considered in tandem with a proposal to appoint a presidential AIDS commission.[42] For staff who were critical of Koop's report, both these efforts offered an opportunity to regain control of the narrative. Bennett and Baur stressed that any such mailing should go through the DPC, to ensure it was in line with "the president's stated beliefs on marriage and abstinence."[43] Baur himself would be responsible for setting up the commission. The President approved the AIDS commission on May 1, 1987, but chose to delay the mailing.[44]

William Bennett, meanwhile, was transforming the backwater of the Education Department, a "quiet department with comparatively limited programmatic responsibilities," into a bully pulpit of his own, not least on issues of public health. Henry Waxman opined that perhaps he had ambitions to be on the presidential ticket some day. When queried by the press, Bennett's response was: "What's the law that says the secretary of education can't talk about other things?" Koop's AIDS report was hardly alone in his crosshairs. He was meantime weighing in on the fate of Supreme Court nominee Robert Bork ("a poker buddy," per the *Washington Post*), and quixotic presidential hopeful Pat Robertson. He certainly succeeding in making Koop's job harder. When asked at a congressional hearing by Chairman Waxman whether he or Bennett spoke for the administration on the issue of mandatory testing, Koop responded, "That is a difficult question."[45]

In parallel, an effort was underway to contain the fallout. Bennett and Koop were asked to work up a joint "Statement on AIDS Education." It received minimal coverage in the press, since it was such a patent effort to paper over disagreement. The statement concludes: "With regard to AIDS, science and morality teach the same lesson. The Surgeon General's Report on AIDS makes it clear that the best way to avoid AIDS is a mutually faithful monogamous sexual relationship. Until it is possible to establish and maintain such a relationship, abstinence is safest."[46]

Weeks after the report was published, Koop woke up a quadriplegic. His old college football injury had re-asserted itself.[47] It was six weeks before surgery at the Bethesda Naval Medical Center enabled him to return to work, "neurologically intact, but not quite as strong as I had been."

When Michael Lindsay writes in *Faith in the Halls of Power* that after the publication of the AIDS report "fellow evangelicals mobilized against Koop with tremendous force," he overstates his case, as the welcome accorded Koop by key evangelical leaders in early 1987 shows.[48] Koop had remained on surprisingly good terms with conservative religious leaders outside Washington, and once he had recovered decided to devote seven weeks at the start of 1987 to getting out the message exclusively to his co-religionists the evangelicals, the grassroots of the "religious right" that Bauer and his other Washington critics claimed to represent. He secured an invitation to Jerry Falwell's influential (televised) pulpit, and Liberty University in Lynchburg, Virginia, and addressed a range of other groups including the National Association of Religious Broadcasters, the radio station network of Moody Bible Institute in Chicago, and key leaders of the Southern Baptist Convention.

Addressing six thousand students at Liberty, Koop said he "resented criticism from fellow conservatives and evangelicals of his call for sex education to prevent the spread of the disease. Make no mistake about it, AIDS is spreading among more people and it is uniformly fatal."[49]

"In those addresses, delivered in full uniform and a neck brace," wrote Philip Yancey in *Christianity Today*, "Koop affirmed the need for abstinence and monogamous marriage. But, Koop would add, 'Total abstinence for everyone is not realistic, and I'm not ready to give up on the human race quite yet.'"[50]

This campaign had much success in enabling Koop to disseminate his message on AIDS directly, in own words, and not through the fog of press reporting. After his February speech to the National Religious Broadcasters, the director of the National Association of Evangelicals, Robert Dugan, wrote in these warm terms: "Contrary to the public allegations of a few folks, I believe you gave a splendid account of yourself both as Surgeon General and as an evangelical Christian."[51] Jerry Falwell, archetypal leader of the religious right who had co-founded the Moral Majority in 1979, wrote to Koop on October 1 of 1987 to thank him for "doing your best to protect the health of every American, regardless of the popularity of your counsel. . . . My thanks for your courage. America is fortunate to have your service during this difficult time." Koop thanked him in turn for his support, "not only on the National scene . . . but also as a source of personal strengths going down a path that I have not always found easy."[52]

But there had been criticism from fellow evangelicals, and he had not found it easy to take. As historian and Koop friend Michael Horton recalled to me, "The thing that I most remember our having a conversation about was how much the evangelical opposition to him during the AIDS crisis crushed him. And he really was hurt by that."[53]

The AIDS report also led to a swift breach with Catholic Carl Anderson, with whom Koop had been close throughout his time in Washington.[54] It was painful on both sides. A mutual friend arranged a dinner between them. Koop wrote of it as "a discouraging occasion." They disagreed about many things in the report, from the focus on sex education to Koop's inclusion of the telephone numbers of homosexual organizations offering help. "He did not buy my argument that an infected homosexual was unlikely to turn to the National Council of Churches or the government to find a place of refuge or a place to die." He remarks: "After that dinner I never heard from Anderson again."[55]

Efforts continued by Koop's critics in the administration to revise the report after the event. On July 31, 1987, he reports to a colleague a visit from Gary Bauer and Nancy Risque, the cabinet secretary, "on the issue of revising the Surgeon General's Report on AIDS." In other words, removing the word condom. "We agreed that there would not be any changes in the report." When members of Congress sought further copies, update issues such as developments in virucides would be dealt with by accompanying letter.[56] Koop's approach was to refuse flat-out efforts of this kind by staff, knowing that it was highly unlikely that staff would be able to persuade the President to speak directly to the HHS secretary and order him to do their bidding. "His staff would call up my staff and say 'My boss didn't like what your boss said.' We had a standard answer; 'When your boss feels that way and talks to my boss, he'll get some action.' Period. He [Reagan] never called about anything like that," Koop said.[57] "To date," notes education aide Robert Sweet in a March 13, 1987, memo to Bauer, "Dr. Koop has resisted attempts by nearly everyone to modify his promotion of condoms as a solution for the AIDS epidemic rather than to promote fidelity, chastity and sex within marriage."[58] But these efforts were curious, since had any substantive change actually been made to the report would have ignited a political firestorm.

Koop told the *New York Times* that he had no regrets about issuing the report but admitted that "if he had to do it over again, he probably would try to be clearer in the section on sex education in schools."[59]

A press conference on March 25, 1987, got Koop into specially hot water with elements of the pro-life movement. He was taking

questions at the National Press Club and offered the personal opinion that while he continued to oppose compulsory testing, "anyone getting married today would want to be tested and would want
to know." One of his greatest concerns, he said, "was the potential threat to the babies of infected mothers. . . . I think no woman
should contemplate a pregnancy without voluntarily wanting to be
tested for the AIDS virus." The next question was about abortion.
As reported in the *New York Times*, "Dr. Koop, a strong opponent
of abortion, answered cautiously." He said: "If you wanted to give
her all the possibilities that were available to her, you would have to
mention abortion."[60]

A major practical issue that soon emerged was condom advertising on television, then prohibited by all three networks. At a congressional hearing before the House Subcommittee on Health and the
Environment, representatives of the networks spoke in favor of their
bans. Ralph Daniels of NBC claimed such ads were "unacceptable to
a significant portion of our audience."[61] But that would soon change,
and irrespective of the position of the federal government the media
would soon be getting out the condom message. So in the *New York
Times* for October 1, 1988, it was announced that all three networks
had agreed to carry public service condom ads. The campaign that
was rolled out involved a huge effort, with amfAR and the National
AIDS Network partnering with the Advertising Council to develop
ads in collaboration with the Ogilvy group. Print media across the
country also joined. While Koop gave his endorsement, he acknowledged that "I know this campaign will offend some people."[62]

President Reagan's longtime aide Edwin Meese III had served initially as counselor to the President, with cabinet rank, from 1981–85,
and then from 1985–88 as attorney general. As we noted, Meese was
seen as the center of gravity of the serious conservatives within the
White House. When I asked him about the emerging conflicts over
AIDS within the administration he acknowledged that "there were
differences of opinion," because "the principal sources at that time
appeared to be relationships between homosexuals, to which many
people had religious and moral objections. And Koop's idea was, this

is a public health problem. And we've got to do everything we can to keep the disease from spreading. The President knew that he had to have somebody as leader [on AIDS], and Koop was the ideal person, both because of his job, and also, of course, the position he took, which was easily consistent with what the President thought."[63]

Koop's old Philadelphia friend Michael DellaVecchia recalled visiting the Koops at the time. "We're having breakfast," he told me, "And Betty says, 'What do you have to do today?' He says, 'Well,' he says, 'I have to go down to Congress, and have to tell people to wear condoms. You know, while they're having sex.' And Betty, being the person she was, she looked over, and she says, 'You know, I'm kind of glad your mother isn't alive to see this.'"[64]

The AIDS Commission

The "Presidential Commission on the HIV Epidemic" proved immediately controversial, since Bauer had been intent on excluding gay members (except perhaps a "reformed" homosexual), and was subject to lobbying from all sides, which slowed the process of setting it up.[65] In the chair initially was Mayo Clinic CEO Eugene Mayberry, charged with producing an interim report within ninety days, and a final report within a year, though he was soon replaced by one of the other appointees, former chief of naval operations (and serious Roman Catholic) Admiral James Watkins.

During a wide-ranging hearing on September 10, 1987, at which both officials and groups testified, Koop was invited to address the commission. According to the *Times*, "The most challenging testimony was clearly that of Dr. Koop, who offered a range of questions that the commission ought to address but offered no solutions. In warning that 'the ethical foundation of health care itself' is in danger, he said he heard more reports every day of some health professional refusing to treat AIDS victims 'or even persons whom they suspect of having AIDS.'"

Bauer had hoped that social conservative Watkins "would have little problem" supporting his approach to AIDS policy. Not so.

"Watkins, like Koop, disappointed his supporters within the administration."[66] And in the process he underlined the lack of uniformity among "social conservatives" on this demanding and complex set of issues. The final report of the commission was published in June the following year, with more than five hundred recommendations, many of them costly, and most in the end ignored, such as the need for three thousand new drug treatment facilities.[67]

The work of the commission expired the following year, and it would be replaced by a separate "National Commission on AIDS," established by Congress in 1988 with a four-year term expiring in September 1993. A chief function of this successor body, with members appointed in equal numbers by House, Senate, and the administration, would be the implementation of the many recommendations of the Presidential Commission, though like its predecessor its only actual power was to write reports. Members would include its chair, Dr. June Osborn, dean of public health at the University of Michigan; HHS Secretary Sullivan; "Magic" Johnson, who would later resign in a blaze of annoyance with the administration; and somewhat oddly Dr. Roy Rowland, the member of Congress who had originally proposed its creation.[68]

Meanwhile, the household mailing idea, proposed and then set aside within the White House, had returned. A brochure entitled *Understanding AIDS* was being developed by CDC, under special authority from Congress, which included the extraordinary requirement that it be issued "without necessary clearance of the content by any [political] official."[69] Bauer and others were naturally concerned both about the likely content of a brochure they could not control, and over the separation-of-powers implications. As Edward Martin, Koop's chief of staff, recalled: "There was obviously a major bar-room brawl, because Bauer and others were doing everything they could to stop it. And of course Koop was supported by Bowen. And . . . Dr. Windom had come in as assistant secretary, and Bob Windom was very, very supportive of Chick . . . as were the other agency administrators."[70] Martin ran interference for Koop on the Hill, on this as on other occasions; "it was important that people like Henry Waxman and Paul Rogers and Ted Kennedy understood that what Dr. Koop was going to be sending out to households was not something that represented the inflammatory, far right point of view."[71]

The President Speaks

Whatever the full explanation of President Reagan's failure to address the gathering AIDS crisis in the early 1980s, the pressure was growing, not least from his wife Nancy.[72] The death of Rock Hudson proved a waymark. Plans were laid for Reagan's first major AIDS speech, to be given at a gala dinner hosted by the celebrity AIDS charity amfAR.[73]

The Reagans had received a letter from Elizabeth Taylor, written April 10—"she writes this letter and makes it personal," as speechwriter Landon Parvin tells it. "She says it would do so much for us to get rid of the archaic stigma attached to the disease and to make people realize that it is no longer a minority disease. It can happen to anyone. It's nobody's fault. Everybody's problem. Elizabeth Taylor says," then, "PS, my love to you. And I hope to see you soon. So I am sure Mrs. Reagan said to her husband, I think you should do this. So he accepted."[74]

As related in Karen Tumulty's biography of Nancy Reagan, Nancy was not confident that the regular White House speechwriters would shape her husband's remarks along the lines she favored. So she lobbied to bring Parvin back. He had been a White House speechwriter in the early 80s, when he had written all her speeches. "She and I just got along," he told me. "One reason Mrs. Reagan asked me to do things is that the White House speechwriter staff were sort of keepers of the conservative flame;" he was not.

Parvin started talking to people and made a remarkable discovery. The President had never had a meeting with Koop to discuss AIDS.

And Parvin said, "This is awful. You can't have the President's major AIDS adviser not having a meeting with the President! So I called Mrs. Reagan, because I knew she would make it happen. And

I said, you know, Dr. Koop needs to meet with the President on this, it is going to be an embarrassment that he's never met with him. And she set it up."[75]

Parvin assumed that this would be a meeting between Koop and the President in the Oval Office. Not so simple. "I can see that the White House staff was worried that if there was a one-on-one meeting with Koop, the President might be too swayed. So there was a cabinet in the Cabinet Room. And there were a lot of people there, you know, White House staff, Bill Bennett, the secretary of education, Koop, I went, there were a bunch of people around the table. I think the inside maneuvering was that he would be outnumbered, basically." Parvin described it as, "Everybody else talking to the President with Koop trying to get some points in." It lasted perhaps thirty minutes.

Once Parvin had a draft speech prepared, "the skirmishing began." There was pushback from White House staff on issues from whether AIDS is transmissible via mosquitoes and handshakes, whether people with HIV should attend school or other routine activities, and whether they can be involved in food service. "The jury is still out on that one," was a common line. So he called Mrs. Reagan and said, "I'm being beaten up," and she told him just to use her name. "And so that's how I kept some of the stuff in. Because I said, Well, Mrs. Reagan wants it this way."

Parvin also met twice with the President and shared with me an anecdote that sheds light on the human dimension of the situation. "All the pressure was in the newspapers . . . the President needs to use the word condom. Well, the fact of the matter is, he was born in the early twentieth century. He's not going to use the word condom in a presidential speech. So I started with where he came from. And for example, you know, one of the things he said was . . . which gives you an idea of the era he was from . . . we were talking about abstinence. And he thought that was important. He told one of his daughters, when she was talking about sex or something—he said, You're gonna find a man you love and want to share your life with, and you'll want to be true to him. Well, you can start being true to him now." Parvin notes that Reagan was well on his way to being eighty. "It didn't fit. I didn't put that in the speech because I knew the audience would just roll their eyes at that. . . . So I tried to keep it on the compassion, as he was a compassionate man."

"It all happened totally because of Nancy. And I was able to keep certain things out. And keep certain things in. Because of Nancy. Otherwise they would have been buried."

The day before the dinner, a cabinet meeting was scheduled at which AIDS would be discussed, so Koop and other colleagues from HHS were present. As Koop recalled, they were nervous, because if discussion went the wrong way the speech and much else could be altered.

Koop found himself seated in the second row round the table, as is conventional for aides and other nonmembers, immediately opposite the President. "By looking between the heads of the two men just in front of me, I had eye-to-eye contact with the President. Unobtrusively, I pushed my chair back about six inches, so I was slightly behind the two men seated on either side of me, James Mason and Bob Windom. . . . No one could see my face easily except the President." Discussion ranged widely. "Whenever the President had a query that I wanted to answer, or whenever a Cabinet member made a statement I wanted to reinforce or rebut, I raised my right index finger beside my nose and almost imperceptibly nodded toward the President. It was like silent bidding at an auction; no one except Reagan could see me. He acknowledged me on each occasion, saying something like 'I would like to hear from Dr. Koop.'"[76]

The American Medical Foundation for AIDS Research (amfAR) Awards Dinner was held in what Koop referred to as a "sweltering tent" outside Washington's Potomac Restaurant on May 31, 1987; Reagan spoke at 8:16 p.m.[77]

After thanks to Elizabeth Taylor and his other hosts, the President opened by lauding the Surgeon General, adding that he is proud that a member of his administration is among the awardees (this brought thunderous applause). Dr. Koop is "what every Surgeon General should be. He's an honest man, a good doctor, and an advocate for the public health."[78] Some of the phrasing that follows is redolent of Koop, and the success of Parvin's efforts to shape the President's emphases and tone. AIDS "calls for compassion, not blame. . . . It's also important that America not reject those who have the disease, but care for them with dignity and kindness. Final judgment is up to God; our part is to ease the suffering and to find a cure. This is a battle against disease, not against our fellow Americans." And then this, adroitly quoting Bennett to anchor his opposition to discrimination: "I agree with Secretary of Education Bennett: We must firmly oppose discrimination against those who have AIDS. We must prevent the persecution, through ignorance or malice, of our fellow citizens."

But there were also lines that left Koop (and some in the audience) less happy. Reagan announced that would-be immigrants will be tested, and those who were positive refused entry, as they are for other infectious diseases (mixed boos and applause at this point). He announced that federal prisoners will be tested, and that there would be a review of testing in veterans' hospitals and in the military (cries of no, plus applause). He encouraged states to test prisoners, and to "offer routine testing" to those applying for marriage licenses (applause) and clients of STD and drug clinics. He stressed a point that Koop did not disagree with: "AIDS education or any aspect of sex education will not be value-neutral."[79] And in a reminder of how things stood back in 1987, he noted the deep uncertainty with which America viewed this silently spreading disease with its long, symptom-free, incubation period. "Just as most individuals don't know they carry the virus, no one knows to what extent the virus has infected our entire society. AIDS is surreptitiously spreading throughout our population, and yet we have no accurate measure of its scope. It's time we knew exactly what we were facing, and that's why I support some routine testing."

Recalling Parvin's sense that Reagan would not be comfortable using the word "condom," it's interesting that he nevertheless slips in the precise point that led Koop to use the word: "Now, we know there will be those who will go right ahead. So, yes, after there is a moral base, then you can discuss preventives and other scientific measures."

As he stepped away from the podium, unobtrusively retrieving a paper clip from his pocket to re-fasten his notes (ever the professional performer), the President was rewarded with kisses on both cheeks from Elizabeth Taylor, who held hands with him as the cameras flashed.

The speech was a masterpiece, with its blend of classic Reagan humor, moving anecdotes, and a staccato burst of policy announcements.

Randy Shilts made his own sober assessment. "By the time President Reagan had delivered his first speech on the epidemic . . . 36,058 Americans had been diagnosed with the disease; 20,849 had died."[80]

Koop was invited to an after-party with Elizabeth Taylor and other Hollywood guests, "in one of the houses along the Tidal Basin." Meanwhile, an anti-gay group from Kansas was in town, burning Koop in effigy. Koop later reflected that "we don't have the right word to describe these groups. People say that this group from Kansas was homophobic. Homophobic means you're afraid of them. But these are people who have unbelievable outrage and hatred. They are not afraid of homosexuals. They would just like to get close to them with a tire iron."[81]

107,000,000 Mailboxes

On January 27, 1988, assistant secretary for health Robert Windom announced at an AIDS conference in London that the PHS would be mailing more than one hundred million copies of an informational brochure, to every street address in the United States.[82] As Brier remarks, the mailer essentially summarized "the ideas first presented by Koop two years earlier."[83]

As we noted, the idea of mailing the country had been brewing in the White House for some time, though the DPC ended up losing control of its content. Now that the mailer was going out, there were various people seeking credit for such an unprecedented effort. Even Windom later claimed that it had been his idea! "I said . . . I don't want somebody coming to me and saying that we haven't told you so. . . . Let's send a letter, a pamphlet, out to every household in the nation. We did. We took 110 million homes that had post office boxes or homes . . . it cost us 20 million dollars out of my budget."[84] But, he added, "It has Chick Koop on there. A wonderful man."[85]

From May 26 through the end of June 1988, a year later than originally mooted, *Understanding AIDS* dropped through every mailbox in America. On the front were Koop's name and very recognizable face. He had not needed to use trickery this time to get the text past his critics in the administration.

"The pamphlet," wrote Sandra Boodman in the *Washington Post*, "which cost $17 million to produce and print, reveals no new facts about acquired immune deficiency syndrome. The pamphlet states unequivocally that the disease is not spread by mosquitoes or other insects, through casual contact in the classroom or other public places, on toilet seats or by contact with saliva, sweat, tears, urine or feces."

In explicit terms that echo those of the Koop report, the pamphlet warns of "the dangers of anal sex, advocates the use of particular kinds of condoms and spermicides and contains advice on how to talk to children about AIDS, which has struck more than 60,000 Americans since 1981. It contains small photographs, including those of two women with AIDS, and urges the public to display compassion and support for those who are infected."

In tandem, HHS produced TV commercials to promote the mailing—and added more than 1,000 extra operators to the toll-free national AIDS hot line.

The *Post* reports, without comment, that "Gary L. Bauer, the White House domestic policy adviser, and Education Secretary William J. Bennett," declined to comment.[86]

Koop had faced challenges with the mailer right down to the wire. Congress voted the funding to print it, but funds to mail it out were lacking. Anthony Fauci, now Director of the National Institute on Allergy and Infectious Diseases, stepped up. "The only trouble," Fauci explained to me, "was that the Reagan administration, which was not particularly interested in doing that, would not give him much of the money to do it. But as an institute director, there is a mechanism called the inter-agency transfer of funds. So I could transfer a certain amount of limited funds, from my budget to his budget, and my budget was, you know, stratospherically thicker than his budget. So we sent out this brochure, much to the dismay of the Reagan administration, because in it he was using words like condoms and gay sex and commercial sex workers and anal intercourse. So that as an example of the kinds of things we did. He and I were very close friends."[87]

In later years, Koop would have much fun sharing another story of Fauci and the mailer.[88] Despite the role of top ad agency Ogilvy and Mather in putting the piece together, when the denizens of those hundred seven million households caught the heading, "What does someone with AIDS look like?" they would find right beside it a picture of . . . Anthony Fauci.[89]

Significance

Michael Gottlieb made history by first identifying the HIV virus in 1981, and went on to cofound amfAR with Mathilde Krim and Elizabeth Taylor.[90] When we spoke, he bemoaned the weakness of the federal response—"we had been voices in the wilderness screaming." Then "Koop stepped in and filled the vacuum. Finally, there is someone at the federal level, who's got his head on straight. So that was impressive to me that he stuck his neck out. Anyone else would have been fired!" But Koop "had the gravitas and the stature to pull it off. That was a ballsy, ballsy thing to do. And I said to myself, Hey, we have an ally here. Koop entered at the right time. I think what he did was extraordinary."[91] For Henry Waxman, who had called Koop "scary" when he was fighting his nomination, he was now "a man of heroic proportions."[92]

Writing in the *Washington Post* shortly after Koop's death in 2013, Joshua Green writes of "An Unsung Hero in the Fight against AIDS." He first reviews Koop's leadership on tobacco control, then adds: "But Koop was also a pivotal figure, and probably saved just as many lives, because he broke a deadlock in the Republican Party that had stopped Congress from addressing the rampaging AIDS epidemic in the 1980s. He did this in two ways: by publicly emphasizing the epidemiological threat the disease posed to all (not just gay) Americans, and by casting himself as a sort of shadow GOP leader at a time when the party's actual leaders were exacerbating the deadly crisis."[93]

National Minority AIDS Council director Paul Kawata, who in the late 1980s was executive director of a coalition of more than 600 community-based AIDS service organizations known as the National AIDS Network, was emphatic: "Dr. Koop was a hero to our movement. His leadership changed the way HIV was viewed in this country."[94] In the words of the *New York Times* obit, he "Almost single-handedly pushed the government into taking a more aggressive stand against AIDS."[95] The authoritative *Forum for Collaborative HIV Research*, in publishing Koop's memories of those days, bills him simply as "the official who . . . charted the nation's policies on HIV/AIDS."[96]

And he proved a gamechanger within the Republican Party. As Thomas Getman, longtime Senate staffer, later reflected, "I distinctly remember being so grateful for the atmospherics that he created in the '80s. I served Senator Hatfield . . . for four years of Chick's service as Surgeon General. And I don't think in the [George] W. Bush administration, we would have had the PEPFAR funding, the PEPFAR attitude, and the great victory in Africa, without Chick's laying the base during that period."[97]

Perhaps the most telling assessment of Koop's significance for AIDS is that of Randy Shilts, in the most celebrated of all books on the AIDS crisis, *And the Band Played On*, penned as early as 1987.

Shilts is reviewing the administration's many failures to engage the crisis, and the President's absence at a time when leadership was crucial. Widespread continuing prejudice against homosexuals lead those with AIDS to keep covering up the nature of their terminal disease, despite Hudson's death. "There were other celebrity patients now, but for all their media cachet, the disease remained fundamentally embarrassing. When Broadway's star choreographer-director

Michael Bennet fell ill, he maintained that he was suffering from heart problems. A spokesman for Perry Ellis insisted the famed clothing designer was dying of sleeping sickness. Lawyer Roy Cohn insisted he had liver cancer, even while he used his political connections to get on an experimental AIDS treatment protocol at the National Institutes of Health Hospital. Conservative fundraiser Terry Dolan claimed he was dying of diabetes. When Liberace was on his deathbed, a spokesman claimed the pianist was suffering the ill effects of a watermelon diet."[98]

Shilts notes a succession of efforts, both voluntary and at the federal level, to shift public awareness and sympathy that got nowhere.

What then? "Ultimately, it was a report issued in October 1986 that turned the tale, galvanized the media and allowed AIDS to achieve the critical mass to make it a pivotal social issue in 1987." Shilts gets to the key to Koop's extraordinary significance. "Koop's impact was due to archetypal juxtaposition. It took a square-eyed, heterosexually perceived actor like Rock Hudson to make AIDS something people could talk about. It took an ultra-conservative fundamentalist who looked like an Old Testament prophet to credibly call for all of America to take the epidemic seriously at last."

He continues: "Unwittingly, the Reagan administration had produced a certifiable AIDS hero. From one corner of the country to the other, AIDS researchers, public health experts, and even the most militant of gay leaders hailed the surgeon general. Koop quickly became so in demand for speeches that he was called a 'scientific Bruce Springsteen.'" Shilts is critical of Koop's failure to engage the emerging AIDS crisis sooner, plainly assuming that the Surgeon General would have been free to act on his own. "Koop's interest was historic for its impact, not its timeliness." Yet: "There was no denying . . . that the report proved a watershed event in the history of the epidemic, and conservatives were stunned."[99]

In David France's recent account of the early days of AIDS, *How to Survive a Plague*, he offers remarkable testimony to Koop's importance to the gay community.[100] He tells how Larry Kramer, playwright, movie director, and leading AIDS activist, was campaigning for the administration to launch a "Manhattan Project" to find a cure for AIDS. France notes that "the original Manhattan Project brought together over 130,000 people at a cost of billions" and "cut through complex bureaucracies" to produce the atom bomb. "If such a monumental campaign were to focus on HIV and the immune system, Kramer had no doubt, a cure would come along just as quickly." As the 1992 election campaign was drawing to a close, with Clinton the favorite, Kramer hosted a weekend in a grand, "castle-sized," East Hampton house he had rented from a friend, inviting lead activists to plot the AIDS Manhattan project.

It was a serious proposal; Kramer had been discussing it with NIH director Bernadine Healey. It would unite the efforts of the brightest and best. Kramer wanted AIDS Commission chair Admiral James Watkins, and FDA head David Kessler, to serve as "ranking officers." They would be "sequestered alongside bench scientists and Nobel Prize winners in a remote desert lab with a towering budget and an Oval Office mandate." Who would be the new Robert Oppenheimer, and direct this Manhattan Project?

According to Larry Kramer, none other than C. Everett Koop, MD, ScD, the dour presbyterian elder whose name had been chanted by eighteen thousand gay activists on Boston Common, one bright June afternoon three years before.[101] [iii]

---

iii   France's book is a puzzle. He tells this story of the enormous regard in which Koop was held by the core AIDS activists of the day, yet at the same time completely writes him out of the history. This is one of only two references to Koop in the whole book, which actually omits any reference to the 1986 AIDS report.

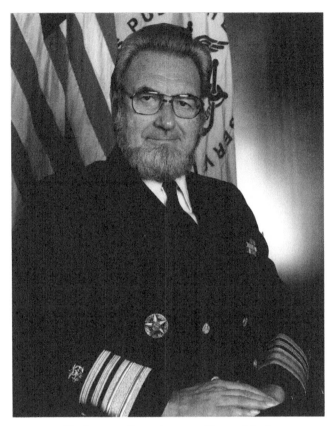

FIGURE 1. The Surgeon General, c. 1982. He was "the first Surgeon General in a generation to wear the uniform."

—National Library of Medicine, public domain

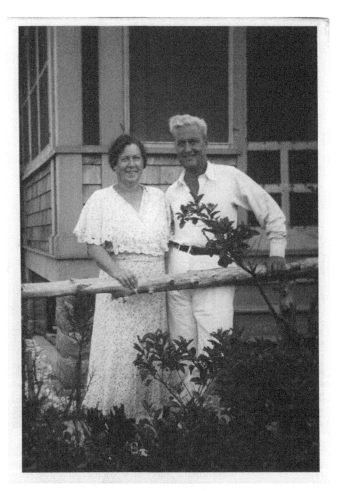

FIGURE 2. Koop's parents, John Everett Koop and Helen Apel
Koop, in the 1930s. His father, Koop said, was his best friend.
— National Library of Medicine, courtesy C. Everett Koop

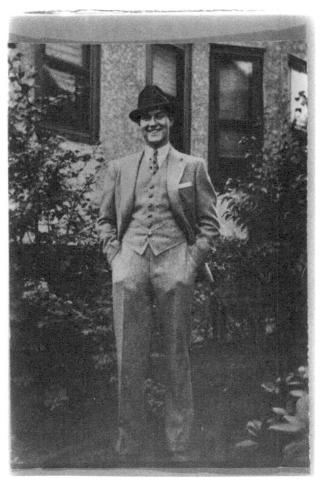

FIGURE 3. Koop on the day he left home for Dartmouth College
in 1933, at the age of 16.
       —National Library of Medicine, courtesy C. Everett Koop

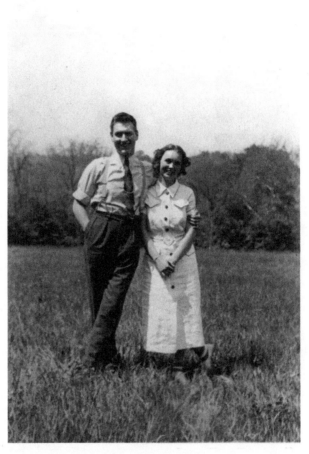

FIGURE 4. Koop with Elizabeth (Betty) Flanagan, c. 1936 in
New Hampshire. They were married in 1938.
   —National Library of Medicine, courtesy C. Everett Koop

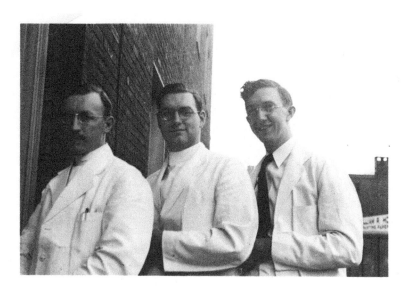

FIGURE 5. Koop with other interns at the Hospital of the University of Pennsylvania in 1941 (he is in the center).

—National Library of Medicine, courtesy C. Everett Koop

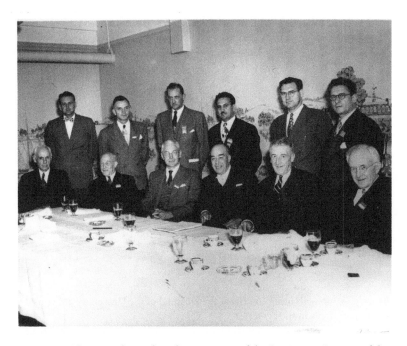

FIGURE 6. The storied 1948 founding meeting of the Section on Surgery of the American Academy of Pediatrics in Atlantic City. Left to right (back): Henry Swan, Robert Bowman, Willis Potts, Jesus Lozoya-Solis, Koop, unknown individual; (front): William Ladd, Herbert Coe, Franc Ingraham, Oswald Wyatt, Thomas Landman, and a representative of the American Academy of Pediatrics. Koop had just had his appointment confirmed as surgeon-in-chief of the Children's Hospital of Philadelphia.

—National Library of Medicine, ©American Academy of Pediatrics

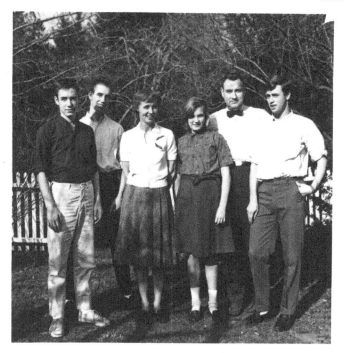

FIGURE 7. The Koop family, c. 1962. From left to right: David, Norman, Betty, Betsy, Koop, and Allen.
        —National Library of Medicine, courtesy C. Everett Koop

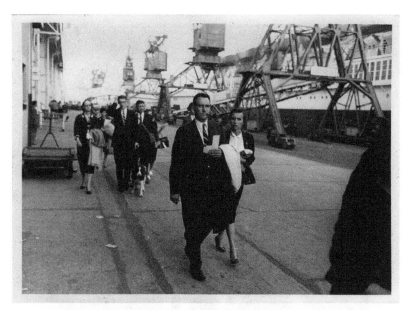

FIGURE 8. Koop and his wife Betty boarding a ship in the port of Rotterdam in the Netherlands, in September of 1964. Koop gave up his pipe a decade later.
—National Library of Medicine, courtesy C. Everett Koop

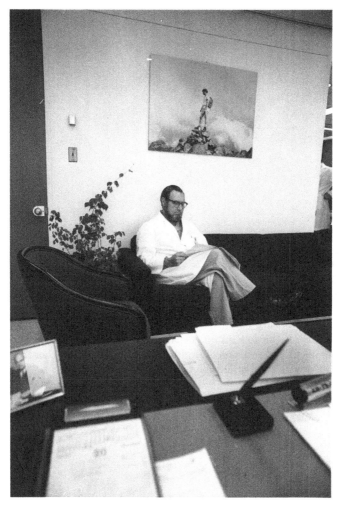

FIGURE 9. Koop in his office at the Children's Hospital, beneath a photo of David. December 1974.
—National Library of Medicine, courtesy C. Everett Koop

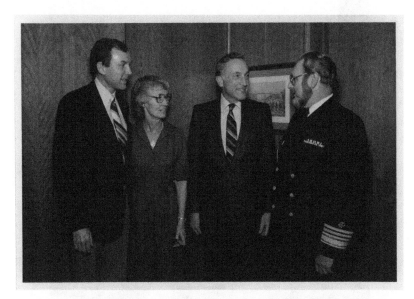

FIGURE 10. Koop's first day in uniform, after he was confirmed by the US Senate, on November 16, 1981, with his wife Betty, his key sponsor, Senator Orrin Hatch of Utah (far left), and Secretary of Health and Human Services Richard Schweiker. He was sworn in as Surgeon General the following day.

—National Library of Medicine, public domain

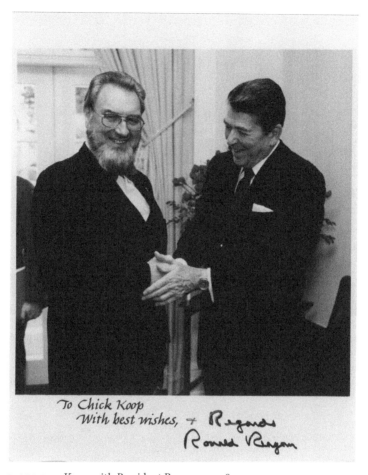

To Chick Koop
With best wishes, + Regards
Ronald Reagan

FIGURE 11. Koop with President Reagan, c. 1981.
—National Library of Medicine, public domain

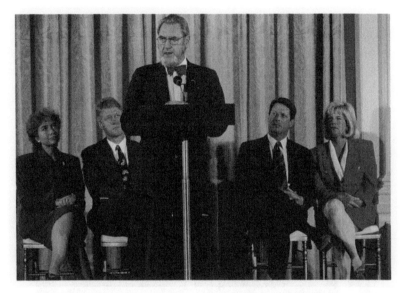

FIGURE 12. Koop speaking at the special White House event convened by the Clintons on September 20, 1993, to showcase his support for their healthcare reform initiative. The Clintons and the Gores look on.

—National Library of Medicine, public domain

Revitalizing the Corps

You can rally people around a uniform.
—CEK

D eveloped in the nineteenth century as an "elite national squadron of disease-fighting physicians," the Commissioned Corps of the PHS had in the view of many devolved into simply a parallel personnel system, alongside the regular federal civil service.[1] Members of the Corps held military ranks, all those of officers; and they had enhanced military-style retirement benefits. From the start, Koop had decided to wear the vice admiral's uniform to which he was entitled—donned first for his swearing-in ceremony. Senior members of the Corps—"flag officers"—would wear uniform for ceremonial occasions. But uniforms had fallen into wide disuse, and more than one-quarter of the nearly six thousand "officers" were bench scientists at NIH and CDC, who didn't have so much as an epaulet in their wardrobes.

Crisis for the Corps

As we noted, shortly after the Reagan administration came into office, the White House Office of Management and Budget (OMB), with a cost-saving mission, shuttered or passed to others the string of seamen's hospitals that were at the heart of the work of the Commissioned Corps, with dramatic impact on many staff—and, needless to say, morale. As Michael Roberts, one-time president of the Commissioned Corps Officers' Association, recalled to me, it "was a big hit and shock to many officers who had chosen a career in clinical health care. Those with less than two years' seniority were de-commissioned and others . . . were reassigned to other positions in the federal prison system, the Indian Health Service or Coast Guard. If they were not pleased where they were to be reassigned, resignation was the remaining option."[2]

Though his role as its most senior officer had become largely ceremonial, Koop took an immediate interest in the Corps. He made a point of spending time with officers at both formal and social events, "particularly during 1981, 82, and 83, when he had more time, with commissioned officers who remembered the history on the esprit of the Commissioned Corps." In Edward Martin's words, Koop "went from being the Surgeon General incidentally, to being, at least from a lot of commissioned officers' point of view . . . increasingly the embodiment of what a Surgeon General stands for, which is a leader."[3]

Despite having no line responsibility for the Corps, as early as 1983 Koop commissioned a task group to come up with recommendations for its future, one of which was that its "operational management" should be placed under either the Surgeon General or the assistant secretary for health, rather than the general personnel management structures of HHS.[4] Martin, who as a fellow pediatrician and senior HHS executive had reached out to Koop during the nomination process, was a member of the group and especially concerned with the malaise that had resulted from lax management controls. He highlighted some problem cases in an "eyes only" memo to Koop. One physician, a Dr. V., "was given orders to Philadelphia and refused to go." When he submitted his resignation, the personnel division reinstated him. Martin's terse observation: "Example of officer controlling the system and refusing to move." Martin sums it up: "We say that the Corps is mobile yet when the time comes to move officers they do not want to move."[5]

Koop shared the report at an April, 1984, meeting of Flag Officers, where three groups were set up to discuss implementation. Also described as a meeting of the Assistant Surgeons General, this twice-yearly event had evidently been initiated in the previous year.[6] "The Uniform for the day will be *Service Dress Blues.*"

The malaise in the Corps was deep-seated. Some took the view that many who had joined the Corps in the '60s and '70s had done so "to avoid service in the real military [the Vietnam draft], giving birth to the derisive description of Corps members as 'yellow berets.'" Kluger quotes former Acting Surgeon General Paul Ehrlich: "The uniform became a symbol of derision. I mean, if I was to have worn my uniform in the '70s through the Humphrey Building . . . I think people would have thrown eggs."[7]

Plainly, the anti-Vietnam War officers did not like the idea of wearing uniforms at all. The Corps was also "pretty much white males." Yet positions in the Corps were attractive, for the same reason that they were also more expensive for the government than the standard civil service conditions of service—because of its military-type retirement system. Meanwhile, the Reagan budget-cutters at OMB persisted in their efforts to do away with the Corps altogether, which they saw as a costly historical anomaly, and the sense of crisis had returned in 1986, just as Koop was settling down to write his report on AIDS.[8] He met with Tom Burke, chief of staff to the recently appointed Secretary, Otis Bowen, looking for support.[9] "Tom Burke was ex-military," Edward Martin recalled. "He was a big guy and smoked cigars. And he was pretty universally disliked except by me. I liked him and Koop liked him. Tom had enormous respect for Dr. Koop. And so he said, if you're going to fight this, you're going to have to do something about the Commissioned Corps."[10]

Martin continued: "His exact words were, you're going to have to kick ass and take names, and make the Commissioned Corps a real uniformed service again. Because it isn't now. And so Chick says, 'Well, how do I do that?'" Burke responded: "Well, I only know one commissioned officer in the Public Health Service who is capable of kicking ass and taking names, and doing what you need to be done. And that's Ed Martin. So Chick called me up to his office. And I said, I think I would be willing to do it. If Dr. Brandt [he meant Secretary Bowen] would agree. And if I could continue to maintain my bureau. So it was done."[11]

As a result, in a highly unusual arrangement that continued until the end of the second Reagan term, Martin continued to direct his bureau while moonlighting as Koop's chief of staff.

He found that Koop's office consisted of only Koop himself, Deputy Surgeon General Faye Abdellah (1919–2017), the first woman to serve at that level and the Corps' former chief nursing officer, and one or two assistants. "Well," he recalled to me, "all of a sudden, you know, I was able to bring in eight or ten extra people that were essentially detailed from my bureau, including Steve Moore, who was a guy who put together functions, and they didn't have anybody to do that. . . . Steve was an expert." How did it end up working? "We met every morning at 7:00 or 7:30. And most of those mornings, I would actually get there at 7:00. And Koop and I would spend fifteen or twenty minutes together, just one on one. Then at 7:30 was the staff meeting."

Interviewed in 1990, when he had become a deputy assistant secretary for defense, Martin recalled the details well. "I can tell you exactly when it was, the first week of March 1987—Dr. Koop's plan was put together." And Koop said: "If you want to hold the Surgeon General accountable for making this particular change, you're going to have to give me authority to do it."[12]

Burke persuaded the secretary to go along with the plan. "Literally, within three and a half weeks—which is a miracle for this department . . . it had gone before the management council of the department, where there was great opposition . . . it had been discussed by the agency heads in the Public Health Service, where there was more disbelief than opposition. . . . Burke with the secretary, just basically cut through it all on the first of April 1987, give a day or two. I mean literally. We're talking about delegation of authorities that were completely changed, revised, a Federal Register notice . . . was on its way." And: "all of a sudden, the commissioned personnel officers division, now called the Division of Commissioned Personnel, reported directly to Dr. Koop. He had been redelegated all the authorities for promotions, for running the Commissioned Corps.[13] In practice, as he told me, Martin was running the show. "I had complete responsibility for what we called the revitalization of the

Commissioned Corps. And the commissioned personnel reported to me, I set up all the advisory groups, changed the promotion system. And Dr. Koop said, 'Everybody gets in uniform.'"[14]

On March 30, a refreshed Office of the Surgeon General was formally established to take on these new responsibilities; and then a detailed reorganization plan for the office was drawn up, complete with timelines and org charts.[15] Maintaining the breakneck speed of the revitalization process—not least, to head off opposition—Koop was ready to announce the new plan by April 6.

He wrote "To All Active Duty Commissioned Officers," that in recent years the Corps has become the object of criticism and at times, ridicule. Serious doubt has been voiced, sometimes warranted, about the Corps' effectiveness as a uniformed service. "As Surgeon General, I have been concerned by the questions which have been raised about the Corps' vitality and effectiveness in carrying out its historic mission." As a result, "major revitalization of the Corps is required." Thanks to Burke, "The Secretary has announced the implementation of the Revitalization Plan as a Secretarial Initiative."

As noted, at the heart of the plan lay handing back to the Surgeon General some of the powers his office had lost in the mid-1960s. Thus, the memo continues, "the office of the Surgeon General will assume direct responsibility for Commissioned Personnel policy and functions, including the administration and management of the Division of Commissioned Personnel." Cooked up by Koop and Martin, the plan held dramatic implications for many officers whose Corps membership had come to mean little aside from enhanced retirement benefits. The focus is on a Corps with mobility—Koop specifies an average of three to five geographic postings during a career. And the revival of the uniform.

There was immediate pushback, particularly from scientists at CDC and NIH, and from their superiors. Koop and Martin held a series of townhall meetings to address the practical implications of the plan. They held "a very difficult meeting at CDC, with literally hundreds of officers who were upset about 'What does mobility mean to me?' and 'What's this bullshit about wearing a uniform?' . . .

'Here I am, a lab scientist. What do you mean I'm going to be sent to the Indian Health Service?'" Assistant secretary Mason took a "very firm, unequivocal and supportive position," if more quietly. Koop was "very forthright and forceful on it, he just said 'This is the way we're going to do it, and we are not just another personnel system.'"[16]

Martin recalled that "the going was terrifically rough in the first four months."[17]

While unease at CDC (588 Commissioned Corps officers) slowly calmed down after "six to twelve months," sustained (and public) opposition emerged from NIH (750).

James Wyngaarden, the director, responded to Windom with a series of withering criticisms of what was planned.[18] His chief concern was to protect "the most successful biomedical science organization in the world," and in particular the creativity of its intramural scientists. He is concerned about the uniform, rotation to other positions, and "most serious of all" required retirement. He foresaw "extraordinary damage. . . . Our objections to compulsory wearing of the unform may seem trivial to you. I can assure you they are not." In the revitalization plan, "I see not a single advantage" for NIH.[19] His deputy director for intramural research, Joseph E. Rall, was quoted as saying: "It is no little hubris for Dr. Koop, in his infinite wisdom, to think he can improve research by making corps members wear uniforms and insisting they move around, perhaps to the Indian Health Service. It shows total ignorance of how modern biomedical research is done." A bruising public meeting followed on the NIH campus on May 18, 1987. One researcher, wearing jeans, said that the general feeling was one of dismay. "I work with animals all day and they're scared enough as it is. A uniform won't help things."[20]

Koop turned on the charm: "It looks like some of you came loaded for bear and weren't sure I was a bunny, so you shot anyway." When the meeting was over, Wyngaarden commented: "We were given assurances that there was flexibility. . . . We'll have to see what is the best deal we can get."[21]

In response to these consultations, Koop decided that, within certain parameters, the head of each agency could work out the uniform requirements for its members. *The Scientist* lists some of the rules that emerged. CDC and NIH: Uniforms only on Wednesdays. FDA: Wednesdays plus another day, by choice. Alcohol, Drug Abuse and Mental Health Administration: Three days a week, by choice. While in the Health Resources Services Administration, Martin's bureau, there would be uniforms every day![22]

Then, "an incredible change occurred." OMB concluded that "Dr. Koop is doing exactly what we said had to be done, so we're going to give you a couple of years to show us you can do it. So," Martin noted with satisfaction, "they completely backed off."[23] The robustness of the Koop-Martin approach left a legacy of anger and resentment in some quarters of the Corps. One senior officer remarked to me, "Ed [Martin]'s thoughts and behavior seem much more akin to the USMC [US Marine Corps] than the health professions. For a revitalization task, sending in the Marines may have been the best strategy, but certainly not widely appreciated from within the Service."

But, he added: "I won't argue with it. It worked."[24]

CHAPTER 13

Abortion Again

To shift the focus of the pro-life movement from the unborn child
to the health of the mother after abortion puts the situation out of
focus and sends the wrong message. . . . No matter what percentage,
large or small, of women are injured in some way by abortion, all the
unborn babies are dead.

—CEK, letter to a critic

He punted.
    —Longtime Koop friend

S uddenly, abortion reared its head. On July 30, 1987, the White
House asked the Surgeon General to write a report on the effects
of abortion on women. As the *New York Times* would later opine,
"Reaganauts hoped that there were enough such effects to discourage
women from exercising their constitutional right," though according to some, there was a bigger agenda.[1] "White House aide Dinesh
D'Souza had convinced the president that by documenting the terrible psychological effects of abortion, Koop's report would lay the
basis for overturning *Roe v. Wade*."[2]

Koop was unsympathetic to the White House initiative, for two
distinct reasons. He had come to dislike the use of political tactics
in the abortion debate. And he was equally unhappy about focusing
the debate on the mother. "In retrospect," says the *Los Angeles Times*,
he saw a dangerous message in continuing efforts to prove psychological damage of abortion. 'It is a subterfuge and I think a kind of
admission of defeat on the part of the pro-life people. . . . If in mid-
stream, they suddenly shift their emphasis to the health of mothers,
they must have forgotten why they got into this in the beginning.'"[3]

This response was curious, since Koop had long nurtured his own concerns about the psychological sequelae of abortion. Back in 1981, before his confirmation, he responded to a letter raising questions about CDC data on abortion mortality that "the one piece of information" we need concerns "the morbidity which is far more widespread and, in the long range, quite crippling."[4] Writing to a friend, he declared that, "If this were not a time of budgetary restraint I would be moving rapidly to do some things that need to be done. One of those is to have a true abortion surveillance program which looks into the morbidity (physical and mental) of abortion. This still might yet be done. We'll see."[5] Plainly, his perspective after years in office had shifted, though his resentment at having to address abortion officially may have affected his response.

But he got to work, seeking needed resources from the assistant secretary for health. He required two staff as "program analysts," plus additional expenses, for a total of $200,000.[6]

It's evident that from the beginning Koop had in mind a substantial, wide-ranging document. On August 31, he responded to a memo from Thomas Burke, the chief of staff, with his section of the agenda for the HHS staff retreat. The subject of the retreat is, "Crucial issues that need to be addressed in the remaining months of this Administration in order of priority." Burke sets the Revitalization of the Commissioned Corps above the list of Surgeon General areas. The upcoming abortion report is a "Presidential Initiative." Koop wrote: "This report can provide a major public health base for future policy decisions with regard to family planning, teenage pregnancy, abortion, and related health and social issues."[7]

Meanwhile, Koop had a private meeting with Cardinal Bernadin, with his friend Roy Schwarz of the AMA in attendance, on which he dictated a lengthy memo to file. He wanted to solicit the Cardinal's assistance in choosing whom he should interview, to explain the scope of the report, and to seek understanding since he will inevitably come out in favor of contraception as a key tool in reducing unwanted pregnancies, and thereby abortions. The Cardinal showed great understanding, even sharing that among the prelates of the church there was continuing discussion of whether the position that had been taken on contraception was correct.

Koop made a revealing comment, in his memo: Contraception is the most important part of this conversation, since it will be "the bottom line of my report, *if indeed I cannot keep it from being written.*"[8]

As with the report on AIDS, Koop had considerable leeway in deciding the shape of the final report. On August 19, 1987, his aide Michael Samuels proposed a schedule of activities. It involved an ambitious consultation exercise, an expanded version of his approach on AIDS, with up to one hundred twenty different organizations and individuals. Seven months was assigned to this process. Then two months for additional data gathering, and two months to write the report. It would be presented to the President between September 5 and 8, 1988. Koop initialed it "OK."[9] So much for the plan.[10]

In the event, the draft Koop report turned more on his analysis of published studies than his engagement with civil society groups and individuals. It reviewed some 250 such studies and concluded that while the physical sequelae of abortion are relatively clear (a death rate of around 0.8 per 100,000; abortion is around ten times as safe as childbirth, for the mother), the psychological effects are difficult to determine. Koop's conclusion was that, "at this time, the available scientific evidence . . . simply cannot support either the preconceived beliefs of those pro-life or of those pro-choice." All the major studies, he concluded, were "flawed methodologically." The "abundance of methodological flaws" included "lack of consistency in the definitions of emotional stressors; failure to control for preexisting emotional problems; absence of control groups; distorted samples; and very low follow-up rates." *Science* magazine cites Henry David, an outside expert, who commented that Koop's approach was "very even-handed."[11]

Koop encountered a series of decisions as his study proceeded. Having concluded that the evidence was not clear either way, he knew he could not give the White House what it wanted. Moreover, as he later testified, he considered that the draft he had worked on went beyond the terms of the President's request.[12] In the end, he decided that instead of presenting the report that had been drafted, he would simply write a letter setting out his conclusion and deliver it to the President. "I regret, Mr. President, that in spite of a diligent review on the part of many in the Public Health Service and in the private sector, the scientific studies do not provide conclusive data about the health effects of abortion on women." The letter was delivered four months later than his own deadline for the original report. Reagan had precisely eleven days remaining in office.

The *New York Times* for January 11 announced that Koop had "confounded the White House and Congress, liberals and conservatives" by telling the President in a letter that "he could not conclude one way or another that abortions were harmful to women. His position has again left him a hero to those who once opposed him and a villain to those who once backed him." His letter of January 9 was "regarded by abortion foes as an act of betrayal." When pressed on the issue, Koop spokesman Jim Brown stated: "He's seen a lot of women who have been depressed after an abortion, but he wants scientific evidence."[13] In a follow-up piece several days later, the *Times* quoted opinions from both sides of the abortion aisle. Former CDC staffer David Grimes claimed that "The data are not only good, they are great. . . . We know more about the safety of abortion than any other operation in the world." Dr. John Willke, president of the National Right to Life Committee, gave a careful response. He agreed with Koop that "most studies on emotional effects were flawed." But he said that anecdotal reports should not be ignored. "We can't fault what he said in the letter, which is basically that we need better and more definitive studies. . . . But I do not agree with Dr. Koop that there is not enough data to draw conclusions."

Looking back, Reagan's Attorney General Edwin Meese drew a parallel with the AIDS report. For all the controversy they both generated, within and outside the administration, he told me that he did not believe that either presented a problem for the President. The effect of abortion "was an issue that the President felt he needed to know more about. And so, again, the President thought highly of Koop, because of his overall honesty and objectivity. And so I think what he came up with was a pretty good, pretty fair and reasonable explanation about the evidence or what he found at the time, on the basis again of the medical aspects of it."[14]

There were two big problems with Koop's strategy.

Plainly, one of his conclusions was that there was no scientifically valid evidence that abortion was harmful. Quoted out of context, it twisted his message. President Reagan noted in his diary for January 13: "1st meeting some talk about Dr. Koop & the mixup of his letter on abortion. It seems he never wanted it made public."[15] Philip Yancey reported that, "when Koop reached his home a short time later, his wife met him in the driveway in a panic. She had just heard Peter Jennings, Tom Brokaw, and Dan Rather quoting from the 'confidential' letter. Moreover, they were reporting flatly that 'the surgeon general could find no evidence that abortion is psychologically harmful.' Koop stayed on the phone until one in the morning trying to clarify his position, and appeared next morning on 'Good Morning, America' . . . . But the damage had been done."[16]

Second, the draft report itself, which he stated he had not formally approved, would end up in the public domain in any case, released at a congressional hearing on March 16.[17] As James Bowman notes in an astute analysis based on contemporary interviews, at one point Koop actually stated that no report existed. "Because the reports of studies of psychological effects would not permit it, we could not prepare a report that could withstand scientific and statistical scrutiny," Koop told a House subcommittee. Bowman summarizes the document: "The draft concluded that abortion is a physically safe procedure and that there was inconclusive evidence concerning its psychological effects. The compassionate but reasoned statement went on to advocate strategies to prevent abortion, including sex education for children, contraceptive research, and subsidies for women to keep unplanned children."[18]

Bowman suggests that "this would prove to be a time when Koop found it excruciatingly difficult to separate his personal beliefs from his professional obligations."[19] Indeed, "seeing a no-win situation, the majority of Koop's inner circle [had] advised him to deflect the assignment to an agency within the PHS."[20] Yet, the same ego that sustained him throughout other controversies prevented him from avoiding this one. "The conflicting pressures were evident: the hope to satisfy the Reagan-Bush administration, the desire to improve relationships with his remaining right-to-life friends, and the obligation not to disappoint the PHS."[21]

Koop's frustration with the situation that resulted comes through clearly and somewhat embarrassingly in the letter he addressed to incoming President Bush a few days before delivering his letter to President Reagan. Addressing him as "Mr. President-Elect," Koop begins: "Although I have no confidence that you will ever read this letter, I do want to set the record straight on a matter which you thought of considerable importance when we talked together at your home in mid-August." He reviews his efforts to keep Bush in touch with developments on the abortion report. "I have made six individual contacts with your designated aide. . . . I left two messages with your transition people. . . . Two calls were unreturned. . . . This has been a very frustrating experience for me."[22]

Plainly, the incoming President's aides did not want him embroiled in the controversy over Koop's report to his predecessor, which Koop seems to have found difficult to understand. Bowman describes the controversy as "the final blow to conservatives who supported Koop within the administration and those outside in constituency groups. They could not believe that he was reluctant to help them."[23] It's plain that he was not reluctant; he was deeply conflicted, at least if the interview that Bowman had a decade later with Koop's aide George Walter—a key drafter of the report—is to be believed.

Koop had evidently met with Gary Bauer at the White House as early as February of 1988 to report that "there were no medical problems with abortion." He informed Bauer that "the best I am going to be able to come up with is a letter explanatory of why the definitive report [the President] wished to be written cannot be written." He wanted to give the President the opportunity to withdraw his request for the report. He says that Bauer asked for time to reflect, then called him and said he should just write the best report he could. Koop then had a further meeting, this time with Nancy Risque, the cabinet secretary, and asked her the same question, with the same result.[24]

The actual course of events was bizarre. Koop, famed for his clarity, determination, and persistence, was plainly flummoxed. After these failed efforts to head off the process with the White House, the fuller report was drafted. Then, at almost the last minute, Koop decided to set it aside. A staff member prepared a draft of a letter. Koop set it aside and decided to write his own version. That was what he delivered by hand to the White House—just eleven days before Reagan left office.[25]

After interviewing several of those involved, Bowman concludes: "Public health professionals, with whom he had functioned so closely, were stunned by Koop's action."[26]

President Reagan noted in his diary for January 10: "The Dr. Koop report is not really a report. It is a letter for me expressing need for research on how to evaluate the abortion setup."[27] Koop's research recommendation was for a study that would cost at least $100 million.[28]

The net result was a mix of perplexity and disappointment on the part of Koop's backers. As Philip Yancey wrote in *Christianity Today* later that year, "those conservatives who had stood by Koop during the Baby Doe and AIDS controversies were rocked yet again in early 1989." He continued: "For some evangelicals, Koop's letter was the last straw, for it appeared that Koop had abandoned the very principles that had gotten him nominated. The controversy left a permanent stain on Koop's career, and may have contributed to his retirement from public service." There were hard feelings all round. "Koop himself feels personally betrayed over the issue," noted Yancey.[29] Charles (Chuck) Donovan, longtime pro-life advocate whose Charlotte Lozier Institute in Washington has catalyzed many peer-reviewed studies on abortion's medical consequences, reflected: "This is a long retrospective observation, but I do think that Dr. K could have done more to deplore the absence of true abortion surveillance (it remains poor to this day) and recognized the institutional interests arrayed against getting that kind of research done. It sometimes seems like he took abortion safety at face value."[30] One old friend of Koop's told me that he didn't want to get "suckered" into the politics of abortion by this indirect effort to discredit it. He saw it as a moral issue about the killing of babies that had nothing to do with their mothers' health.[31]

The *New York Times*, which back in 1981 had welcomed the Surgeon General nominee as "Dr. Unqualified," embraced "Dr. Koop's Abortion Advice" once the House of Representatives had finally made the draft report public. In that draft, alongside discussion of the paucity and unreliability of data on abortion sequelae, Koop "took the occasion to offer constructive advice for those on all sides of the debate on ways to reduce the abortion rate." The *Times* noted that Koop had been "eloquent" on AIDS and smoking. "This latest prescription deserves to fall on equally receptive ears." The editorial singles out three of his recommendations: Sex education, greater access to contraception, and subsidizing the costs "for women who bear rather than abort unplanned children."[32]

Koop's call for research was picked up years later by a group of openly pro-choice researchers, which authored the oddly named "turnaway study," of women who had sought and for various reasons been denied abortions (they were "turned away"), later published in book form.[33] They write: "In Koop's 1989 letter to President Reagan, he called for more and better research of abortion's effects, specifically a five-year prospective study analyzing all the many outcomes of sex and reproduction, including the psychological and physical effects of trying but failing to conceive; having planned and unplanned, wanted and unwanted pregnancies; and delivering, miscarrying, or aborting pregnancies. His call for better research would go unfulfilled for twenty years."[34]

Brian Wilcox of the American Psychological Association (APA), "who contributed his own literature review to the [draft Koop] study," had pointed out that "there are no good studies anywhere comparing women who have had abortions with the most relevant control group: those who have borne unwanted children to term."[35]

So in 2007, Diana Greene Foster and her colleagues took on the challenge of studying the outcomes of both birth and abortion for women with unwanted pregnancies. She writes: "The strength of the

Turnaway Study's design is that women just above and just below
the gestational limit are women facing the same circumstances—
sometimes just a few days determines whether a woman can access
abortion. . . . Over the course of three years, 2008 through 2010, we
recruited more than 1,000 women from the waiting rooms of 30
abortion facilities in 21 states. Facilities set their gestational limits to
reflect their doctors' level of comfort and ability, as well as comply
with state law. . . . At each site, for every woman denied the abortion, we recruited two woman who received an abortion just under
the gestational limit and one who received an abortion in the first
trimester."[36]

The most interesting outcome of the study may be its stunning
finding that in women denied abortions, and therefore carrying
unwanted pregnancies to term, "the trajectory of mental health
symptoms seems to return to what it would have been if the woman
had received an abortion." Foster adds: "I admit I was surprised
about this finding. I expected that raising a child one wasn't planning to have might be associated with depression or anxiety. But this
is not what we found over the long run. Carrying an unwanted pregnancy to term was not associated with mental health harm."[37]

Meanwhile, Koop received a letter that brought him solace, from
what might have seemed a surprising source. Udo Middelmann was
a son-in-law to Francis Schaeffer.[i] Koop had had no contact with him
since a decade earlier when he and Schaeffer were filming *Whatever
Happened to the Human Race?* Writing to the Koops' home address
at 4 West Drive on the NIH campus, Middelmann begins by noting that it has been years since their last contact. But "I have followed you from a distance," through articles and videos and family
updates. "Last night Edith [Schaeffer's widow] and I were watching
a sub-committee hearing on your report to the President here in her
home. I wanted to . . . let you know how much I appreciated your
clear and courageous testimony, your evident commitment both to
the scientific standards required of any clear mind as well as to your

---

i Who had died in 1984.

moral/cultural convictions about human being at any age, in and out of the womb."[38]

He sums up: "Thank you for your efforts both on behalf of a suffering human family and on behalf of rightful thinking and practice."

Koop replied: "I don't think you realize how welcome your letter of March 17th was and at what an appropriate time it came. . . . It seems that no matter what I do that the well meaning press alienates me more and more from pro-life people. . . . Thank you so much . . . it was a boost at a very needy time."[39]

CHAPTER 14
Stepping Down

Long-time supporters of Doctor Koop are bitter and depressed. . . .
An atheist would have performed just as effectively for the Left.
                                   —CAL THOMAS, prominent conservative journalist

Midway through Koop's second term, a group of friends decided to pull together a classic Washington dinner in his honor—with sponsors and hosts festooning the invitations, and a guest list to die for. The Salute to the Surgeon General was planned for May 19, 1987. In the six months since the release of the AIDS report, controversy had been swirling among key players in the socially conservative "pro-family" movement. Leading those most critical of Koop was formidable campaigner Phyllis Schlafly, famed for her remarkable defeat of the Equal Rights Amendment, teamed with Paul Weyrich, one of the core founders of the "religious right." On May 1, the *New York Times* gave half a column to "The Koop Testimonial." Here's the lede: "Republican Presidential hopefuls are scrambling to disengage themselves from a testimonial dinner honoring Dr. C. Everett Koop . . . who was once a favorite of conservatives."[1]

Under pressure from Schlafly and others, three key presidential hopefuls, Jack Kemp, Bob Dole and Pete du Pont, pulled out, though George H. W. Bush—who would of course emerge as the victor in the election—confirmed his support, even though he did not actually attend.[2] Kemp was first to jump, then Dole, then the largely forgotten du Pont. Some saw this as the beginning of the end of his career in government. The Salute certainly backfired as an effort to honor Koop, though, as Edward Martin drily noted, not entirely without benefits. "He would never have gotten the kind of attention for that [AIDS] report if he had not had these crazies going after him every single day. It also consolidated the department behind him."[3]

Unsurprisingly, the household AIDS mailer, sent out a year later, added salt to the wounds. "The last straw" in Koop's reputation with many conservatives, reported the *New York Times*, "was the household mailing on AIDS. . . . James P. McFadden, chairman of the Ad Hoc Committee on Defense of Life, reacted with fury. 'Here is a guy who looks like an Old Testament prophet—who ever would have imagined that he'd end up selling the gospel of sodomy to the entire country with a mailing of 107 million advertisements for condoms!'"[4]

"Koop was angered by the conservatives' attacks," reported John P. Judis in *The New Republic*. When Weyrich bumped into him soon after, Koop refused to shake his hand.[5]

Then came the abortion non-report.

Koop's friend, theologian and ethicist Harold O.J. Brown, with whom he had helped found the Christian Action Council (CAC) back in 1975, wrote a critique of "The Strange Pilgrimage of C. Everett Koop," raising questions, such as, why Koop had not decided to spend his final months in Washington, when he had nothing to lose, going after abortion. The executive director of the CAC, Tom Glessner, had asked Koop on April 28 why, if he stated that "Smoking by pregnant women is dangerous to fetal health," he could not also say, "Abortion by pregnant women is fatal to fetal health." Koop responded, "I would be laughed out of office."[6] Brown continued to hold Koop in high esteem, which added to his distress. "Never in American history has a man of higher professional qualifications than Dr. Koop's been called to so high an appointive post. . . . Hardly any official of Dr. Koop's rank, or indeed any rank, has been exposed to such a torrent of concentrated vilification as that Dr. Koop had to endure during and after his confirmation hearings." As one Reagan administration official put it to Judis, during the confirmation he was "mau-maued."[7]

The Bush Administration

As the new administration took over in January of 1989, Koop hoped, at a minimum, to be asked to remain in office as Surgeon General. According to Fauci: "I remember having conversations right here in my office, with him. Saying, this isn't about you. It's nothing personal, this is purely business. This is the way that Washington works. When new presidents come in, they pick their own people. The President wanted to pick his own Surgeon General. But Chick was really deeply hurt by that, because he felt he had done such a great job. He thought that that was unfair. Chick took it very personally. Yes, took it as if it was an indictment of him. And he even had hopes that he might be made the secretary!"[8]

Koop had been speaking with friends and colleagues for some time about his high hopes of getting the job. In his memoir, he recalls a dinner hosted by secretary of state-designate James Baker III and his wife Susan, whom the Koops knew socially. He "boldly took Susan aside and told her that although I liked the Surgeon General's job, I had come to the conclusion that I could best help the President and the nation if I were the secretary of Health and Human Services. . . . I had understudied the job for eight years [and] could hit the ground running and accomplish a lot very quickly." Koop says that Mrs. Baker's "eyes lit up, and she said 'Of course, you'd be just wonderful in that job.'"[9]

Whatever Susan Baker politely said to him, what Koop's candid friends were telling him was a very different story.[10]

Edward Martin summed it up for me. It was "totally unrealistic." He and Koop had discussed it a number of times. "I was always very sanguine about telling him that it wasn't going to happen." And he explained why. "When you hire a secretary of HHS . . . these people are senators or governors, people that bring substantial constituencies to the administration." Koop? Well, "Chick's basic constituency he had alienated! The right-to-lifers. So he didn't have a constituency. He wasn't value add. What he thought he had was integrity, discipline, honesty, and he was a great physician, and he thought that ought to count. Well, that's not how they make these decisions."[11] Martin continued: "The other thing is . . . he would not 'work the Hill.' If you're a secretary, you're making deals on both sides of the aisle all the time. And Chick didn't do that, he didn't make deals. I mean, Chick didn't make deals."[12]

Meanwhile, someone had called Koop with "inside information" that he was indeed under serious consideration. But he "would have to assure George Bush and his team that I would not be as active and independent as a Cabinet member as I had been as Surgeon General." Koop adds: "I knew I would not want the job with those constraints."[13] Jack Henningfield, a colleague in tobacco control who like Martin and Fauci became a long-term friend, was equally candid. He told me: Koop was the only person in Washington who didn't understand that Bush was "not going to hire somebody to work for *what they thought was right*."[14] Koop was pretty clear that those would be his terms.

Years later, speaking with his trainee Moritz Ziegler, Koop still thought that his mistake had been not to have been "bolder" in asking for the job! "I wanted to be the secretary of health. I probably was wrong in not going to George [H. W.] Bush and saying, 'These are the reasons why I think I should be secretary of health: (1) I've been understudying the job for eight years; (2) I could hit the ground running; (3) I know my way around; and (4) I can do some of the things that you want to accomplish in the way of health care reform.'"[15]

This really is a remarkable statement, since it demonstrates—as the friends with whom he had been discussing the situation had in their various ways been gently saying to him—that despite his extraordinary experience as Surgeon General, and the political adroitness he had shown at some key points during that time, he did not understand some very basic facts about Washington politics. In his memoir, he proves the point with barbed remarks about President Bush: "In spite of his repeated statements that he wanted Cabinet members who spoke their minds, George Bush, like most presidents, required team players. . . . I think my independence was anathema to the Bush administration."[16] That lack of understanding becomes even more clear, when we read that Koop's plan had been to tackle healthcare reform, a task fraught with political hazards that engulfs close to one-fifth of the entire American economy.[17]

In another reminiscence he confirms yet further his bizarre failure to grasp one of the essentials of how politics works. "I went down to Washington with a label. It's a great mistake that people are picked because of their label. . . . I don't know whether Reagan sat down with some henchmen and said, 'Let's pick Koop because under these circumstances, you can expect he'd do that.'"[18] Without such a "label," why on earth would anyone be picked for a political appointment?

"Before Christmas," *Nova* tells us, he knew "he would not be the new Secretary, neither had he been asked to stay on as Surgeon General beyond his present term."[19]

Meanwhile, Secretary Bowen had received an abrupt call from the White House asking him to clear his desk by the following noon.[20] Bowen pinned the blame on John Sununu, Bush's incoming chief of staff, known for his brusqueness.[21] This is how the new administration was dealing with a cabinet officer, two levels above Koop.

But since the Surgeon General was in the unusual position of holding a political appointment with a fixed term, he could not easily be dismissed. It may seem surprising that he did not just go of his own accord, though he will have noted that CDC director James Mason, with whom he got on well, had been made assistant secretary for health in the new administration, and therefore his new immediate boss. Koop wondered whether it was his pro-lifer critics who had persuaded the Bush people to do away with him. If that were so, it would have an amusing side: Koop had been appointed to please this community; now he was being shown the door to please them.[22] But it is hard to believe that that had been necessary. Koop was a determined loose cannon and had made it very clear that if he was retained within the administration he had no plans to let them tie him down, which was an act of political suicide.

So, in classic bureaucratic fashion, he was made to feel unwelcome. He was cut from a staff retreat. His scheduler was taken from him.[23]

And the unkindest cut of all: His access to the secretary's private dining room was withdrawn.[24] Per *Newsweek*: "Relations between Surgeon General C. Everett Koop and top Bush officials were far more sour than generally reported."[25]

Through all this, Koop will not have forgotten sharing with his longtime friend, Harold O.J. Brown, that during the election campaign he had been quietly approached by representatives of the Democratic presidential candidate, Michael Dukakis, with an offer to keep him on as Surgeon General if Dukakis won.[26]

Koop writes in his memoir that the day Louis W. Sullivan's nomination as secretary of HHS was announced, he called him. He was offended when Sullivan failed to return the call.[27] For his part, Sullivan, in a later interview, recalls an initially difficult relationship. "Chick Koop, of course, the Surgeon General . . . actually had been one of the candidates to be Secretary. It was a strained time when we met, after I had become Secretary, and I think it was harder on him than on me. . . . *Here's this guy, comes up from nowhere and he has the job that I want . . . .* I was trying to reassure him, because . . . I hadn't hungered after this position. It was almost by accident that this had happened."[28]

Resignation

Koop's May 4 letter of resignation to the President is brief to the point of terse.[29]

"Dear Mr. President,

"On February 15 I wrote you to say that I would not serve out my full term as Surgeon General. Effective July 13, 1989, I will be entering terminal leave status. I will be on terminal leave through September 30, 1989 and will enter retirement status on October 1, 1989.

"During the time that I am on terminal leave, the Assistant Secretary for Health will name an Acting Surgeon General.

"Sincerely yours. . . ."[30]

The letter includes no expression of thanks for the opportunity of service, and no good wishes for the future of the administration. Nevertheless, the President's response is adulatory. "In your seven and one-half years as surgeon general of the United States, you have redefined and invigorated that crucial job. Your very personality has come to symbolize the dedication and selfless devotion of the Public Health Service, whose uniform you wore with pride and distinction."[31]

Sullivan too is fulsome in his praise. "You have been a voice of honesty, integrity, compassion and plain good sense."[32]

In their syndicated column, Jack Anderson and Dale Van Atta tartly observe: "President Bush and Human Services Secretary Sullivan didn't have the backbone to ask Koop to leave. They simply gave him the silent treatment until his own self-respect forced him to resign. . . . Koop's curt letter of resignation to Bush earlier this month covered a mountain of hurt." They add, astutely: "First a surgeon, Koop never bothered to master politics."[33]

Why had Koop chosen to resign, so near to the conclusion of his contract in mid-November? It doubtless gave him a sense of agency. This comes through clearly, if misleadingly, in the *Nova* that aired in October of 1989. Koop declared that "I did not resign because I wasn't made Secretary. I did not resign because I wasn't approached about being Surgeon General. I resigned because I have bigger and better things to do, and there comes a time in government when you have expended all that you can expend." Had the *Nova* been less adulatory (and better journalism), Koop would have been challenged for making such a claim. Six weeks after he stepped down, his job was set to disappear.

And it is also clear that had he been offered a third term as Surgeon General, as he discussed with Fauci, let alone the secretary's job, whatever "bigger and better things" he had on his mind, resignation would have been out of the question.[34] As the inevitability of leaving government percolated through his thinking, plans were developing for what would come next. As Betty Koop ruefully remarked many times, retirement was not among his gifts. Indeed, his trainee and friend Howard Filston reflected that, "to some extent he looked down on folks who retire."[35]

The *Nova* crew had followed him to Geneva, where he was making his final visit to the World Health Assembly in May of 1989. Then they joined an add-on family trip—with his wife and daughter Betsy—across the border to France, where there was a monument to his son David, dead now for more than twenty years.[36] In a stark reminder of frailty and loss, the Koops had to cut the trip short and hastily returned stateside. Betty had developed pneumonia in both her lungs. It turned out to be Legionnaires' Disease.[37]

There's a curious coda to the *Nova* program that shows how insensitive Koop could be. He was particularly pleased with the show, a televisual obituary that gave him full marks. As a result, he wanted to award his Surgeon General's Medal to producer Susanne B. Simpson, and her colleague Gretchen Berland.[38] He called Paula Apsel, the storied Senior Producer of *Nova*, who tactfully replied in a letter that this would not be appropriate. *Nova* maintained a rule—a garden variety principle of journalistic ethics—that "nothing of value may be accepted from people or institutions on whom they are reporting," since it might be seen as a quid pro quo for positive treatment. Koop could be tin-eared; and he was not used to being thwarted. "That film should portray a press that recognizes the Surgeon General—as do the public—as being a man of integrity that would not stoop to influence a documentary," he huffed. "NOVA also has the distinction of being the first to refuse a Surgeon General's award for exemplary service to the Office of the Surgeon General."[39] It was an embarrassing exchange.

As the Koops began to make their plans, they faced the fact that for eight years they had occupied government housing on the NIH campus. So Koop wrote to James Wyngaarden, the NIH director, with whom he had lately arm-wrestled on the Commissioned Corps revitalization project, to ask if they could stay in the house for a time after his fall retirement date. Wyngaarden's answer was no. Koop is requested to forward to one of his subordinates the date at which his retirement will take effect so they can repossess the property. Koop replied direct to Wyngaarden, "I think it's best to assume that I will not leave a day before I have to which is October 1st." (There's an annotation on the letter that he intends to discuss the matter further with assistant secretary Mason.)[40] Meanwhile, he wrote to the Membership Services Department of the AMA on April 14, asking if he could be excused from paying his dues since he was stepping down.[41]

As news of his retirement spread, the encomia and awards poured in. Senator Kennedy, whose hand he had refused to shake after the Senate confirmed his nomination back in 1981, commended him as "an exceptional public servant and courageous Surgeon General" with an "outstanding record of achievement."[42]

And on June 11, 1989, Dartmouth College, his alma mater, conferred on him the honorary degree (Doctor of Science) he had failed to secure all those years back for I.S. Ravdin. The presentation speech ended: "Your candor and fearlessness in meeting your responsibilities have demonstrated, with refreshing force, that the Surgeon General of the United States can be hazardous to this nation's complacency."[43]

Then he had what must have been a bittersweet experience—to receive the American Health Foundation's "Salute to C. Everett Koop" at their twentieth anniversary meeting—complete with a speech from Louis W. Sullivan. It's a powerful tribute, elegantly expressed. "The American people," Sullivan remarks, "have an uncanny knack for separating wheat from chaff in those who serve them. Dr. C. Everett Koop was pure wheat." Switching from the Bible to that other most American source of metaphor, he adds: "[W]e at the Department of Health and Social Security will be retiring Chick Koop's number later this year. For like Baby [sic] Ruth, Ted Williams and Willie Mays he is, and has been, one of a kind."[44]

And then this: "At times like this I wish that we, in public life, did not have to settle for eloquent but never eloquent, enough *words*. Because our *words* are juxtaposed against *deeds*. Chick's deeds of leadership, of inspiration, of insight of integrity those words, try as we might, reflect only the shadow and not the substance of the man, we honor tonight."[45]

Looking Ahead

While nursing hopes of continuing as Surgeon General or becoming George H. W. Bush's secretary for Health and Human Services, Koop had nevertheless begun to explore alternatives. Even before the presidential election, September 6 of 1988 had found him in New York City, at the offices of the William Morris Agency on 55th and Avenue of the Americas.[46] This visit would bear fruit for both parties in a press release, dated May 8 of 1989, announcing that effective July 13, when Koop would go on terminal leave, Morris would represent him—in publishing, broadcasting, lectures, and film.[47]

Koop had carefully prepared for the meeting, including a brainstorm with Morris's Norman Brokaw, three days before, on which he made notes.[48] Top left of his first page is "Money." Top right, "Credibility." And on the following page: "I am most believable doc in America, but also internationally." The *Nova* program would be broadcast in October. "What follows?" He enthuses about television opportunities: "Biggest returns for all my goals for time and energy spent!" And he notes three questions he needs to address. First, his relationship with friends and former colleagues Gans and Gorsuch. Second, "How do I take ideas in my mind re video to fruition?" Third, "How to keep credibility."[49]

After his trip to the office in New York he dictated his reflections on the visit. He had liked all the people he met. He has an upcoming meeting with Brokaw in California for a further discussion. Everything is on the table—television, the video series he has in mind, lectures; and indeed "Advertisements are not out of the question for money." Morris takes 20 percent of his fees, and claim their competition typically takes 30 percent plus. "In short," writes Koop, "I was impressed, came away with a sample contract . . . and probably have no compunction about signing with them."[50]

By June 26, 1989, before Koop had even stepped out of his office in the Humphrey Building, Brokaw was handling a plea from celebrated TV host Phil Donahue that he appear on his program. The Koop show was on the road.[51]

Farewells

There were many farewells as Koop stepped down.

Time magazine called on dying, gay photographer Robert Mapplethorpe to take Koop's photo for their April 4 cover. It would be Mapplethorpe's final commission.[52]

The Commissioned Corps said farewell at the Bethesda Naval Officers Club, "Open to all uniformed PHS Officers. Uniform of the day: Summer Whites, Salt and Pepper."[53] The State Department hosted him in the James Madison Room, where Ted Kennedy and former Surgeons General were among the guests.[54]

Edward Brandt, his first boss at HHS, missed a farewell in the Humphrey Building since he had managed to confuse his schedule. Brandt had originally considered the office of Surgeon General an anachronism ripe for abolition. Now dean of the medical school at the University of Oklahoma, Brandt wrote that, "It is a great honor to know you."[55]

Koop's own farewell to Otis Bowen, warm colleague and HHS secretary throughout Reagan's second term, was also fumbled. "I wanted to call you and say good-bye," wrote Koop, "but didn't have a number and decided not to try it through the White House in view of the change in Administration." He continued, "you couldn't have been more generous than you were with me."

Bowen framed the letter and hung it on his office wall.[56]

Part V
CITIZEN KOOP

In earlier times, when an individual achieved great things, he or she might be rewarded with a knighthood, a throne, perhaps even can-onization. Today, when an individual has achieved the pinnacle of his or her profession, the reward is becoming a brand. When a person becomes a brand—think Madonna, Michael Jordan, Martha Stew-art—he or she has made the transition from individual to icon. The mere mention of the person's name evokes not just an image of the indi-vidual, but impressions of the values for which the individual stands.

— "Dr. Koop: The Brand," *People Reputation Management* magazine

The one thing that I leave office with is credibility, and when you sell it, you've lost it, and when you rent it, you've lost it. I'm trying to find a way to lease it, and get it back.

—Nova, *The Controversial Dr. Koop*

Koop retained his prominence in American public life after he stepped down from office, bolstered by the high-profile NBC television series he anchored on healthcare. George H. W. Bush would soon be defeated after one term by Bill Clinton, ushering in a new period of influence for Koop at the highest level of government as he found ready access both to the Clintons and to Vice President Al Gore.

Meanwhile, developments in technology offered fresh avenues for health education. The video cassette now seems hopelessly dated but offered in the 1970s and after the first opportunity for video commu-nication that was asynchronous—not determined by broadcast list-ings. Driven by movie rentals, the video cassette recorder was adopted near-universally in American households by the 1990s. As we shall see, Koop was determined to exploit this technology for health messages.

At the same time, the commercial internet was catching on as busi-ness models emerged for online entrepreneurs, and a rush of start-ups

dazzled users and markets quite as much as their starry-eyed develop-
ers. They also dazzled the investment banks, who were the only players
actually guaranteed to make money out of the game, as IPOs popped
like champagne corks.[1] The rising tide of a NASDAQ that shot up 85
percent in 1999 raised pretty much all the boats, just as it dashed them
hard in the first three years of the new millennium in successive falls of
39 percent, 21 percent, and 31 percent.[2] Never was there such a winnow-
ing of the commercial deployment of a new technology.[3]

On July 13, 1989, Koop left room 710G, his office on the 7th floor of the
Hubert Humphrey Building, at 200 Independence Avenue, a free man.

He was done with his government job. Indeed, he was done with
employment.[i] His campaign for America's health would continue,
but on his own terms—"with no governmental portfolio and no
governmental constraints," as he told Sarah Boxer of the *New York
Times* soon after.[4] "I can be as outspoken as I wish."[5]

Koop had also woken up to the fact that, while he had not come
into government intending to make money afterward, as many did,
there was certainly money to be made. Nearly nine years on a federal
stipend—it had risen to $90,934 by 1989—had not been pleasant.[6] But
he knew that his reputation was for integrity. It was in his interests
to be prudent. He had no plans for making easy money by endorsing
Japanese condoms.[7]

One wonders what was going through the mind of Citizen Koop,
as the *Los Angeles Times* dubbed him, as he fought the rush hour
crush on the Red Line train up to Medical Center, the NIH's own
metro station, and walked home across the campus to Betty—and,
no doubt, a dry martini.[8] One rather prosaic concern certainly was.
The Koops had received notice to quit their government housing at
4, West Drive, by October 1.[ii]

Ten days into retirement, Koop would be celebrated in the highly
complimentary PBS *Nova* film, "The Controversial Dr. Koop."[9]

---

i   After thirteen weeks of accumulated vacation time, on October 1 he would become a
federal retiree.

ii   Home was soon just two miles away, at 5924 Maplewood Park Place, Bethesda.

CHAPTER 15

In Washington

I think I belong here. I think that's where my skills are. I think it's an
address I ought to have if I want to do the things I want to do.

—CEK, to writer Philip Yancey

One of Citizen Koop's first discoveries was that he had ready
access to some of the biggest names in American life, from
business to sports to television.[1] He's soon having breakfast with Bill
Cosby, pitching a favorite project to Amway billionaire Rich DeVos,
and collaborating on a book with Magic Johnson.

In May of 1990 Koop found himself at breakfast before the University of Pennsylvania's commencement with Cosby, star of one of
television's most family-friendly shows.[i] Koop took the opportunity
to pitch him on a project involving adolescent health, and in a follow-up note lays on the flattery.[2]

Koop was chairing the board of a new museum of medicine, destined
for the Washington Mall. One of the big money people he knew was
Richard DeVos, who headed up both Amway and Gospel Films.[3] When
DeVos invited Koop to join him at a meeting with Billy Graham on the
west coast, flying in DeVos' private plane, Koop took his opportunity to
pitch the project. Though DeVos signs his letters "Love ya!" it's plain he
doesn't know Koop well. He addresses him with the giveaway "Everett,"
Koop does not sign "Chick," and DeVos never funded the project.

Meanwhile, Koop's wife Betty had a heart attack, and he has to cut
his trip short to hurry home.[4] On May 9, Koop wrote to his friend
Tim Johnson that she is "recovering nicely."[5] Meanwhile, Koop and

---

i   Lately scandalously fallen from grace.

Johnson are working on their book of letters, *Let's Talk*, debating issues like abortion.[6]

On November 7, 1991, basketball star Earvin "Magic" Johnson announced at a press conference that he had contracted HIV. Together with Rock Hudson's death, Magic Johnson's announcement was a defining moment of the early AIDS era. Koop was immediately in contact with Johnson's publicist, agreeing to serve on the board of the Magic Johnson Foundation, and to help "this young man" in any other way, not least, curiously, to "protect him from exploitation."[7]

It was announced on December 6, less than a month after the diagnosis became public, that "Magic Johnson has agreed to write three books for Random House," including an autobiography. "C. Everett Koop, the former Surgeon General, is to work with Mr. Johnson on the safe-sex guide."[8]

Meanwhile, as his dance card filled up, he was busy turning down no fewer than thirty offers of honorary degrees.[9]

As he moved among celebrities, Koop still found time to socialize with his staff. A month before the frenzy of Magic Johnson activity we find him in Saint Louis, hometown of his assistant Mary Ann Geoghegan. He was speaking at Washington University's centenary, and has taken Mary Ann's family out for dinner, at the celebrated Nantucket Cove restaurant—her travel agent mom Judy ("I will use no other agent," he said), and four other relatives.[10] Koop was on his second Absolut vodka martini when local gossip columnist Jerry Berger stopped by for a chat about his newly-published memoir. Koop ordered his shrimp unpeeled and was looking forward to a Nantucket Platter.[11]

Opinion Maker

By the early 1990s, Koop had moved on from many of the great issues that had consumed energy and vision for most of his professional life, and in both his careers. After stepping down, he would say little about AIDS, or abortion, or pediatric surgery, or the rights of the handicapped.[12] He continued for a time to participate in debates about tobacco control.[13] The one substantive health issue to which he devoted fresh energy was obesity, an issue he regarded as a leftover from his time as Surgeon General.

After losing his institutional support at HHS, he immediately began to put together a fresh team. His history professor son Allen arranged a year's leave from Dartmouth to work on his memoir.[14] Former medical colleagues Paul Gorsuch and Stephen Gans were recruited to help with the network TV series that kicked off these efforts, together with other projects—an arrangement already in place by May 1989, when Koop submitted his resignation. One of the many approaches that arrived in the mail was for a column in *Good Housekeeping* magazine. He sent it on to Norman Brokaw with the comment, "This might be something to think about particularly as we have the assistance of Steve [Gans] and Paul [Gorsuch]."[15]

"I want to be seen as an opinion maker," he told Paul Dean of the *Los Angeles Times*. Freelance writer Philip Yancey was preparing a profile. They met at Princeton, where Koop was to get an honorary degree. "I had several hours with him for the interview," Yancey later told me; "he was a mellowed man compared to the person I knew from twenty years before, did not have that kind of imperious demeanor at all. He had been wounded, but survived, and had broadened his view, and had a more compassionate side that I had not seen before."[16] He wrote in his notes on the meeting, "skin pale, wrinkled, shows age." "Tan slacks, pull-on cotton shirt, blue canvas shoes." "Overweight."

Koop needed rapidly to "transition from title to person," as the *Los Angeles Times* put it, interviewing him a few weeks later. "Home is no longer red-brick government quarters. Koop, like ordinary folk, has a new huge mortgage on a small house in Maryland."[17]

He worried that stepping down from the job would turn him into a mere "former Surgeon General." By engaging the William Morris Agency—"Hollywood agent for Marilyn and Elvis," said the *Washington Post*—he had secured the best. "For the first time since leaving his federal post in July," reported the *Times*, "Koop is talking to the media—but only to interviewers selected by the Beverly Hills agent he now shares with Gerald and Betty Ford." Koop is quoted as stating: "I have to be very careful not to be overexposed."[18] But he need hardly have worried. A household name is a household name. "I am very pleased," he went on to remark, with characteristic immodesty, "to see news reports, headlines and magazine things talking about C. Everett Koop and not talking about the former surgeon general."[19] He had received around two hundred invitations to affiliate with academic institutions.[20] Yet what he most wanted was to devise ways in which he could continue to be "the nation's healthcare conscience," essentially to serve as a Surgeon General cut loose from government.[21]

The NBC specials offered him a remarkable opportunity to do just that.

The "Bulliest Pulpit"

Koop's eponymous network television series featured five hour-long documentaries filmed on location around the country.[22] The *Los Angeles Times* described him in the first episode, on "Children at Risk," as "like [veteran TV journalist] Mike Wallace with a stethoscope. . . . One moment he is interviewing a mother who used crack cocaine during pregnancy, the next moment he is hugging a terrified young boy after administering him an immunization shot."[23] According to the *Deseret News*, "C. Everett Koop tried to change the world of health during eight years as surgeon general. . . . He now thinks he may do even better at the task as host of five one-hour TV specials airing on NBC over the next few weeks."[24]

Koop had plainly enjoyed making the *Whatever Happened to the Human Race?* series; here was a further opportunity to make movies, but for a much wider audience and under his new branding—as the most trusted name in American medicine. In October of 1992, he reported to Brokaw at William Morris, he had enjoyed a visit to the International Health and Medical Film Festival in San Francisco, where he gave the keynote, and picked up two Freddies, "one for the NBC film on aging and one for the film on adolescence. That makes five awards counting the Emmies. Not bad for my first television venture."[25] As we see later, Koop's connection with the festival proved also a key stepping-stone to his ill-fated involvement in DrKoop.com.[26]

Koop had long been in negotiation with NBC about the series, in which he offered unvarnished commentary on America's healthcare system, its woes and opportunities. He told the *Los Angeles Times* that he was very critical of the Bush administration's efforts on the healthcare front. "There's nothing happening with health in the current Administration. Our biggest healthcare problem is that we have no health system. I knew I would not be able to accomplish anything in that Administration, so," he adds disingenuously, "I got out."[27]

Writing

Once his memoirs were out of the way, Koop was considering all kinds of writing projects. Back in 1988 Henry Waxman had sent him a novel by Steve Pieczenik. "Dear Henry," Koop wrote back, "I know I'm going to enjoy it when I get a chance to read it and it might even stimulate me to write the medical mystery I've always wanted to do."[28] Around the same time, Koop wrote about a book on medical ethics, that evidently ran into the sand.[29] Religious publisher Multnomah Press had approached him. "It is entirely possible" that in the future he will be writing a religious book.[30] Meanwhile, Jacqueline Kennedy Onassis pitched him from Doubleday. Koop's priority has to be work on his Random House memoir, but, "When that is finished . . . perhaps there are some things we could accomplish together."[31]

A slew of other book ideas never saw the light of day. One was on leadership (and AIDS). Yet another was partly written, in cahoots with his college roommate, Michael A. Petti; working title, "Your Health: Fact and Fiction." He got as far with this one as to share half a dozen chapters with the William Morris Agency.[32]

But he was soon much too busy to sit down and follow through on writing anything.[33]

Speeches

Meanwhile, Brokaw and the agency were busy building his career on what Koop liked to call the "distinguished lecture circuit." Koop is candid with the *Los Angeles Times* that he needs the money. He can't build an inheritance for kids and grandkids "on a federal pension." His base speaking fee is $25,000 a shot (the equivalent of around three months' pay as Surgeon General).[34] As his trips ramped up, without federal aides to cushion him, a banker friend provided him with a pseudonymous credit card, so he could book his travel incognito.[35]

Koop had a specific goal in mind, as he began to spread himself around, with "television specials, his book, the speeches and interviews." They are all intended to be "conduits . . . to the commercial videotapes" that he has planned for the elderly and is "just aching to do . . . health videos directed at people like you to buy for your mother. There are three one-way tickets to nursing homes that don't have to be. Fractured hips. Diabetic amputations. Incontinence. And I have a good answer to all three."[36] That was back in 1989, well before Time Life came calling with their video pitch.[37] It helps explain how readily he fell for it, a top-branded, funded, model to deliver exactly what he had wanted to accomplish for years.

Nonprofits

Among the nonprofit projects he took on soon after stepping down, three stand out: The Safe Kids Campaign, the Carnegie-sponsored National Ready-to-Learn Council, and the National Museum of Health and Medicine.

The National Safe Kids Campaign, founded in 1988 by his trainee and long-term friend Martin Eichelberger, offered Koop an office base after he left government at Washington's Children's National Medical Center.[38] Koop had been in at the start with Eichelberger, writing him on May 5, 1988, that he would be pleased to serve as honorary chairman—during his time in office, it was all that federal rules permitted. "This is an important and unprecedented effort because it has a foundation of injury prevention programs at the grassroots, communications and education for both the public and the professions, and initiatives in public policy at all levels of government."[39]

As Citizen Koop he could be chairman proper, and remained actively involved, chiefly in soliciting funding for a cause in which he had actually been engaged since the 1950s.[40] Looking back, Eichelberger told me, "Safe Kids Worldwide is in all the states, and thirty-four countries. We went from nothing. . . . And Chick was key to this whole thing."[41]

In September 1992, *Education Week* announced the formation of a "national council to promote school readiness," an effort under the umbrella of the Carnegie Foundation for the Advancement of Teaching, with Koop as co-chair. Council members included the AAP and the National Governors' Association.[42]

The third major commitment involved taking the helm of an effort to develop the National Museum of Health and Medicine in Washington, DC, that he had tried to pitch to DeVoss. Koop had agreed in July of 1989 to chair its foundation, saying that "it doesn't make sense that the nation's capital, which shows its citizens everything else imaginable, doesn't have a health exhibit."[43]

The existing Medical Museum of the Armed Forces Institute of Pathology was currently on the grounds of Walter Reed Army Hospital out in Bethesda. "No matter what you put out there, the average tour group coming to Washington hasn't got the time to travel out there."[44] Later, he explained: "My reason in the beginning for being interested in a museum in Washington that had to do with health, was that I used to stand in my office up on the top floor of the Humphrey Building and see all these kids standing by one of the reflecting pools, getting their pictures taken, when they came on their senior trip to Washington, and I kept thinking about the wonderful opportunities that they had, and then it occurred to me that they could be stimulated to be almost anything in the world by what they saw in Washington, except something in medicine and health. Because there's no place to see it."[45]

Koop was also free to rejoin two nonprofit boards that held important symbolic significance from his life before public office, and from which he had withdrawn as a result of his nomination to the office of Surgeon General. We have seen how even in office he found ways to help AUL, the pro-life public interest law firm based in Chicago, in their fundraising efforts. "I would be most happy to serve again on your board of directors," he wrote to executive director Guy Condon, volunteering his service.[46] This is particularly interesting in light of the public spats that Koop had had with various pro-life leaders, and widespread disappointment within the movement about the outcome of the abortion report saga.

Soon after, historian Michael Horton, then president of the Alliance of Confessing Evangelicals, the Philadelphia-based successor group to Barnhouse's Evangelical Foundation, persuaded him to rejoin the board a half-century after he had first served on it in 1952. "When Koop spoke, that was the end of the story." Horton recalled him as a friend as well as an ally. They had first met during Sunday morning service at Tenth Presbyterian Church when Horton was a child. Now he found himself spending time with him as an adult. "I was actually on the receiving end for my cigars," Horton told me. He punched back at Koop: "What about your single malts?" Horton observed that, "there's an element of selection in the way he would use the statistics." He got quite a concession from the former Surgeon General. "He says, 'Well, I guess we pick our vices.'"[47]

Meanwhile, Wheaton College in Illinois, the elite evangelical institution where nearly two decades earlier Koop had launched his crusade against abortion, was keen to build a relationship with him. On February 22, 1990, Koop was invited to campus to give the first Penner Lecture.[48] It proved a memorable event. A reporter from the *Chicago Tribune* relished the unusual match-up of the famously conservative school and Koop's candid AIDS talk.

> He was addressing topics not normally discussed on the campus, where smoking, drinking and social dancing are prohibited, for heaven's sake. So when Koop started talking frankly about balancing the ethics of being a Christian and facing the problem of AIDS, the

audience didn't know how to react. When Koop talked of condoms, most of the audience tittered like schoolchildren. . . . But finally, the man who used to be the nation's doctor got a big round of applause. Dr. Marcia Lipetz of the AIDS Foundation of Chicago told the group that 'I think it's great that we're talking about gonorrhea, anal sex and condoms at Wheaton College.' Koop quipped, 'You can't dance here, but you can talk about that.'[49]

Later in the year, college president Richard Chase invited him to take the chair of an advisory board for their emerging Center for Applied Christian Ethics (CACE). In the process, Koop developed a touching friendship with Alan Johnson, the Wheaton professor heading up the project, and his wife Rea, which would outlast their respective involvements with CACE and end only with the Johnsons' deaths.

After Johnson's retirement, Koop—acerbic as ever—feels free to observe that, "we need a Board that makes CACE a top priority and not just a meeting that might be attended if there is nothing more important going on." An effort in the mid-90s to establish a Koop ethics chair embarrassingly fizzled.[50] At eighty-four, Koop considered stepping down: "I am in a precarious cardiac situation and have taken some heroic slices out of my life so that I can get rid of some of the stresses." Meanwhile, "Betty has had a very difficult year and is barely holding on by her fingertips. We don't have a diagnosis, but she is constantly depleted and exhausted." What's more, the DrKoop.com situation is unspooling. "It has also been a very stressful year for me as you might read from the financial news and I am not in the position that I had hoped to be in at this time, when I could do some major giving to Christian things."[51] In 2004, after he had finally stepped down from CACE, Koop shared with Johnson in a handwritten note that he has had two heart pacemakers fitted.[52] Later: "I'm having too many death encounters—but the Lord granted another reprieve. I cherish your friendship—we'll meet on the other side if not here."[53]

Koop kept finding time both for old friends and at least some of the many individuals who sought his attention. To his old friend from the pro-life movement, Herbert Ratner, he wrote that "I really thought I had moved on to a new plane in life, and not have to deal with the life issues, but then along came assisted suicide."[54] A former Senate staffer shared that she has had a distressing letter from a friend at whose wedding Koop once officiated. Unfortunately, she has lost the letter, and can remember neither her friend's address nor her married name. Can he help?[55] And he found time to respond to a woman whose only connection was once having cleaned for a friend of Betty's. She asks for a blurb for her religious tale of a goose with one foot, and he responds with enthusiasm. "Bet you never expected to learn anything from a goose! . . . It is a simple tale, but I found myself thinking of it day after day."[56]

The Corporate World

In parallel with his extensive nonprofit commitments, Koop began to avail himself of lucrative and useful opportunities in the corporate world. In December 1990, for example, he joined the board of BioPure, a company working on blood substitutes, the field in which he had done his doctoral research and also contract work for the US Army during WW2, and in 1998, he joined the board of First Circle Medical, working in the same field.[57]

From 1992 he also worked with Life Alert, the trailblazer in alarm systems for the elderly living on their own; he remained their spokesman until his death.[58] On March 24, 1994, MBf USA, Inc., confirmed a contract in which Koop would serve as "consultant and advisor" to a company in the "personal health and nutrition" field. He would give four speeches a year that they could use for promotional purposes, chair their advisory board and foundation, and be available to advise as needed. The fee over four years would be one million dollars.[59] Among other companies whose boards he joined were Nutragenics, Neurocrine, and Bionutrics—where fellow directors included the chairman of the Salk Institute and the former chairman of American Express.[60]

Time Life Medical

"Next on Koop's agenda is a series of videocassettes for the elderly," noted the *Chicago Tribune* shortly before he stepped down from office.[61] In a collaboration with his former HHS colleague Thomas R. Burke, he made a video on smoking cessation, and a nice fee.[62] Another project followed, with Cal Covert from a Virginia communications company and his colleagues Paul Gorsuch and Stephen Gans, on "Getting the most out of your hearing aids." In July of 1995, Covert shared that it has won a Telly award, its third after a Bronze Chris and being a selected Finalist at the Academy of Medical Films.[63] Soon after, he is back in touch about a mooted video on diabetic foot. But things have suddenly changed, and Koop is no longer free to take on these ad hoc projects.

Time Life grandly announced: "This initiative merges the medical leadership of Dr. Koop with the marketing savvy of Time Life, a brand synonymous with high quality, accessible information throughout the world."[64] The *Washington Post*'s jaunty response: "Take two videotapes, and call me in the morning." Koop would not simply be making medical videos, but chairing Time Life Medical, a spin-off company using Time Life branding under license.[65] "That may be the new prescription from C. Everett Koop . . . for patients getting the runaround from their doctors."[66] The *Wall Street Journal*, taking a more business-focused angle from the start, headlined: "Time Warner Unit to Invest in Firm Planning a Series of Medical Videos."[67] Bloomberg offers the cautionary observation that it's "Koop's first venture into commerce."[68] From a business angle, it's apparent that this structure was designed to limit the risk to the parent company, which in the event proved a wise move.[69]

The plan was to produce dozens of television-quality thirty-minute tapes, under the overall title, "At the Time of Diagnosis." An initial series of seventy-five was projected. When the doctor gives you the bad news, you stop by the pharmacy and pick up the relevant tape to get a better idea of what's in store. Koop appeared at the start of each video, introducing leading physicians from across the country. They would have "high production values" (in other words, cost a lot of money to produce), and the retail price was set at $19.95.[ii] The first batch of tapes was set to be in pharmacies by early 1996.

The idea for the project had not actually been Time Life's. An advertising executive, J. Keith Green, had made an approach to the company early in 1994. As vice-chairman of a top New York agency, he was considered a "superstar," per the *Wall Street Journal*.[70] Green networked his way to a meeting with Koop, and the deal soon followed. Green was somewhat coy in disclosing its terms. According to Bloomberg, Koop would collect "more than what he made as Surgeon General . . . but quite reasonable for someone who brings as much to the project as Dr. Koop does."[71] Koop was actually paid $750,000 a year. Green hired an "accomplished video producer," Nan-Kirsten Forte, to run production.

"Quickly, it became apparent that spending would be lavish." Forte urged Green to rely on contractors as much as possible, as is customary, to contain costs, but Green wanted to hire people. "Soon, about 150 employees and contractors were at work, often laboring late into the night." The set too was on the grand scale—a two-tier effort, that required a discreet elevator for Koop's use. "A board member told Mr. Green that he was building a shrine to himself."[72]

As the *Journal* looked back from February 13 of 1997, it employed a newsier headline, "Health Videos Starring Koop Took Sick, Saw Dismal Sales."[73] "Dismal sales" was an understatement. According to the *Journal*, Green had projected that inventory would turn over two and a half times in the first year. As it turned out, "sales were progressing at such a slow pace that only about half of the inventory would eventually be sold." The revenue projections were therefore exaggerated by a factor of more than five. This was no marginal situation.[74] Time Life promptly pulled the plug.

"Dr. Koop was perplexed and upset. He placed a call to Time Warner Chairman Gerald Levin, who referred him to Mr. Logan. The decision to pull out, Dr. Koop learned, was irrevocable."[75] Bizarrely,

ii   The equivalent today of around $40.

a venture led by a marketing guru and chiefly funded by one of the world's most careful companies had done insufficient market research on how much consumers were prepared to pay. They sold much better at $9.95, as the company scrambled to unload inventory, but by then it was too late.[76] "The business side was hard for him. Either he was too trusting of other people or just didn't have the savvy," was how one colleague summed things up.[77]

Koop and the Clintons

Koop had long been in favor of radical healthcare reform that would facilitate universal access—a concern dating back to his days as a medical student in New York City, when he found himself delivering the babies of the very poor. He did not favor accomplishing this goal by means of a "single-payer" system akin to those in Europe.[78] He had hoped in vain that President George H. W. Bush would appoint him secretary of Health and Human Services, with sufficient latitude to take such a project forward. But when Bill Clinton won the White House four years later he had fresh hopes of influence.

During the presidential campaign in 1992, Bill Clinton had reached out to Koop on the healthcare reform agenda. Koop recalled nine separate phone conversations. Initially, he was able to call Clinton direct, but the campaign placed an intermediary between them. He was a medical student; Koop refused to speak to him, and the conversations ended.[79] Once the election was done, Koop met with Timothy Westmoreland, on loan from Waxman's office to the Clinton transition team. Bizarrely, Koop wanted to be named Surgeon General in the Clinton administration.[80]

Westmoreland had worked with Koop on various fronts, respected him greatly, and grew fond of him. But he recalls the embarrassing manner in which Koop made the request, "in front of a roomful of people." Koop "point blank looked at them and said, I am the most trusted person in America. The polls say that the American public trust me more than anyone else." Westmoreland commented, "This is not the way to introduce yourself to these people, you're asking them for assistance. You're almost asking them for a favor. And instead you're saying, Take me, I'm the most important person you could possibly be talking to. And of course, it didn't go any further."[81]

Initially, Koop was publicly critical of the Clinton healthcare effort. He characterized the secrecy of the task force's work as "reprehensible." "Koop said the letter he sent Hillary Rodham Clinton detailing his suggestions was never acknowledged."[82]

These criticisms were noted in the White House, where in April of 1993 two advisers to Mrs. Clinton wrote her and healthcare czar Ira Magaziner a memo headed "C. Everett Koop Strategy." After quoting Koop's critical remarks, they conclude: "When our plan comes out, it will likely succeed or fail based on what third-party people with credibility on health care—like Dr. Koop—say about the plan. We need Dr. Koop's support for the plan. Because he is the doctor with perhaps the most credibility with the American people, we cannot afford to continue to ignore C. Everett Koop." What to do?

Magaziner met with Koop, and the "strategy" moved ahead. On June 30, senior policy adviser Lynn Margherio briefed the First Lady—in five single-spaced pages! The goal? "To engage Dr. Koop's support of the plan." The strategy? "We will need to continue to . . . do our best to make him feel an important and welcome contributor." The memo outlined a plan for July 1, when he would be given very special treatment at the White House. First, he would have two hours to review the latest, confidential version of the reform plan. Then, lunch with Magaziner in the White House Mess. Later, a meeting with the First Lady. And finally, at 5:30 p.m., a meeting with the President in the Oval Office.

Carol Rasco, director of the DPC, clarified that Clinton would meet with Koop to discuss his role in educating the public about the plan. "We believe Dr. Koop will ultimately support the plan, once he feels invested in the process." He's also a "logical choice as the chair" of a health information infrastructure commission. "From this visible position, he could educate the public on the merits of the plan as a whole and the specific aspects of building an information infrastructure."[83]

Koop later recalled that the President said, "I know you can't be my salesperson . . . I realize that we have differences of opinion about some things and what I'd like to reform . . . but what I'd like to ask you, would you be willing to be the moderator of a conversation between the medical profession and me and/or the First Lady?" His response: "I could not possibly turn that down."[84]

Less than three months later, on September 20, the administration hosted a breakfast event in the East Room of the White House, for physicians supportive of the reform plan. It was centered on showing off Koop. "The event is intended to highlight the support of Dr. C. Everett Koop and a wide range of other prominent doctors."[85] The President and Vice President and their wives were all there. The choreography was impeccable. The four of them entered the room. The First Lady welcomed everyone, the Vice President spoke, Mrs. Gore spoke, then Koop delivered his own remarks, and introduced the President. After Bill Clinton's speech, they formed a receiving line so the doctors got to shake their hands before breakfast in the State Dining Room. The President and Vice President would be in the Red Room. Mrs. Clinton told the crowd they are all invited to join them and chat. And the press were present.[86]

Two days later, on September 22, 1993, the President addressed a joint session of both houses of Congress. Eyebrows were raised when Koop was seen seated with Mrs. Clinton in the gallery. Then the President included him in his speech. "Now, nobody has to take my word for this. You can ask Dr. Koop. He's up here with us tonight, and I thank him for being here."[87] There was applause.

In a broad if soft endorsement of the Clinton effort, Koop wrote in the *Chicago Tribune* for September 29, 1993, that "Since I left office as surgeon general four years ago, I have dedicated most of my time and energy to speaking out on the need for health care reform. A few weeks ago I told President Clinton that without passing a single law or issuing a single regulation, he had accomplished more on health care reform in the last four months than all of his living predecessors put together. He has done this simply by accepting the challenge of putting healthcare at the top of the national agenda."[88]

In tandem, Koop and the First Lady traveled the country, addressing medical audiences and seeking to sell the plan. Koop was plainly
in his element. "And we would come home from someplace, Atlanta,
and I'd sit with her and her chief assistant in the plane, and we'd just
outline—I'd say, 'This is what you learned today. This is what you
found is going to be hard to push the medical profession on,' and so
forth. And we'd get back to the White House late in the day, and her
devoted staff would be waiting, at 12:00 midnight or 1:00 o'clock, and
she'd say, 'You do this, and you do this, and you do that.'"[89]

Once he was in the inner circle, Koop proceeded to pepper Magaziner with faxes, day after day, on all manner of topics, including the museum! "Although this should not be part of the health
plan," he acknowledged, "I think it would be very apropos if the
President supported this legislation which is attached."[90] In one of
at least four faxes dated September 8, he asked detailed questions
about the upcoming forums and ended with "could I have a prompt
response?"[91] Koop's energy—and impatience—are particularly evident in these hectic months.

He had a more relaxed relationship with Vice President Gore. Following up a call on April 26, during which he had pitched a series
of tech-related healthcare reform proposals, he got a friendly reply
(Dear Chick, Sincerely Al). "It is always great to hear from you." Sadly,
he cannot take Koop up on an invitation to visit Dartmouth—at ten
days' notice![92]

In her memoir *Living History*, Hillary Clinton describes Koop as
an "adamant foe of abortion," yet "an invaluable adviser and ally,"
who, as Surgeon General, had "witnessed the failings of the system
as both a clinician and a policy maker."[93] She writes of their travels
together. "To keep up the momentum, Dr. Koop and I hit the road
again," she writes.

> On December 2, we addressed eight hundred doctors and health
> care professionals attending the Tri State Rural Health Care Forum
> in Hanover, New Hampshire. Dr. Koop had become an increasingly
> enthusiastic advocate of our health care plan. When he spoke, it was
> like listening to an Old Testament prophet. He could deliver the hard

truth and get away with it. He could say, 'We have too many specialists in medicine and not enough generalists,' and an audience filled with specialists would nod in agreement.[94]

Soon after, Koop was prepping her for a January 20 presentation to the Association of Children's Hospitals, where of course he was back on his home turf.[95]

The Clinton plan would be slowly defeated in a series of negotiations and votes, in both houses of Congress, amid disarray among Democrats and pushback against the kind of "big government" that the proposals were widely held to represent.

Shape Up America!

On September 26, 1994, as the healthcare reform initiative was petering out, the First Lady and Koop held a catch-up meeting at the White House. Koop opened with his plan for Shape Up America! (SUA!).[96] He "wants HRC to do event kick off press conf in W House. Early Dec. (before 12th when he gets knee replaced)," records the meeting note. Next, the Vice President has asked for briefings on the Health Information Infrastructure discussion; Michael McDonald and Koop will join departmental briefers. Next, he reports on his New England "test bed" pilot effort on bioinformatics, and notes that he is developing a public/private partnership that he will chair. Fourth, he wants to discuss Haiti health issues. He also updates her on his role with the international aid organization the Medical Assistance Program (MAP), that he had helped found many years before; he has oddly agreed to be their spokesperson on dental health.[97]

Koop reflected later that if he had had another four years as Surgeon General, he likely would have focused on the rising challenge of obesity.[98] SUA! was launched on the South Lawn of the White House, in December of 1994, with the requested help from Hillary Clinton.[99] "I am undertaking my final crusade," said Koop.[100]

Bloomberg summed it up like this: "He has enlisted 60 medical groups and 30 corporations to back 'Shape Up America!' Companies such as Kellogg, diet-food peddler Jenny Craig, and drugmaker

Johnson & Johnson are putting up as much as $1 million each for Olympics-style sponsorships. The aim is to pound home the virtues of moderate exercise and incremental weight loss." Koop's message: "You're going to die 10 years early, taking blood pressure medicine and insulin and worrying about cancer. If you call that a high-quality life, then fine, be fat."[101]

Sponsors were free to use the Shape Up logo (which included the name of the Koop Foundation) on their products.[102]

One reviewer was impressed: "At first glance, the *Shape Up America!* home page is a promotional vehicle for products and sponsoring corporations, but it actually provides useful information via quizzes on fitness, portion control, and the pitfalls of eating out; a body-fat lab; a childhood obesity assessment calculator; family fitness tips; recipes;" and so on.[103]

The *New York Times* carried a detailed report of the launch, followed soon after by an editorial endorsement.[104] "*Time* magazine gave Shape Up America! eight free pages in its May 8, 1995 issue: this amounted to $1.2 million in unpaid advertising."[105] *Shape Up America!* outlived Koop by several years, retaining the Koop Foundation name on its logo.

Jan Strode was then the chief operating office for Jenny Craig. She recalled that SUA! had two significant effects. It had an impact on corporate America. As he had a decade before on smoking, Koop was pressing corporate leaders on what they were doing to help their employees live healthier lives—in the corporate interest, as well as that of the individuals themselves. It also re-introduced Koop to the public arena, five years after he left government.[106]

Policy

Despite his entrepreneurial "third career" with its myriad projects, Koop remained for several years a significant presence in the policy community in Washington, DC. Free now to speak his mind, his interventions were forceful, whether addressing the newly formed

AIDS commission or committees of Congress. Initially, his main focus was on tobacco.

Koop's near-decade-long anti-smoking campaign, and in particular his focus on converting nonsmokers into anti-smokers, had helped foment an increasingly febrile situation in which the industry had lost control of the narrative. His call for every nonfederal actor to take the initiative—from party hostesses to corporations to city and state governments—progressively undermined the relevance of the tobacco lobbyists' influence in Washington. That was the context for two seminal legal cases in the immediate aftermath of his tenure.

In 1991, the cigarette companies were sued by Norma Broin, a nonsmoking flight attendant from Miami who had developed lung cancer. The suit morphed into a class action on behalf of 60,000 FAs, and on October 11, 1997, the companies agreed their first ever class action settlement, for $300m (the plaintiffs had asked for $5 billion), which was used to establish the Flight Attendant Medical Research Institute.[107] Sarah Milov observes wryly that since research funded by the settlement would be used in subsequent cases, "the nonsmokers' rights movement had its own secondhand influence."[108] The companies also agreed to support the 1990 smoking ban on domestic aircraft.[109]

Meanwhile, the State of Mississippi sued in 1994 to recover Medicaid costs and settled three years later for payments of $3.4 billion over twenty-five years—the first settlement of any of the more than forty states that had filed similar suits.[110] Mississippi was one of a handful to settle ahead of a major negotiation involving dozens of states, focused on $368.5 billion in payments and an acceptance of FDA oversight, that would require approval from Congress. In return, the companies would get immunity from future liability, and it was the immunity provision that drew the strongest criticism from those in the anti-smoking movement who were critical of the bill, Koop included. Yet immunity was the only factor that made the companies willing to do a deal. What looked from the outside like a punishing dollar penalty in fact meant that the companies had insured their operations for a quarter-century, at a predictable cost that could be passed on to consumers. Henry Waxman, who was managing the process in the House of Representatives, asked Koop and former FDA Commissioner David Kessler to convene a group of public health leaders to review the proposed settlement, and report back to Congress. In response, according to the *Wall Street Journal*, "They urged Congress to write a fresh bill pursuing public-health goals and incorporating their task force's findings."[111]

Much congressional discussion followed, including a bold effort by Senator John McCain to stiffen the package and remove the immunity provision.[112] But nothing passed. "In the end, the attorneys general and the industry settled the state lawsuits privately for $246 billion, to be paid out over twenty years, and a more modest set of marketing restrictions that did not require federal legislation.[113] There was no immunity clause."[114]

Koop had plainly been in two minds about the whole process. In June, 1997, he stated on *ABC Nightline* that "I have often been misquoted that I am adamantly opposed to a settlement." Many antismoking activists, he noted, "want to see the culprit, the tobacco industry, flogged in public, and I understand how they feel. I feel that way myself. They are very guilty. But flogging a company in public, if it does not produce something for the health of the American people, is a futile gesture."[115]

Controversy

Later in the 1990s, Koop jumped into a series of controversies about potential environmental and other chemical threats. He broadly sided with manufacturers and attacked environmental campaigners, whom he accused of exaggerating risks. Gregg Easterbrook, author of *Surgeon Koop*, came to his defense. "Koop is taking the rational position on a lot of these things. . . . Everything he says is very strongly grounded in a decent body of research—it's just a body of research that the environmental left doesn't like."[116] The *Washington Post* noted that he had "become an increasingly high-profile ally of a major player in many acrimonious public health debates: The

American Council on Science and Health (ACSH), a nonprofit organization that gets extensive funding from chemical and manufacturing industries—and is widely seen as an industry front group."[117]

Back in September of 1988, when he was beginning to make plans for leaving government and consulting the William Morris Agency, Koop had noted as a key concern, "How to keep credibility."[118] We might wonder whether he had discussed these interventions with Norman Brokaw, who had helped him carefully craft his initial public image.

What made things more serious for Koop's image was his lack of sensitivity to potential conflicts of interest, and his tin-earned response to criticism.

For example, he testified before a House subcommittee that latex gloves, which had been criticized on allergy grounds, were a victim of "borderline hysteria." It emerged that some time earlier he had signed a consulting contract with a major manufacturer of the gloves, which had paid him $650,000. Koop was quick to point out that his work was with another division, but his failure to disclose this information caused a furor, and it led to his first sustained criticism in the mainstream media since his confirmation. The *Chicago Tribune* was unforgiving. He was guilty of a "blatant conflict of interest. . . . More shocking still is his apparent inability to understand what the problem is."[119] As in the case of *Nova*'s refusal to accept Surgeon General medals for its journalists, Koop seemed, as the *Tribune* says, just not to get it. He was horrified by the suggestion that he could be corrupt. He naively believed that the wider world should simply take his word for it which, needless to say, it did not. His taking sides against powerful environmental groups served as an accelerant to the controversy.

The *Post* quoted former FDA Commissioner David Kessler, who had worked closely with Koop on tobacco issues and greatly admired him.[iii] "The shame of it," Kessler comments, "is he doesn't have people who can say, 'Hey, Chick, that's not a smart thing to do.'" Koop

---

iii   Kessler told me that he had never felt comfortable calling him Chick! David Kessler interview.

believed in making up his own mind, and as his HHS chief of staff, Edward Martin, said, once he had, there was no one who could challenge him to think again.[120]

It was particularly unfortunate that these spats calling his ethics into question blew up just as the visionary website DrKoop.com began to make the news, with its own potential for controversy. As the decade drew to a close, Koop's reputation was on the line.

CHAPTER 16

At Dartmouth

The Koop Institute is dedicated to health care reform in any way possible, but we're concentrating now on the reform of medical education
to achieve that end.

—CEK

O n May 19, 1992, the president of Dartmouth College, James O.
Freedman, announced, with much fanfare, "an event of national
importance."[1] The college was establishing "an institute dedicated to
medical education, to reshaping the nation's health system." It would
"inform the Dartmouth Medical School curriculum." What's more,
Freedman continued, "the Institute will contribute to the betterment
of medical education and practice across the country."[2] Freedman's
grandiose language suited Koop and his vision very well. Dartmouth
Medical School would be the test bed for a revolutionary approach to
the training of doctors, which would echo around the nation. Dartmouth "was excited when he came, with his incredible reputation
in pediatric surgery and his accomplishments as Surgeon General,"
said Woodie Kessel, former HHS colleague and soon a fellow of the
Koop Institute.[3]

This vision was never realized. Little did Koop know at the time,
but the dean of the medical school, Andrew Wallace, was not on
board.[4][i] These sweeping, visionary terms did not suit Wallace in the

---

i Anyone who has worked in an American university is familiar with the situation in which
the president pushes for change, the faculty resists, and the dean acts as a broker between
the two. There were some special elements in this case. As one candid observer told me, "the
grand promises made by Dartmouth were thwarted by the dean of the medical school, who
hated Chick and felt eclipsed by him. And by Chick's own ego." Confidential interview.

least. He had been on vacation when the plan was announced. When he got back he complained that Freedman had re-written the agreed press release after he left. He demanded that Jane Bassick, director of public affairs, show him the paper trail. "I learned about it over the phone," he told her; "I became disturbed when major modifications were made without including me in the process."[5] Koop was walking into a minefield.

The Institute and the College

So it is small surprise that right from the start there was a rocky relationship between Koop and the Dartmouth administration. There were seriously differing expectations. Koop's sense of the strategic significance of the Institute, and of his own importance, and the corresponding resentment that some administrators and faculty felt, proved a recipe for disaster.

A faculty colleague who became close to Koop, Joseph O'Donnell, summed up why Koop came back to Dartmouth, and what his first hopes had been for this new relationship. "Koop came to Dartmouth to found the Koop Institute because he wanted to change medical education. He wanted to celebrate the lineage of the profession he loved by forming what he envisioned as a guild. Undergraduate pre-medical students would be welcomed and mentored by those further down the line, helped by medical students, housestaff, faculty, and wise 'elders' such as himself. He wanted to build bridges between public health and medicine, attack some of the most vexing behavioral problems facing the nation, preserve rituals such as the physical exam, use the arts to teach the art of medicine, foster careers in service and advocacy, embrace technology without letting it detract from the doctor-patient relationship, and promote a sense of community among physicians."[6]

Koop's extensive vision built on the remarkable sweep of the May 1992, press release. "The intricate plans for the C. Everett Koop Institute are still aborning," he wrote to a correspondent in the summer of 1992.[7]

In an illuminating article published the following year in *The New Physician*, a magazine for medical students, under the perceptive title "General Koop," Stephen C. George writes of the Institute's lofty goals. It "aims at nothing short of changing medical school curricula nationwide, solving the primary care shortage and creating a 'new kind of doctor for the 21st century'—at once adept with high-tech tools to control the explosion of medical knowledge, and more competition in such low-tech skills as doctor-patient communication and health education."[8] The journal *Medical Economics* picked up on what Koop was trying to do, asking: "Can 'America's family doctor' reshape medical education?"[9]

This grand model of the Institute plainly existed in Koop's mind, and also in Freedman's, but apparently nowhere else. "Most of the people thought the Koop Institute was going to be a place for Dr. Koop to keep up with his correspondence and entertain visiting dignitaries. And that would be it. And get money into the college."[10]

The relationship was also soured by problems around John Duffy, whom Koop had recruited to run the Institute on-site from its beginnings. Duffy was a psychiatrist and a distinguished Commissioned Corps career officer, who held the rank of two-star admiral and had served as Chief Physician Officer of the PHS.[11] Just over a year after his appointment he resigned in rather public fashion, quoted in the college newspaper as claiming a "lack of direction and real programs in the institute."[12] It was plain that the relationship between Koop and Duffy had broken down; an inauspicious beginning. Duffy felt that he was "stuck spinning his wheels" at the Institute, trying to manage political issues within the school, while Koop was generally not there.[13] Koop was troubled by the situation, which he saw as "a disaster," telling his old friend surgeon Paul Brand that he would like to talk it over with him.[14] Given Koop's ego, he was likely uneasy when in February of 1993 both he and Duffy were awarded honorary MAs by the college.[15] Then the cover of the Summer 1993 edition of *Dartmouth Medicine* had a cartoon of Koop and Duffy *together* sculpting "the doctor of the 21st century." Given Koop's approach to management and his ownership of the Institute, it appears to have been a misjudgment all round to put in place a director who was a senior figure in his own right.

Just six months after Freedman's announcement, it's plain that Koop's expectation that the medical school would embrace his ideas for reform of the curriculum had already run into the sand. He tells Dean Wallace that if Dartmouth does not "come up to the expectations" of their initial agreement, it will have egg on its face. In the National Academy of Sciences and the Institute of Medicine there is a high level of enthusiasm for what Dartmouth can accomplish in curricular reform. Wallace has been pushing back, saying that while he agrees with the Koop "ideals . . . it is important for us to implement curricula [*sic*] reform thoughtfully and carefully, and not under undo [*sic*] or unrealistic pressure." Koop is plainly frustrated. "Believe me, Andy, I would not have come to Dartmouth to affect [*sic*] the curriculum changes that you and others seem so enthusiastic about, if it were not for the assurance that changes would be made in the curriculum in order that innovations might be substituted for time redeemed." His final paragraph makes clear that the core issue is not simply that of "commitment to curriculum changes," but "the acceptance of the Koop Institute" itself.[16]

Koop's correspondence with the president, too, constantly has an edge. "Apropos our recent conversation of using me, as an asset . . ." he began one letter. The previous Saturday, as part of the "Dartmouth-UNH Game Day Festivities," there had been an hour-long Health Care Forum. Sans Koop. "If we were trying to put Dartmouth's best foot forward, might it not have been a good idea to have that member of the Dartmouth family who spent three hours in the White House last week on health care reform say a word or two?" He closed: "Believe me, I am not looking for places to speak. . . . I only raise the questions in light of making hay while I enjoy this position of national prominence."[17]

Alongside the dean's resistance on the curricular front, Koop faced frustrating restrictions on fundraising. Target donors had to be approved, and Dartmouth often had other plans for them. Once funds had been raised, the medical school would take off a big slice for institutional overhead.[18] Administrator David R. Serra recalled to me constant struggles. "Every time that we got in line for something, to leverage Dr. Koop's good name, Dartmouth was already in line for some other purpose, and so we would be warned off. It became almost comical, like we couldn't even go after the low hanging fruit. So it was very, very frustrating for Dr. Koop."[19]

As early as February of 1993, Koop wrote to Freedman that he "can not adequately express" his disappointment that he had not approved an approach to the Pew Charitable Trusts. Koop is frustrated in part because of his long-standing relationship with the Pews. "No one can claim that I have not thrown my energy, enthusiasm, and talent" into the Institute, "initially so strongly supported by the Dean of the Medical School and you. Indeed, it was your unusually strong enthusiasm and promise of support that proved critical in my decision to return to Dartmouth." He continues: "On the other hand, as you know better than anyone, the actual reception, once I arrived has not been nearly as energetic or enthusiastic, and I have labored up hill every step of the way." There has been a "less than cordial climate." He concludes: "More than ever, this month I return to Hanover with less enthusiasm and a greater burden."[20]

In pursuit of funds, Koop continued knocking on every (approved) door he could find. He had even tried NASA, with an imaginative pitch seeking their interest in a "large-scale trial of telemedicine." The administrator explained that NASA's interests do not include "resolving problems of medical practice on Earth."[21]

Meanwhile, the Institute was operating with thoroughly terrestrial budgets. On January 13, 1994, a memo to the CFO Adam Keller noted significant mid-year variances from the budget set for financial year 1994—an unrestricted budget of just over $400,000, three-quarters of which was a hangover from a gift during the previous year, plus a little over $200,000 in restricted funding. The funding from Koop's McInerny Chair flowed to him through the Institute, so the latter would have been three-quarters his own $150,000 emolument.[22]

The donor clash is surprising, since shortly after the press conference announcing the Institute Koop had met with Dartmouth's Office of Development to brainstorm potential solicitations. The clash over overhead is also a surprise. Koop had spent forty years in academic medicine and knew exactly how the system worked. They are both evidence of an early fraying of relations, as grandiose expectations went unfulfilled and Koop became increasingly frustrated.

Succeeding Duffy as leader on the ground was young lawyer David R. Serra—whom Duffy had hired as an administrator just three days before his own "resignation." When Duffy stepped down, Serra took over with the title of executive director.[23]

Two years later, in October 1995, a new director was appointed, William (Bill) Culp. Culp was a dean in the medical school, who would supervise the programs of the Institute and "build bridges" with the faculty in tandem with his other duties and stabilize the relationship between the school and the Institute.[24]

Culp did not stand down until February of 2011, when faculty member Joseph O'Donnell was appointed Koop's successor as Senior Scholar.[25] O'Donnell summed up the situation like this: "The Dartmouth relationship was difficult. Bill Culp said that it was like being at the dock when the Queen Mary's coming in, and the dock was the Dartmouth administration putting its foot out to stop it." Of Koop, he added: "He was just, he was big, you know, big, big ego, big person, done a lot, famous. And, you know, he was hard to control."[26]

There was plainly a basic difference of focus. Joseph Walsh commented that Koop "wanted a light shone brightly on his projects," whereas "Dartmouth wanted attention on its programs and the involvement that Dr. Koop could bring to the educational and research mission there, and the notoriety that he could bring."[27] As one colleague candidly observed: "Dartmouth was looking for him to bring money to the institution, at least that's what the dean wanted. Koop wasn't interested in that. He wanted to do his thing, and have people leave him alone—not just leave him alone, but love him! He was disappointed that he wasn't as big a figure here as he thought he should have been. The bottom line—nobody could figure out a way to turn the Koop name into something that donors would support."[28]

So what emerged from early turbulence was a space on campus for a welter of creative initiatives that had only occasional connections with the curriculum, and so caused little controversy. Some were focused on Koop's ideas for reform of medical education and the wider healthcare system, but they generally bypassed the medical school.[29] Meanwhile, Koop lectured to groups across the campus, engaging with students in settings formal and informal.

For the first few years, Koop commuted to Hanover by train, for one week a month. One former director of the Institute recalled that "it was very convenient for him. A limousine picked him up and took his gear and he didn't handle anything. And he got on in first class. People recognized him and he worked during the commute. I'm not surprised at all that he didn't move."[30] Joseph Walsh, who served as coordinator at the Institute for some time from 1992 and was involved in development efforts, recalls that "in actuality, he would be in Hanover probably ten days a month, because he'd come in on Friday for the weekend, and then stay the full week, and then depart the following Sunday."[31] In light of early frustrations with the Dartmouth administration, the Koops' decision to remain in Washington was hardly a surprise.

As Koop tells the story, what finally triggered their move was his exasperation with negotiations over the tobacco settlement. "He recalls talking with his wife Betty in their kitchen in Bethesda, Koop railing against the intransigence of the industry and the lawmakers he felt betrayed the cause. 'I stopped to catch my breath, and we said in unison, "Let's get out of here."' The next day they put their house on the market. . . ."[32] Their new home at 3 Ivy Pointe Way was just a few blocks from the medical school, and it was there that they would spend the remainder of their long lives.

By then, things had settled down at the college, and Koop had other projects on the go. He wasn't going to give up on the Koop Institute, but in the scheme of things it mattered less. George wrote that the Institute "serves as a convenient command post for Koop's post-surgeon general agenda. Faxes and phone calls pour in from around the world, all vying for his attention. He has been consulting with the Clinton administration on health-care reform since May and is currently traveling the country touting the president's plan. At an age when most doctors are content to play the back nine, the septuagenarian surgeon is a blur of activity."[33]

As time passed, "the medical school leadership changed, and events changed, and there were promises kept and not kept."[34] Woodie Kessel reflected: "Some of it was related to who the deans were, who the presidents were at Dartmouth . . . some promises were not fulfilled. What he expected never fully operationalized itself. I think fiscal reality overtook the laudable promises that were made. And I think he was somewhat surprised."[35]

Yet from Koop's point of view, while he was frustrated that his agenda for reform of the curriculum soon ran into the sand, Dartmouth provided him with a salary and an office for the rest of his days, together with a base for a range of other endeavors.[36] He soon pivoted to a different approach, which offered him the best of both worlds. Institute director Serra was an attorney, and helped him set up a separate, nonprofit, "sister institution," the Koop Foundation Incorporated.[37]

The foundation gave Koop freedom to raise funds from whatever source he chose, and to develop projects that would not fit the Dartmouth campus context. It also offered a mechanism to evade the overhead institutional "tax" on grant income, which in Dartmouth's case was 40 percent.[38] Since Koop was going after large grants, some with matching corporate funds, the sums involved were substantial.[39]

Colleagues like Serra and McDonald had roles in both. The brands could be commingled, or projects switched between the two. Koop had placed himself in the ideal position to secure funding and develop his initiatives, taking advantage of high-level relationships in Washington, DC that would not easily translate into the culture of an academic institution.

Projects

A succession of projects was developed at the Institute during the more than twenty years of Koop's time at Dartmouth.[40] "Every time he came to town, he wanted to talk about a new project."[41] They bear witness to the astonishing fertility of his imagination, since they were nearly all developed from his own ideas. Joseph Walsh recalls "projects that weren't necessarily all knit together, they weren't related, they were a bit disparate. But they were all great, great projects." They included Partners in Health, which "put medical students into the schools, public schools to teach them an ethic of prevention, that they could then take home to their parents."[42] "HealthSTART" was an extension of the Partners in Health program using the same pedagogical model. As former Koop Fellow Sean P. David, MD, explained, family medicine residents "went into elementary schools in rural New Hampshire towns to teach about health promotion and health hygiene, avoiding smoking, and cultural sensitivity to third and fourth graders."[43]

Another project involved developing cartoons that would later feature in the Koop Institute animation, "Smoky Lies." This was a 20-minute anti-smoking movie made for schoolchildren by producer Monica Wilkins, with Koop and many others involved. Using digital animation technology, technical lead Joshua Nelson worked with family medicine resident Sean David and a team of students to introduce the Fall-Down Brown characters, including "Smoking Joe Moose," to a James Bond inspired anti-tobacco action/adventure feature. Wilkins spent three years at the Institute, from 1997–2000, as an animation director and graphic artist.[44] At the height of the Institute's activities in 1999, the *New York Times* reported that in a "small back room" of the Institute there were "crammed" thirteen computer screens and a fish tank. Students are working on an animated children's James Bond parody film called "Tobacco Never Dies." "Now, at 82, [Koop] directs his army with the animation, fire and bluntness that seem to make him a formidable opponent for Mr. Moose and the tobacco industry and for a list of other forces he believes threaten the nation's health."[45]

Faculty members Christopher Jernstedt and Virginia Reed remember the Institute as an incubator of projects like their Center for Educational Outcomes that were later spun off. Walsh, then working with the Institute, invited them to help evaluate the Partners in Health program that placed medical students in local schools. The center took off from there. Jernstedt recalled: "The core idea from a psychological viewpoint is really sound . . . because when medical students have to describe things to a fourth grader, they learn how to communicate, and I believe that will change how they communicate with their patients."[46]

The center's name later changed to the "Center for Program Design and Evaluation," and it moved to a new home in the Dartmouth Institute. Jernstedt and Reed recall teaching a senior seminar of a dozen students who then presented their research to Koop. They met in the faculty lounge at the top of the Hopkins Center, in "a small room overlooking the campus, his beloved campus. And he sat in front on a stool. And they came up one at a time and presented their senior thesis in this class to him. They couldn't believe they were presenting to the former Surgeon General. And then we would come to our house for dinner. And he's there. It was the kind of thing he loved, and it made an impression on the lives of these people."[47]

A highly innovative program hosted by the Institute for several years was on healing and the arts, under director Naj Wikoff. Wikoff had originally served as program director of Dartmouth's Hopkins Center for the Arts, and as early as 1993 Koop set out to build a collaborative program with him. "A first step," wrote Koop, "is to establish a program of regular musical performances at the Dartmouth Hitchcock Medical Center—which should bring comfort and enrichment to patients, staff and visitors. . . . Let me express my wholehearted support to your proposal to establish three performance/residencies for violinist Jamie Laredo; Richard Stoltzman performing with the Tokyo String Quartet; and the Lark Quartet in the 1994/1995 season."[48] Wikoff later joined the Institute staff.[49]

The Institute also served as Koop's base for an ambitious initiative on biodefense, in which he collaborated with Dartmouth colleague Joseph Rosen, writing in detail to the White House and also calling in aid Anthony Fauci.[50] A string of further Institute initiatives followed, from healthcare videos, web-based health education sites, and the visionary Koop Village—which anticipated the later commercial development of DrKoop.com.[ii]

One faculty member recalls financial difficulties developing at the Institute in the late 1990s and assumed that it had ceased to operate. When invited to be interviewed for this book, she responded that "I didn't realize it was still there."[51] When I asked if she thought Koop had any lasting impact, she answered: "I don't know that he ever had a particular impact on the curriculum, per se, except" the schools elective; adding, "I'm not sure when that program stopped being offered."[52]

The Koop Building

Freedman had followed up the expansive announcements of the spring of 1992 with a plan for a new education building that would bear Koop's name. This was the first of several occasions, over more than two decades, when a Koop building was discussed, or promised, or planned.[53] Woodie Kessel looked back on these troubles. "They made all sorts of promises." But "the red and the black of the accounting office overtook things, and the internal politics of the institution. The president of Dartmouth would turn over, or the dean of the medical school would turn over, and his relationships were with the old people not the new people. Chick had this way of saying, 'They want me to pay for myself.' I think the fiscal realities overtook the laudable promises that had been made."[54] When, less than a year before his death, Dartmouth announced that they were naming the medical school for Theodor "Dr. Seuss" Geisel, Koop "nearly went through the roof"![55]

The building issue would haunt Koop's time at Dartmouth.

In 1994, a memo mentions plans for the C. Everett Koop Conference and Education Building of ninety-seven thousand square feet, costing an estimated $16.4 million.[56] But there were delays, and the idea of a Koop building went off the boil. As one longtime faculty

---

ii See next chapter.

member recalled, "For several years at least we heard the conversations about getting a building, raising the money for the building and naming it the Koop Building at the med school and for a while it looked like it's going to happen. But my memory is that it was about *his* raising the money, not the college. . . . You've got to raise the money for the building, you, your friends, or your family, that's how buildings get built. Certainly my memory is that he was going to raise it and thought that he could [but] that didn't develop."[57] This was plainly not Koop's original understanding with President Freedman. But it was a theme of his conversations with various administrators over the years. "He was very bitter about the failure of Dartmouth to follow through," Walsh recalls.[58] As O'Donnell notes, "to Koop's credit he would say, use me, use me for fundraising or whatever. And they never quite could figure out how to do that."[59]

Yet, fourteen years after the Institute was founded, in November of 2006, it was finally announced, to much razzamatazz, that there would be a C. Everett Koop Medical Science Complex—in the event, more than three times the size of the original plan for an education building. It would house in one wing Dartmouth's Center for Evaluative Clinical Sciences, and in the other, the offices of physicians working in neuroscience and other specialist fields—for a total of nearly three hundred thousand square feet.

For the ground-breaking, President Clinton sent his greetings. Koop's life story was celebrated in a film. In a series of speeches, James Wright (Freedman's successor as Dartmouth's president from 1998) and his colleagues paid homage to Koop, who had just turned ninety years of age. Construction was scheduled to begin late summer of 2007, with the Koop Medical Science Complex to be completed by fall 2009.[60] O'Donnell ruefully reflected, "They had him out with a hard hat with all the big shots, picturing the first shovelful, and so he really thought that meant it's gonna happen."[61] But "he got the rug pulled on that one too."[62]

On September 15, 2008, New York investment bank Lehman Brothers failed.[63] The global economic meltdown had begun.

There is still no Koop Building on the campus of Dartmouth College.

CHAPTER 17

Tomorrow's Medicine

I sit and talk with the parents of my tiny patients. We have sweated out the hours together in recovery, and been on the phone together with community agencies to see what kind of help would be there when the family takes the baby home. I have visited them at home and served with them on committees for neighborhood improvement. My patients and their families know me on the same terms that I knew my family doctor.

—CEK, *Pennsylvania Medicine*, 1975

I don't think the most visionary person sitting before you in that audience has any concept of the tremendous changes that are going to take place in the practice of medicine because of the communication possibilities of the Internet. It is the communication of the future, and it combines our three present forms of communication: television, telephone, and the computer.

—CEK to the American College of Chest Surgeons,
by satellite hook-up, 1999

K oop's vision for the future of healthcare involved a pair of rad- ically contrasting components: The transformative deploy- ment of digital tools, coupled with humanistic reform of the medical school curriculum. As he peers into the future, he is also haunted by the past, and those early memories that thrust him into a medi- cal career and defined his vision for how medicine should be prac- ticed. "Why did we have such respect for our family doctor?" he asks, then offers several reasons. "For one, he cared about us. When we were sick, he came to see what he could do. Not to see 'what could be done'—but to see what he, personally, could do." He would talk with the patient and the family, and "then, after a quick and usually

289

accurate diagnosis, he explained in layman's language just what the trouble seemed to be and what he thought we—that is, he, the patient, and the family—could do. He made us his allies in the fight against disease. We weren't just part of the problem: we were part of the solution."

What's more, back in the 1920s and 1930s, "we didn't expect miracles. We hardly expected cures. Nevertheless, we genuinely loved and respect[ed] our doctors." Today? "We *do* expect miracles, we *do* expect cures, and the public is coming to hate its doctors."[1]

As the *Dartmouth Alumni Magazine* summarized Koop's thinking: "The cornerstone of Koop's vision is the primary-care physician, a general practitioner who is committed to preventive medicine and the doctor-patient relationship, but also able, at the push of a button, to consult with specialists hundreds of miles away using the latest in video and communication technologies."[2] His "vision of health care is both futuristic and nostalgic—an unlikely hybrid of *Marcus Welby* and *Star Trek.*"

The Digital Agenda

Joseph V. Henderson, who directed Dartmouth's Interactive Media Lab and subsequently spun off his company World 2 Systems, spoke fulsomely to me of Koop's grasp of the significance of the emerging digital technologies. "He got technology in the sense that he knew . . . how to use media really, really well. And a humanistic element to media. . . . He got it immediately."[3][i]

In parallel with his push for more humanistic medical training, Koop was constantly pressing for the curriculum to take technology more seriously. On May 14 of 1993, John Duffy sent a memo to Dean Culp headed "New Directions," reporting on "the need for a more aggressive intervention in the curriculum with regard to computer skills." Incoming students need to be "computer literate," and the curriculum designed in such a way as to take advantage of those skills.

---

i   As a Koop Fellow working in the Institute, Henderson had helped develop the Koop Village, discussed later in this chapter.

Three particular ideas: Incoming students should own a computer; there should be a test for incoming students of their computer "competence and literacy;" and a "short, intensive remedial course" for incoming freshmen who need it.[4] In tandem, Koop was pushing hard on the boundaries of advances in technology, and seeking to develop models that would deliver benefits to patients, with a sustained focus on the profoundly disruptive implications of the core emerging technology of the day: the internet.

Through the 1990s, with varying degrees of success, Koop led five strategic initiatives, all intended to exploit "the communication possibilities of the Internet" for tomorrow's medicine.[5]

"Telemedicine will revolutionize care," *USA Today* headlined his argument in August of 1993.[ii] "The shortage of primary-care physicians and coverage in rural areas are key health-reform concerns. A former surgeon general says high-technology can help."[6] The "managed competition" model favored by President Clinton "may work" for the 60 percent of Americans in denser areas, but Koop was skeptical about the 40 percent in rural America. Telemedicine will be the key—"a combination of computers, two-way television and interactive video," with primary care doctors' offices linked to major medical centers. It also offered one of the keys to the cost containment he knew would be crucial to enabling universal access.

Koop's interest in the potential cost savings from telemedicine arose from a more profound focus—on the developing merger between medicine and information technology, known as bioinformatics.

Addressing the 1999 annual meeting of the American College of Chest Physicians—by satellite link—Koop laid out his view of the dawning future. In conversation with the president, Dr. Allen Goldberg, he made the sweeping claim at the head of this chapter. At that time, Goldberg recalls, "34% of U.S. adults were using the Internet, and in 1998 22 million Americans had used it to search for health information."[7]

---

ii   This has a curiously contemporary ring, thirty years on in the 2020s, after Covid forced medicine and every other profession to put to practical use communications technologies that had long been little valued.

1. Health Information and the Clinton Administration

Before the Clintons invited Koop to join their healthcare reform effort he had been lobbying them on the need for a bipartisan commission on bioinformatics. In the event, he was soon involved in the "health informatics component" of the task force, the sole listed presenter at a White House working meeting on May 25, 1993, for a dozen "outside participants" and Clinton staff. His topic: "The Role of Health-oriented Telecommunications Applications in Health Care Reform."[8]

Koop quickly immersed himself in a series of high-level discussions of the implications of digital advances for healthcare. In early October of 1993 he is co-chairing "a very important committee at the National Academy of Sciences" over three days, on the "interface between super communication and the healthcare system" in the Clinton healthcare reform effort.[9]

At the Vice President's suggestion, Koop convened a consortium of twenty private sector CEOs to collaborate with the interagency task force operating inside the administration (by John Silva of ARPA, the Advanced Research Projects Agency).[10] The consortium had its first meeting in mid-April of 1994 in Washington. Koop reported to the First Lady on April 19 that it had not gone well, owing to serious differences of perspective between some of the private sector companies. The plan was to bring Koop's group together with the interagency task force by the end of May.[11] The group was headlined as the C. Everett Koop Foundation National Health Information Infrastructure Consortium.

On July 20, 1995, Koop wrote to the consortium members to follow up the July 11 meeting inviting them each to write to the President, First Lady, and Vice President on the importance of their efforts.[12] Meanwhile, unease was being expressed within the administration about the prominence of this "Koop effort." It cannot be seen as "THE" focus of public/private vision, since "that's what the Vice President wants the Advisory Committee to be on an overlapping set of issues (data standards and privacy)."[13]

2. The Koop Foundation: Bioinformatics Research

In December of 1993 Vice President Gore asked Koop "to help identify and stimulate private sector leadership to make an impact on
building the health component of the National Information Infrastructure (NII)"—by applying for a substantial research grant. Koop
persuaded Michael McDonald, a pioneer in the field who had been
invited to make a presentation to the healthcare reform team on bioinformatics, to lead this effort.

Koop decided to take this project forward through the Koop
Foundation, which soon secured two substantial grants from the
Department of Commerce.[14] The first was for nearly fifteen million
dollars, on a joint effort that would also pull in matching funding
from corporate partners, totaling $30,868,943 (without, of course,
the institutional overhead charge that awards to the Institute would
attract).[15] The "Health Informatics Initiative" was set to run for two
years from January 1, 1995, to "analyze the healthcare industry from
the point of view of modern information management . . . to support
the task of re-engineering the industry to take best advantage of the
developing National Information Infrastructure."[16]

The second project began a few months later and garnered almost
twenty million dollars, again one-half of that from the federal government.[17] McDonald led these projects from the foundation.[18]

3. The Northern New England Health Informatics Initiative

As the Institute moved toward its first anniversary, in spring of 1993,
Koop began to leverage his connections with the Clinton administration and launched an ambitious effort to develop the "Northern
New England Health Informatics Initiative," in the process pulling
together several existing Dartmouth projects and key people.

The local *Valley News* reported in April of that year that there was
growing excitement over the potential local impact of the "information superhighway," and the opportunities for Dartmouth and
its hinterland of "a White House committed to fundamental health
reform." The Institute issued a promotional video "dramatizing such a

scenario," with Koop introducing its "futuristic vision of healthcare." Among the Dartmouth resources to hand: John Wennberg's Center on Evaluation, Joseph Henderson's Interactive Media Lab, Joseph Rosen, "who is involved in several public and privately funded research projects in virtual reality," and the Dartmouth Telecomputing Laboratory at the school of engineering. The video has been "sent off to dozens of key players in the White House, Congress and the Department of Defense, and to corporations that could fit into such a joint effort."[19] As he secured substantial grants for bioinformatics research, tracked through the foundation, Koop positioned this Dartmouth-based network as a case study. To manage the project, he hired telemedicine expert Michael Caputo, regarded as one of the pioneers in the field.[20]

"Through meetings, focus groups, conferences, and pilot projects, NNEHII served a leading role in the advancement of informatics and telemedicine in the New England medical community," though in the event it went well beyond the original northern New England area.[21] The kick-off event brought together academics from several other New England universities, together with health information groups. Following a pattern familiar from his Surgeon General workshops, Koop kicked off with a "charge," and then moderated the closing discussion of reports from breakout groups—on communication, education, and manpower.[22] The project director, in turn, was tasked with "synthesizing" information from this event and turning it into a feasibility study and then an action plan.[23] A further conference, on December 11, 1995, focused on issues of privacy and electronic data handling; Koop again gave the keynote.[24]

4. The Koop Village

When Koop was first approached about the project that would become DrKoop.com, he was already developing a prototype internet-based source of medical information and communication. It was called the Koop Village and comprised an imaginative set of health resources.[25] "The Koop Village, which is currently under development, will be a World Wide Web based conference and discussion center. A rich graphical environment depicting a turn of the century New England village, the Village will contain a variety of buildings, each dedicated to a different subject in human health. Together, these buildings will house a multitude of topic-based meeting rooms."

Elsewhere, the site stated: "A few locations within the Village will provide active textual information for the user presented in an exploratory, hyperlinked format, including a personal library and biography for Dr. Koop, and a monument of Hippocrates on the town green with information about the Hippocratic oath. In addition, clickable animations may be added to the graphic environment to enhance the exploratory feel of the Village." And: "The communication tools within the Koop Village will be quite sophisticated and easy to use, representing a blending of existing technologies. They will also allow for the visual communication of emotional (facial) expression as well as text, which is intended to add depth and feeling to text-based communication."[26] This last reference reminds us of some of the limitations of the 1998 internet.

While the text quoted looks to the future, some features of the Village were already accessible. Sean David, now on faculty at the University of Chicago medical school, was an early part of the team developing the Village. "There were demonstration projects that used the Koop Village . . . I guess this was back in 1996. So it was a little ahead of its time, in a way, the chat room. And it was a chat room that with some planning you could build meetings around. And so we thought since tobacco control is a global issue and very fragmented, this could be a way to bring people together in a new model of activism." David went to the University of Cambridge, as a visiting family medicine resident, and set up a "Trans-Atlantic Conference on Tobacco Control" between tobacco experts at Dartmouth and the Institute of Public Health at Cambridge. "We did a Trans-atlantic test session; we set it up, we invited people to come to it and did a proof of concept. There were other projects that used the Koop Village as well, I'm not sure how many people took full advantage of it. And eventually, ten years later, there was social media."[27]

Also emerging from the Koop Village initiative, Koop and McDonald established in 1995 the Health Initiatives Foundation, now flourishing under McDonald's leadership as Resilient American Communities with over 800 member communities across the United States.

"RAC provides frameworks upon which a community builds resilience from within and in ways that equitably sustain and enrich all people," and has been specially active on the Covid front.[28]

Meanwhile, the Koop Institute was generating a succession of stand-alone projects offering web-based healthcare information. In the summer of 1996, a visiting professor from Penn State, Gregory Caputo, spent six weeks as a Visiting Fellow at the Institute developing *The Diabetic Foot Clinic*, consisting of accessible diagnostic algorithms for the use of physicians and other healthcare professionals. "The project's efforts were focused on the development of a World Wide Web-based resource for the prevention of lower extremity complications—such as amputation—in patients with diabetes."[29]

A freestanding site was developed to focus on the threat of *Hepatitis C*. Koop was deeply concerned about its spread, which he regarded as a graver threat than AIDS. Epidemic.org was devoted to alerting the public to key details.[30] "Hepatitis C already infects three times more people than does AIDS," he warned in a video on the site. "And by the turn of the century, it will kill far more people than AIDS each year. By working together, we can help to reverse the spread of this terrible disease."[31]

A further project integrated initiatives on the Dartmouth campus with nationwide resources on *Computer-Based Instruction* in medical education. "Multimedia computer-based instruction (CBI) is a vehicle to reform medical education: to make it less passive, more interactive, more realistic, and more relevant to 21st century medicine. The Koop Institute was instrumental in first developing medical CBI programs and is now involved in establishing CBI on the internet to promote wider access to this important source of medical education."[32]

5. DrKoop.com

"I've had two major messages that I've tried to get out to the public all my professional life. . . . One is to take charge of your own health. The other is that there is no prescription I can give you that is more valuable than knowledge. . . . I've tried the non-profit world, and the non-profit world is not interested in supporting those messages on the Internet or in any other way."[33]

While the young staff of the Institute were busy writing code for the embryonic Koop Village, Koop himself was talking with entrepreneurs about a potentially game-changing web-based development that would turn their Koop Village thinking into a great Koop Metropolis.

Koop had first encountered actor and entrepreneur John F. Zaccaro in 1991, when Zaccaro persuaded him to join other well-known figures, including violinist Itzhak Perlman and *Good Morning America's* Nancy Snyderman, on the advisory board of the International Health and Medical Film Festival, home of the Freddie awards. In 1994, Koop was invited to be the celebrity speaker.[34] It was Zaccaro who introduced him to Donald Hackett, described by *Fortune* as a "20-year veteran of the health information industry." Together, at Hackett's urging, the three of them brainstormed "Dr. Koop's Personal Medical Record System," a modest effort to enable patients to manage their own medical histories and costs on their home computers.[35] So, on July 17, 1997, the company was founded as plain "Personal Medical Records Inc." (PMRi).[36] On October 1 of that year Koop was in post as Chairman of PMRi, with a three-year contract, at a fee rising to $150,000 in the third year.[37] Meanwhile, trademark filings were being made for "Dr. Koop's Community"—and "drkoop.com."[38]

This original, modest, business model rapidly evolved into a web-based strategy, in which medical record-keeping would be online, and just one of a wide range of offerings. "Personal Medical Records Inc." became "Empower Health Corporation." The site launched in July 1998. Six months later, we find Nancy Snyderman hosting a Q and A on spastic colon, there are twenty-two facts to discourage holiday drunk driving, and one of the "interactive communities" is discussing healthy aging.[39]

Once the site was up and running, the company moved to raise capital by selling stock in an IPO[iii]—with what some observers regarded as unseemly haste. Bear Stearns, the merchant bank, was happy to take the company into the public market, and the IPO was, initially, a success. On Tuesday, June 8, 1999, they sold 9.4 million shares

---

iii   IPO: Initial Public Offering, the first sale of stock in a new company, which can provide capital for rapid expansion.

at $9 each, raising $84.4 million for the company.[40] The stock briefly hit an all-time high of $47.75, rendering Koop's slice of the pie a theoretical $119 million. Meanwhile, one friend told Koop that he had wrung his hands when he heard there was an IPO on the horizon, because "People don't want Dr. Koop to be a multimillionaire. They want him to save babies, blow the whistle on AIDS, and take on the tobacco industry."[41] Another friend, former chief of staff Edward Martin, had pointedly declined Koop's invitation to join the board of directors.[42]

In the *Wall Street Journal*'s memorable turn of phrase, the company's core strategy was "to tap the credibility of the feisty Dr. Koop." The plan was to deploy this singular name to "establish an identifiable brand in an increasingly crowded field of health and wellness concerns."[43] The *Washington Post* made a similar point. "New Internet stocks have a reputation for pulling off stunts like that, though in fact recent ones ran into a bit of trouble as investors have grown wary. But Drkoop. com restored the magic. It has something that none of the others do: Koop."[44] As CEO Donald Hackett put it to me, "Dr. Koop's insights, ethics, and principles set a standard everyone at the company aspired to live by."[45] Empower Health's modest ambition to host personal health records on home computers had morphed into a towering offering that briefly made DrKoop.com the world's top health site.[46]

So, as web magazine *Zdnet* asked, "How could a venture headed by the most recognized physician since Marcus Welby MD fall so far so fast?"[47]

In a telling observation, the *Washington Post* noted that the day after the IPO, far from hunkering down in the company's Atlanta offices planning next moves, Koop spent the day in meetings working on the Health Museum, before heading out to dinner with the board of *Shape Up America!* He told the *Post* apologetically that he hoped "to become more involved with the site 'if I can ever get the rest of my life straightened out.'" So it is no surprise that staff in Atlanta saw little of him. "It was a crazy time," one recalled to me. "Koop would fly into town very infrequently with his entourage of security. It was amazing. . . . Honestly, the exposure to Koop was incredibly small."[48] Said another: "His name was on our product," adding candidly that "the people he entrusted his name to had varying levels of skill and ethics."[49]

There followed a series of questionable business decisions that quickly spent a large slice of the capital they had just raised. In just the three following months (July, August, and September), Hackett, Zaccaro, and company signed checks for $24 million, against income of a mere $2.9. What's more, less than a month after pulling in the $84 million, the company decided to commit a further $89 million, more than their entire take from the IPO, to AOL—America Online— Steve Case's internet "walled garden" that for many users in the '90s *was* the internet and therefore a critical marketplace. DrKoop.com would shell out the funds over four years, without even securing the right to be AOL's exclusive health provider. AOL had a tough reputation. Their lead negotiator had been known to swing a baseball bat at meetings to underline the point.[50] Meanwhile, the NASDAQ was beginning to recover from its "irrational exuberance" over internet stocks and start to head south.[51]

Fortune quotes analyst Stephen DeNelsky of Credit Suisse, who summed up their deadly situation neatly: "These deals boxed them into a corner very early on." They would be forced to go back to the markets to raise further tranches of capital, which plainly could not happen if their stock price was flagging. In April of 2000, just ten months after pocketing their $84 million, the company announced they had only enough cash to stay in business for four months more; they were looking for rescue from a buyer. Months before, buy recommendations had been flowing—the bearish Bear Stearns had issued a fifty-seven-page report with the title "The Doctor is In." Now they were thrown into reverse.[52] PriceWaterhouseCoopers, the company's auditors, decided the time had come to raise a red flag over whether DrKoop.com could survive.[53]

Meanwhile, their core value proposition—"you trust Dr. Koop, so you can trust DrKoop.com"—had been coming under threat. The magic of the Koop name that lay at the core of the company's offering was being turned upside down by a series of blunders.

For one thing, several breaches were being reported of the "short-swing profit rule," a basic prohibition on the sale of stock by insiders for six months after they buy it.[54] Director Richard Helppie sold his three days after the IPO. A month later, the husband of another director, ABC medical correspondent Nancy Snyderman, sold some of his.[55] Koop himself, and CFO Sue Georgen-Saad, had failed to file details of small purchases by members of their families. *Fortune* reports analyst Josh Fisher of W.R. Hambrecht rolling his eyeballs: "These were just some of many small things that undermined my confidence in management. . . . It seemed strange at a public company with a major investment bank behind it."[56]

Controversy grew when two particularly embarrassing facts came out during that momentous summer of 1999.

"Until recent days," wrote Holcombe B. Noble in the *New York Times* for September 5, "the Web site did not give notice of an arrangement that entitled the company and Dr. Koop himself to a commission on products and services sold because of the Web site. Dr. Koop gave up those commissions on Aug. 27."[57]

The second embarrassment was potentially more serious, over the blurred line between ads and information on the site. Noble quoted an ethicist who had been exploring a "DrKoop.com Community Partners Program" that "contained a list of hospitals and health centers described as 'the most innovative and advanced healthcare institutions across the country.' In fact, the list was an advertisement for 14 hospitals, each of which had paid a fee of about $40,000 to be included."[58]

Koop was stung by these criticisms, and responded swiftly, though reputational damage had already been done.

He realized that the advertising issue was a fundamental one for the industry, and could be addressed on a wider front, since it affected much of the revenue-focused activity on every health site. Ethics guru Arthur Caplan put the situation in the fall of 1999 in context: "The current tempest over the DrKoop.com website is revealing not so much about Dr. Koop's own ethics but about the lack of ethical consensus concerning medicine on the internet. It is very important that those who use the internet know when conflicts of interest exist, what financial ties are present, and who is vetting the accuracy of the information." He concluded: "Most of the websites now operating will, and should, address the issue of how to keep editorial credibility in an age of big money and high stakes."[59]

So Koop convened the top twenty health sites in a project called "HI-Ethics"—for "Health Internet Ethics"—that on May 8, 2000, released a set of principles addressing the thorny issues concerned.[60] But by then the stock of DrKoop.com was way down.

These were both adroit moves on his part. Meanwhile, he had been doing some rethinking. In late 2000, while the company was still afloat after refinancing, Koop was asked whether he had regrets. He replied candidly, "Seeing the way it's come out and what it has cost me emotionally and intellectually, I wish I had done it differently." Differently how? "I would not use my name. I think my mistake was to use my name."[61] He plainly did not understand that the company's entire value proposition, which distinguished it from every other in the crowded healthcare space, lay precisely there.

An effort to put in new management and new money failed to shore up the site.[62] When runway runs out, the end is swift. "Shortly before the bankruptcy filing, DrKoop stock was worth less than a penny a share." You get bargains at a fire sale, and Florida e-commerce company Vitacost, hawking discount vitamins, snapped up the website URL and its brand for $186,000—together with nearly one million registered email addresses that came with it.[63] That was the ultimate indignity for Koop. A zombie DrKoop.com website would long outlive Dr. Koop himself,[iv] and he could do nothing about it.[64] As required by law, at the foot of every page it states: "This website is not associated with C. Everett Koop, M.D., former Surgeon General of the United States." The problem, of course, is that, after all these years, it *is* associated with him, a living monument to the failure of his venture.[65] DrKoop.com went down with accumulated losses of $207 million.[66]

Some contemporary assessments were unforgiving. *Fortune* fumed about "Dr. Koop and the Greed Disease," accusing the company of "mediocre leadership, a huge burn rate, and a flimsy business plan."[67] The online magazine *Tedium* offered a gentler assessment. "DrKoop.

---

iv   DrKoop.com remains live as of this writing, selling vitamins and oils, and also, in at least an echo of the real doctor, weight-loss cures and quit-smoking programs!

com . . . could have really worked out well, and everyone working with that company knew it."[68]

Koop later reflected ruefully to his Wheaton friends Alan and Rhea Johnson, "I guess the Lord never wanted me to have a lot of money."[69]

A Vision for Medicine

In a remarkable address at the New York College of Medicine's commencement exercises for 1985, Koop set out his philosophy of the physician.[70] Koop was a physician first, and for him, paradoxically, that was the key to understanding his success in the surgeon's role.

After the usual pleasantries, reflecting on changes in medicine since he graduated from Cornell in 1941, when "scientists were [merely, even then] predicting that 'antibiotics' would revolutionize the treatment of infectious disease," he set out "Koop's Five Principles of Practice"—"the best graduation gift I can give you." They shape a humane understanding of the physician's role, that same vision that impelled his effort for curricular reform at Dartmouth nearly a decade later.

"My first principle for the practicing physician is to make the families of your patient your allies. . . . Tell them as much as you can. This is what 'informed consent' is all about—the bond of trust and understanding between physician and patient vital for the success of any treatment regimen." He notes that "This principle forced me to communicate with ordinary people who were under great stress. It forced me to know what I was doing so completely and in such detail that I could rephrase what I was doing in simple language, passing on the information to people who did not have my medical or scientific background. They were people, though, who had the right and the need to know what was happening to their child. When they still did not understand, I knew it to be my fault, not theirs."

It's to this that he attributed a remarkable fact. In forty years as a surgeon, he had never once been sued by a patient or family.[71] And why? "They were my patients, but they were also my friends and my allies. Friends and allies do not sue each other. They should have no reason to be that angry."

Second, "be ready for surprises." Koop took great joy in his work, and the people with whom it brought him into contact. Be ready for "the excitement [that] comes in the interactions you have with your patients or with their friends and families or the warmth you feel when you share ideas, problems, sorrows and achievements with your colleagues . . . other doctors, nurses, technicians or administrative personnel."

He had found great joy in the operating room, yet "over the years I was surprised many times by the joy I felt when I was able to address the anxiety of a youngster or the child's parents and turn their fears into courage or their despair into hope. I felt joy when I got to know someone well who was a special kind of person—one of my patients, a mother or a father, a guardian, a clergyman. . . ."

Then he turned to money, "but not the money you are going to make. I don't care about that.[72] Instead, you will find that money is far more important to your patients than it will ever be or should ever be to you." Patients are deeply concerned about the cost of medical care. "Talk to your patients and their families about the costs of the care they are about to receive. Work out with them if possible what might be covered by insurance and what might have to come out of their own pockets."

His fourth principle is "a corollary of the first." Focus on your colleagues, all of them. "Whether you are receiving or delivering a consultation in the form of a lab report or an opinion or whatever, give it time and attention."

And finally, ethics. "Remember that you are the embodiment of medical ethics and standards of practice. . . . There is no room for a middle ground in the life-and-death work in which we are engaged."

Koop closed with a celebrated quote from Ralph Waldo Emerson. "There is properly no history, only biography." Because "the real story of this world is the aggregate life stories of every man and every woman who has ever lived. . . . Your biographies will be medicine's history."[73]

Part VI
PERSPECTIVE

To strive, to seek, to find, and not to yield.
                    —TENNYSON, *Ulysses*

Betty Koop passed on February 18, 2007, almost exactly seventy-one years after a brash young man of nineteen, right here in Hanover, New Hampshire, had sent a Valentine to his roommate's seventeen-year-old girlfriend.[1]

Their long love story was finally ruptured. Betty's lengthy, bedridden decline, touch-and-go for years, was over at last. Shortly before her death, Koop had asked pastor friend, Kenneth Larter, for his aid, "in this very long dying process."[2] Larter told me, "I think she suffered from a lot of sadness, and depression."[3] She had long been sick, including a series of bouts with pneumonia. Toward the end she needed attention round the clock. Koop would sometimes go into her room during the night so he could sit with her and hold her hand, telling her carer to lie beside her on the bed and get some sleep.[4]

Two years earlier, Koop had written to an old friend that "she is now very debilitated, weighs 82 pounds," and is "a much better sport than I would be under the same circumstances." Yet, "she would rather move on."[5] In an undated memo to himself at around the same time, after noting her three concurrent chronic diseases, he noted that "physicians have suggested that she starve herself to death. . . . If I had an incurable disease . . ." he wonders, but leaves the thought incomplete. "Having lived with my pro-life position for so many years—that goes against the grain."[6] As Betty weakened and he prepared for her passing, he felt alone in ways that surprised him. Their children, "seven grandchildren and now four great-grandchildren . . . seem more remote than I thought relatives would be."[7]

As daughter-in-law Anne later told me, Koop "didn't do well with people who are sick, like, grownups. He's so used to them being there. Mom was the backbone to Dad."[8] Betty's long illness troubled him for another reason also. As trainee Howard Filston put it, "I'm also an evangelical Christian. . . . But I don't believe quite the way he did. I think he really believed that everything that happened, God . . . orchestrated. And I think when Betty was sick for so many years that shook his faith considerably."[9]

Soon after Betty's passing, Koop invited a handful of friends, including the Larters, to join him aboard the Queen Mary II on a transatlantic cruise. Larter shared caring duties with aide Sheryl Bailey.[10] Koop was an inveterate fan of the sea, in large boats and small. Over many years, a cruise to London would be an annual treat for him and Betty. "He loved friendship, and he loved companionship. His health was failing, but in his mind he was still incredibly clear."[11] And he loved the shipboard attention, as Larter pushed his wheelchair around the deck and fellow passengers recognized him. "He was on stage!"[12]

By then, Koop was ninety, his own health continuing to slip. "Until I was 86," he had shared with a friend, "I could keep up with much younger folks, in the following year I aged 10 and now I find I have very little ambition . . . very little stamina."[13] Even then, he found it impossible to let go; he plainly had ups as well as downs. In August of 2008 we see him agreeing to lecture at Harvard, sharing with his friend Howard Koh that the current year is his busiest ever! "Who do you know who was offered two jobs, each carrying six figures, in his 91st year?"[14] Three months later, he wrote to Hillary Clinton, designated Obama's secretary of state, to offer his services. "Don't be misled by my age, I still have all my marbles."[15]

Yet his long, driven life, one headlong burst of energy and vision that had brought not merely success but celebrity, was finally fading. Once, it had been said, to walk with him through the streets of Philadelphia was like walking through Memphis with Elvis.[16] The limelight, in which he had lived for much of a hundred years, was dimming.

CHAPTER 18
The Long Diminuendo

We talked about when Koop couldn't be Koop. What was going to
happen? But that's what he wanted to be, Koop.
—JOSEPH O'DONNELL, Dartmouth professor and friend, interview

L ester Gibbs had first met Koop when he and Betty moved to
Hanover back in 1997. On Sundays, the Koops worshipped at
son Norman's nearby church in Woodstock, Vermont; Gibbs, a former military musician, was the organist. "I was invited to the Koops'
house for Thanksgiving," he recalled, "and that became a tradition
every Thanksgiving and every Christmas Eve." Years later, after Betty's passing, Koop "came up to the organ after service. And he said,
'You know, I've had some of your food that you've cooked for Christmas, and you're a pretty good cook. I need more.' And I said, 'Okay,
I'd be glad to come and cook some.' 'Well, no, this is going to be a
deliberate thing. You're actually going to live right in the house. I
really need help at night. I've got a daytime person. But I need somebody to cook supper and breakfast. So why don't you just move in
upstairs?' I said 'Okay,' so I did. And we just clicked and he started
talking about recipes like chicken and dumplings. Chick liked his
food."[1]

On September 12, 2008, in his role as chauffeur, Gibbs had driven
Koop down to Philadelphia for a special event at Tenth Presbyterian
Church.[2] A new organ was being dedicated, a four-manual Aeolian-
Skinner, a gift "to remember the debt I owe Tenth Church for what it
has contributed to me and my family over the years, and at the same
time, to commemorate the life of my recently deceased wife and the

life of our own third son, David, who went to his heavenly home in 1968."[31][i]

After the ceremony was over, they first stopped for dinner at a favorite restaurant where, Gibbs recalled, "everyone knew him." Then they set off for the long drive north, and at around 2:00 a.m. Gibbs thought Koop was talking in his sleep, "because he had a habit of doing that. And he said, 'I'm going to get married.' And I'm thinking yeah, really? I'm not sure what dream he's got going right now but this one is really out there. He reaches over and he touches my shoulder. 'Are you listening to me?'" Gibbs asked for more details. Koop said, "she was the pretty one" they had met at the church. "How is this going to happen?", Gibbs asked. "I'm going to call her up tomorrow and tell her." Gibbs responded, "I don't think that's how things work these days."

Cora

Cora Hogue had long served as a missionary in Italy, later joining the pastoral staff of Tenth Church where she had responsibility for small groups, teaching, and counseling. She had never been married. And she did not know Koop, having arrived at Tenth when he was already in Washington.

In fact, it would be the best part of a year before Koop made the call. But he had seen her that one time, and—for him—that had been enough. When they put his call through to her office, she was wondering what on earth he might want of her. He first said he needed to confirm that she was the right one, that she had been the woman in the "shimmering green dress."[4] Then, he had two requests. Would she have dinner with him when he was next in town? And, would she give him her private phone number? Somewhat to her surprise she said yes to both requests. She told me she was especially surprised

---

i   Koop cannot have forgotten the part he had played in acquiring an earlier organ for the church, as far back October 26, 1952! There had been controversy in the congregation about the purchase, and Donald Grey Barnhouse had arranged for a debate, with Koop recruited to speak in favor. See Chapter 2.

by the latter, since she was involved in counseling disturbed people and kept her private details very private. And then Koop began to call, sometimes every day, for weeks. He was persistent, but also very funny; she remembers laughing much of the time. One night he called and told her that he was falling in love with her. The next night she told him, "I think I can say I love you." Meanwhile, an unexpected practical issue had arisen. Thanks to the vagaries of early 2000s cellphone billing, Cora felt she had to tell Koop that she couldn't afford these long calls anymore.[5]

Come the new year, Gibbs was tasked with a secret mission, to drive Koop and Cora to New York City for the weekend. The household staff and Koop's assistant at the Koop Institute, Susan Wills, were inquisitive, but they were told nothing. Gibbs spent much of the weekend with Koop and Cora, including their meals together. They stayed in separate suites at the Waldorf Astoria, and toured Koop's old haunts from Coney Island (a Nathan's hotdog was compulsory) to his childhood home in Brooklyn, where Gibbs was instructed to mount the steps and knock on the door. The householder was astonished to see the famous man waving from down on the sidewalk. "After dinner on the last night," reported the West Lebanon *Valley News*, he asked Cora to marry him "almost casually." ("Almost like a business proposition," was how she put it to me!) "She answered in the same light-hearted tone."[6]

Michael DellaVecchia was a friend from Philadelphia days. He recalled a particularly dull meeting at the College of Physicians, where by chance he had been seated beside the very recognizable Koop. Koop had turned to him and whispered, "this is BS, let's go out and talk." Decades of friendship later, he was a regular visitor to the Koop household.[7]

Then, one February morning in 2010, "I'm driving in to do surgery in awful weather. My cell phone goes off. And I'm saying, what's this about? I'm on time for surgery and everything. I looked down and it's Koop. And you know, it's about six in the morning. And he starts with some small talk. And finally, he goes, 'What are you doing on April 17?' I said, 'I don't think anything.' And he says, 'Can you do me a favor?' I said, 'Yeah, absolutely.' He said, 'Will you be best man in my wedding?'" DellaVecchia quipped in response, "Got a house in a good school district, Chick?"[8]

There was context to the marriage surprise. In a note to trainee Michael Gauderer just three weeks after Betty's death, Koop had written of his loneliness, and that it would get worse; and he ended with the enigmatic remark that it's "very hard to imagine a new arrangement."[9] In other words, he had been trying to imagine it. And he will not have forgotten that three of his longtime friends, Jonathan Rhoads, Peter Paul Rickham, and Robert Zachary, all widowed (Zachary twice) in their 70s and 80s, had gone on to remarry.[10] One friend who knew the Koops for decades shared with me that, perhaps ironically, his closeness to Betty helped explain his decision. "She was fantastic. . . . She was an unbelievably good adviser, and he missed her terribly. And he was a very lonely person, because he didn't have a great relationship with his kids. So he was looking for somebody to fill that loneliness. And Cora filled the bill."[11]

When Koop sprang the news that he was getting married on April 17, sons Allen and Norman both had other plans. Norman and Anne had booked a vacation a year beforehand, timed to fit in with their jobs (he was a pastor, she a school principal). Norman's widow Anne is a shrewd observer of the dynamics of the family. "Dad being the impulsive kind of person that he was," he had just picked a date— "instead of asking the boys, Are you going to be around?" Norman responded, "Dad, you know, you need to let people know. . . . But we can't just go and jump because you've decided to go and get married." Of course, that was not all of it. "In the beginning we thought, what ninety-three-year-old man really needs to get remarried? I guess he was of the generation where you always thought you had to have a woman on your arm."[12] But he had made up his mind and expected the family to fall in with his plans. As Gibbs put it to me: "He liked to be in charge. It was the thing he knew best, in public life, in private life. He was the boss." He kept his emotions "very private." Indeed, "I don't think anyone in the church even knew about it until they actually announced their wedding." His sons were upset that he had not confided in them, he added; not least Norman, who was also his pastor.[13] Neither of them would be at the wedding.

Koop was so upset that he actually considered disinheriting his sons, though his lawyer and a friend succeeded in dissuading him.[14] Best man Michael DellaVecchia told me, "Chick was very hurt. I think they felt that at his age he should not be getting married. . . . The ministers who presided at the ceremony felt that Chick is a cognizant, feeling person who definitely wanted to marry Cora. So let's make it a good day."[15]

A packed crowd turned out for the ceremony at Tenth Presbyterian Church in Philadelphia on April 17, 2010, where Larter's wife Evelyn, an old friend of Cora's, served as matron of honor.[16] Daughter Betsy and her husband flew up from Texas, and were particularly warm in their welcome of Cora into the family.[ii]

Linda Boice recalled, "Our ministers were like big brothers to Cora. They were so supportive. It was lovely. It wasn't O, Dr. Koop's getting married again, attend! It was with rejoicing. Cora is wonderful. And it's so wonderful she's marrying Dr. Koop, with such support from the people who knew Cora."[17]

3 Ivy Pointe Way

Needless to say, Cora's arrival had a dramatic impact on the life of the Ivy Pointe household. Gibbs continued to serve as cook. Since Cora was a vegan, and Koop had no plans to become one, he found himself preparing two sets of meals. There were several staff around the house—Gibbs combined cooking with night duties, driving, and bill-paying; there was another carer with daytime responsibilities; others had cleaning and secretarial roles; and more than once a Dartmouth student lived in to help out. Later, of course, skilled nursing services were needed.

Best man DellaVecchia was a frequent visitor. On one occasion, a friend had made some "very delicious chicken matzah ball soup,"

---

ii The sons would also be absent from the National Memorial Service that followed his death. Betsy was there, and her husband spoke on behalf of the family.

and he took it along. "Well, we all sat down at the table, and this thing was just eating its way up your nostrils. Chick was totally salivating over it, had like three bowls. And [vegan] Cora said, 'Well, let me try.'"

"Chick was used to having people answer to him and Cora didn't fit that mold," observed DellaVecchia. "So they had their differences. But that's not to say that she didn't love them. And she did. She took care of him very well to the end. You know, we jumped in and we changed diapers together."[18] Cora had lived an independent life as a missionary and then as part of the ministry team at Tenth Church. She had her own opinions, and a strong personality. As her friend Linda Boice pointed out to me, Koop found that hard; sometimes sparks would fly. But, "My impression is that she was really good for him. That she kept him going. They did social things. She believes in prayer up to her eyeballs. I suspect that he grew spiritually having her as a wife. O yes, there were tensions. She was committed to supporting him, but she was not a doormat."

Around eighteen months after the wedding, Koop was chatting with an old friend in Philadelphia. "Suddenly, he said, 'Marrying Cora was the best decision I made in the second half of my life.'"[19]

Woodie Kessel recalled one of Koop's last visits to Washington, with Gibbs as chauffeur. Koop and Cora were staying at the Willard Hotel and had dinner with Kessel and his wife. "And he says to me, 'Hillary, tell her I want to see her tomorrow.'[iii] And I said, 'Chick, you know, I'm obviously going to call but you think, you know, first of all, we're not sure if she's in town.' And he looked at me like, 'Well, are you calling?' I said, 'Okay. You know, I'll call.'"

And Kessel called, and talked his way through to someone who took a message. "Eventually, her special assistant calls me back. And we get a driver, we go over there, and it becomes a to-do, because he's got the wheelchair. . . . But then Chick, and I, and Cora and Hillary are in the little room off the secretary's office. And it's funny. Chick is telling jokes, and Hillary's telling jokes. And Cora was bemused. It

---

iii   Hillary Clinton was secretary of state in the Obama administration from 2009–2013.

was really quite amazing to see a side of him, and a side of her, grand friends, despite their political differences. . . . The belly-laughing between the four of us was just amazing."[20]

The Koops were again in Washington for his ninety-fifth birthday in 2011, when friends hosted a party in a museum, against the curious background of an exhibit on infectious diseases. Guests included Fauci, Surgeon General Regina Benjamin, and Koop's friend and former colleague Jack Henningfield. Koop and Betty had been keen swing dancers, so at Cora's suggestion Henningfield, and his wife Lucy, performed a dance in his honor.[21]

One of his final trips was in February 2012, just a year before his passing, when he and Cora were driven the six hours down to Philadelphia to watch the reading of a new play—and take part in an after-action discussion. Back in 1977, *Philadelphia Inquirer* writer Donald Drake had covered the agonizing case of Koop's separation of the twins who could not both survive because they shared a heart, and whose rabbi grandfathers had insisted on debating the ethics of their case.[22] Now Drake had written a play based on the case. After watching from the front row, "Koop had no reluctance addressing the audience. . . . The reading brought back to mind his own 'religious' moment during the surgery. . . . When I tied off one carotid artery and killed a child," Koop said, "I'd given no thought about what would happen to the body . . . I had one dead baby and one live baby; I separated them. One of the nurses took the child who was now dead and carried it to the door of the operating room. The door opened and there stood the rabbi."

"He continued: 'The fact that he was there seemed almost like God's blessing on what I had just done.'"[23]

Meanwhile, the Koop household continued to be hospitable. One night, Gibbs was accompanying Koop to a concert at the College, when a student asked, "Is that Dr. Koop?"[24] During the intermission, Gibbs introduced them, and Koop invited him over. "It turns out that his mother was a gynecologist, and his father was a heart specialist, and they will be visiting for homecoming." Koop had them all round for dinner.

Koop was given to acts of great personal generosity. Joshua Drake was a student who lived in as aide for a year. Koop offered to put him through seminary. Drake told me that he was hardly alone— Koop funded "many Dartmouth students he met, especially those going to medical school or seminary."[25] Gibbs adds, "he [also] put a lot of kids through college." These efforts were kept private; "very few ever knew this." One Sunday in church Koop overheard a couple in conversation with their daughter. "They happened to be sitting behind Dr. Koop, and she was talking with her folks about wanting to be a nurse. And her father said, 'Well, we just don't have the financial means to do it.' Koop turned around and said, 'Don't worry, I'll take care of it, what's the school?' A couple of days later he called the school and said he would pay her tuition." And that was that. "In fact," Gibbs told me, "she and her husband attend the church where I'm playing the organ."[26]

Despite his growing frailty, Koop remained keen to undertake what public engagements came his way. They energized him. Best man DellaVecchia put it to me bluntly: "It's pretty clear that you or I would not have done it," before commenting on the problems of Koop's incontinence and growing forgetfulness.[27]

Gibbs was once asked by a boy at church if he would come to his Civil Air Patrol (CAP) promotion ceremony and put on one of his bars. He checked with Koop to see if he could be free that evening. Koop had met the boy, as Harry and his brother had done yard work for him. "We'll both go!" he replied. "And we'll dress up like Christmas trees." Gibbs told Harry to inform his commander that Koop would be joining them, "because this guy was a vice admiral, three stars!" In response, the CAP felt obliged to turn out their highest-ranking officer in the state to welcome him. Koop was invited to speak to the forty or so kids present, and their parents. "He marched up to the podium and spoke for about twenty minutes. He had eye contact with every single one of those kids, encouraging them to become leaders, to get educated to know what was going on in the world, to go on to further education—and let the military pay for it!

And when he got done, all these kids just got up and they were wolf whistling and clapping and cheering."[28]

Larter, pastor and former nurse, was sometimes called on to help out during his visits. "There were still occasions when he would be asked to give a short speech. And so here, you know, we would be struggling to get him in the car! But then when he was called to go up, out of the wheelchair, with his cane, all dressed up in his bow tie and everything, he would walk to the podium and deliver these short talks with absolute clarity and precision." Larter recalled a "gaggle of young women" medical students surrounding him after a speech, "looking up, adoring," as they peppered him with questions, "and he responded with sometimes intimate details about medical issues that were probably not completely appropriate for that setting." Larter turned to Susan Wills, Koop's assistant from the college: "if you could see what he was like, before we got him into the car, this is a different person entirely." She smiled. "You and I know what's going on behind the scenes. But when he's on point, and there's an audience . . . ." She photographed the scene, and Larter's wife Evelyn sent Koop the picture on a fridge magnet.[29]

Henningfield recalled that, in the spring of 2012, "Cora called, and said Chick really is poorly. I'm not sure how long he's gonna be around. So I said, I'll be there this weekend. And so I bought two orchids, one for me to start a Koop orchid collection and one for him. And they let me take it on the plane. And when I got there, he wasn't looking really very well. And he said, Well, what would you like to talk about? I put an orchid on the table, and said I'm going to start an orchid collection. So tell me how to take care of them."[30]

Meanwhile, despite tensions over the wedding, granddaughter Tina Bazala remembers that "towards the end of my grandfather's life my dad [Norman] was just there every day; their relationship was always one of the closer ones of the kids. But at the end, they were very close, and it was good for my father to have that, that newfound intimacy with him."[31]

A Man of Great Friendship

At the National Memorial Service that followed Koop's death, Carroll Wynne, on staff at Tenth Presbyterian Church, summed him up as "a man of great friendship."[32] Over many years, Koop had cultivated many, many friends. Some were close, and their friendship became yet more significant for him as his celebrity, and his health, slowly ebbed.

Josh Drake, the student who lived in for a year, made breakfast and accompanied Koop on trips, recalled "getting stories of all the political cartoons that he had saved. . . . I got to enjoy him gloat over the various walking canes that sort of became one of his fashion components." As they traveled together, they would often end up "in a group dinner at some restaurant with six or seven doctors sitting around him reminiscing . . . or, in a couple of cases, even pulling out X-rays and MRI pictures." Back at the house, "he'd have his nightly martini or two, or glass of scotch; he had quite the liquor cabinet for sure."

Once, on a trip to Philadelphia, Koop took sick. "Him on the other end of things was never enjoyable," observed Drake drily. Late at night he got a call from Koop. He was going to sneak out of the hospital. Drake was to take a cab to the airport, rent a car, and pick him up. They drove through the night to the Dartmouth Hitchcock Medical Center, in which he had a lot more confidence.

Koop and Cora would be guests at the Drakes' wedding in 2011. Two years later, Drake was invited to speak at the private family funeral. The family gave him Koop's desk.[33]

Four friendships Koop was denied in his final years were those of fellow evangelicals with whom he had worked closely in earlier times, all dead to cancer in their 60s and early 70s. His brothers in the 1970s fight against abortion, Francis Schaeffer (Fran), and Harold O.J. Brown (Joe), died at seventy-two (lymphoma) and seventy-four (sinus, then a decade later the throat), respectively.[34] Fran had died at his US home in Rochester, Minnesota, with his family around him, on May 15, 1984. His widow Edith recorded: "It was 4 a.m. precisely that a soft last breath was taken . . . and he was absent. That absence was so sharp and precise."[35] Three weeks before Joe's passing, at 8:25 p.m. on July 8, 2007, friends had gathered in his Charlotte, North Carolina, home with his wife Grace to sing hymns and thank him for all he had done. This brilliant but self-effacing man could no longer speak. He jotted a note for Melinda Delahoyde, his former student who had taken leadership of the Christian Action Council two decades before. "I really do not think of myself the way these people speak of me."[36]

On Good Friday, April 21, in the year 2000, Tenth Church's longtime pastor James Montgomery Boice was diagnosed with advanced cancer of the liver, dying just eight weeks later, on June 15, at sixty-one—imaging the life of his predecessor Donald Grey Barnhouse, who had also been called young to the church (at thirty-two; Boice had been twenty-nine) and had also died rapidly and in harness—in his case of a brain tumor, at sixty-five.[37] Koop had been close to Boice from the very start of his ministry, when back in 1968, on the morning after their son David's death, the fresh-faced new minister had turned up at the Koops' home with a bowl of his wife's dessert.

Michel Carcassonne, leading French pediatric surgeon and a close friend from the 1950s, had also been taken by cancer. It was Carcassonne who had secured for Koop the *Légion d'honneur*. In a moving letter, five years before his death, he told Koop that he has been his best friend. Koop replied: "I was very touched by your letter . . . as we look forward to the waning years of our lives."[38] Carcassonne passed on March 12, 2001, at seventy-three, after a "long bout" of lymphatic leukemia and metastatic cancer of the prostate.[39]

Others who were close and had predeceased him lived longer: Robert Zachary (February 1, 1999) died at eighty-five,[40] Peter Paul Rickham (November 17, 2003), at eighty-six, and Jonathan Rhoads (January 2, 2002), at ninety-four. I.S. Ravdin, to whom he owed his career, had died way back in 1972 (August 27, at the age of seventy-seven, after what the Royal College of Surgeons described as "chronic illness which incapacitated him mentally and physically").[41] Koop's colleagues and close family friends Erna Goulding and Louise Schnaufer had also lived long: Schnaufer until eighty-six in 2011, and

Goulding until ninety-one, dying on November 19, 2012, just three months before Koop.

Of Koop's friends who survived, several stayed close in these waning years.

Tony Fauci, director of the National Institute of Allergy and Infectious Diseases from 1984, with whom he had worked on AIDS, had become Koop's personal physician as well as a close friend. He was a regular Hanover visitor, as was "Dr. Tim" Johnson, ABC's medical editor. Johnson was also a minister of religion.[iv] He first met Koop in a Washington hotel suite to interview him for the iconic ABC news show 20/20. Johnson pressed Koop on his seeming shift from his conservative roots. While Koop was used to being criticized by conservatives, and lauded in more liberal and progressive contexts, Johnson proved a more complex interlocutor. Like Koop, he straddled evangelical religion and public life. So their interview turned into a much fuller discussion, and then a friendship.[42]

Woodie Kessel, the HHS colleague (and pediatrician) who had befriended Koop early in his time in Washington, became a key collaborator at the Koop Institute.[43] Koop's widow Cora spoke to me warmly of Kessel's relationship with her husband; his "closest friend" in the final days. A shared sense of fun sparkled through their friendship. In former times Kessel would drive Koop around Washington in his open-top sports car. Later he raced his wheelchair around Ivy Pointe Way. "We would get in the automated wheelchair, he and I, we'd drive around the cul-de-sac on, you know, on nice days, and just talk and chat, just around and around in the cul-de-sac. You know, I miss him terribly, we were just incredibly good friends."[44]

Larter had first met Koop early in the 1990s, when working for Tenth Church in a ministry to AIDS patients. Koop had been signing copies of his memoir at Tenth, and Larter lined up for an autograph. He was surprised to find that Koop knew all about the ministry. He had just been awarded a medal by the city of Philadelphia, and he told Larter he would donate the accompanying check to the ministry.

---

iv   Of the Evangelical Covenant Church, a small and relatively conservative denomination

The encounter sparked a growing friendship. They met again at a celebration of James and Linda Boice's silver anniversary in 1993. Larter wrote to the Koops "one of the most thoughtful and beautiful letters we have ever received," Koop replied.[45] "As the years rolled on from that point, our contact increased. . . . He had this gift for making friends, and for reasons that are still not clear to me he reached out to myself and Evelyn, and initiated a process that deepened friendship, and the amount of time we spent together."[46]

Michael Fiore, who would become one of the nation's lead experts on tobacco control, was a young researcher with the HHS Office of Smoking and Health when he first met Koop. Over time, "we became personally closer." Then Koop invited him to Dartmouth to teach for a week, and to bring his son, offering to spend an hour a day mentoring him. "And that was a very memorable week for my son and me . . . we had family events with all of his family. It just was very special in a lot of ways. And as he got older and older, I began to visit him more often. So, at least every three months or so, I would go up and visit with him. It moved from me being his mentee to us being very close friends. And of course, one hard thing for a lot of people is when you have to step off the stage. You kind of see who are truly dear friends and stay with you. And I know that meant a lot to him."[47]

A Shrunken Stage

Larter delivered the homily at the close of the National Memorial Service, a stark account of his time with Koop during the final stage of his life.[48] Commenting on the many tributes that others had given, he said that "most of those words and the tributes focused on what I would call the strong years of Dr. Koop's life. . . . My own intimacy with him was not in those strongest years. They were years spent in a long diminuendo. When the parades were over, and the fanfares were silent. In many ways, I got to know Chick best in what I would call the house of mourning, the house where the losses of his life became more obvious and very, very painful." Larter continued: "In April of 2012, when I went to spend some time with him and Cora, he was hideously depressed. And at one point I asked him, 'Why, what is it that makes you the most sad?' And all that I could get out was that 'I've lost control.' And then I asked him, 'What comfort do you have, knowing that you have lost a great deal of control over the trajectory of your life at this point?' And he looked me in the eye and said . . . his comfort was in the redefining of our brotherhood."

He turned to address Betsy, the Koops' daughter, who with her husband was there to represent the family. "I had neither the privilege of growing up in your household," he said, "nor did I have to face the challenges of being raised and living with a formidable, single-minded, and ruthlessly determined father and husband. I was only a friend, who came late on the scene."[49]

Then Larter told of his final visits. "I would go up occasionally to help out with his physical care . . . there was a large bedroom that he and Cora shared and the people who were there looking after him, particularly at night, because latterly he went on hospice care. There was always a caregiver around 24/7." And he continued, movingly, "There were a lot of very precious and very significant moments with him, in this progressive decline, even in his dying. He was a man who physically could no longer maintain the charismatic presence that was so much a part of who he was. . . . The circle within which the dying individual moves diminishes. But for those of us who were allowed into that circle, at the end, there was a poignant vulnerability and intimacy that he had never allowed until then. It was very important that he be on stage, but that stage shrank to a home, and finally a bedroom."[50]

Ten days before his death, Koop said to one of his carers, "I am getting ready to go to a place I've never been before." And, soon after, to Larter, "I want my father."[51] Larter continued: "My guess is that even at the very end—I was with him within twenty-four to forty-eight hours of his dying—there may have been occasions when his intellect was clouded, I think his awareness and his ability to still connect remained with him until he became unconscious just very shortly before he died." Linda Boice recalled, toward the very end, "Cora was sitting at his bedside holding his hand while she talked with me on the telephone."[52]

Gibbs had all along refused to call Koop "Chick." He was ex-military, and despite their familiarity could not get over the fact—as he told me—that Koop was a vice admiral! There was much banter between them, as Gibbs drove him around and cooked for him and helped him into bed and out of bed. In return, Koop called him Captain. "It wasn't until shortly before he died," Gibbs told me, "that I actually referred to him as Chick for the first time. It was in prayer."

Then a couple of days later, on February 25, "I was preparing lunch for Cora. By this time his kidneys had failed and he was not taking food. I called Cora, she came out and we sat down at the table, and the nurse came, and said, 'His heart has stopped.' And we went in, and sure enough. And I called Allen."[53]

CHAPTER 19
A Life

Coming down from the little girl's room, he sat on the sofa and wept, repeating, "Why is it taking her so long to die?" Karen Kelso called Koop's home two nights later to report that Jane was gone.... Karen would later reflect, "Koop had buried his own child, so he knew some parts of life are unbearably awful."

—GREGG EASTERBROOK, *Surgeon Koop*

I remember so many things that this wonderful man did. He became one of the most popular people ever in the history of government. And we all love him to this very day.

—SENATOR ARLEN SPECTER, at Koop's ninetieth birthday party

Everything he believes in, he believes in fiercely, and to sit in a room with him is to be infected with that fierceness, whether you agree with him or not.... His experience gives him a great deal of viewpoint, and it's hard not to foist it on others.

—STEPHEN GEORGE, *New Physician* magazine

The AIDS report "hit the country with the force and the illumination of a lightning bolt."

—SENATOR EDWARD M. KENNEDY, quoted by James Bowman, *Exemplary Public Administrators*

Many people outside his circle of friends were put off by his ego; but I think he was misunderstood. He used his ego as a bullhorn, a platform to reach vast, diverse, global audiences; and yet he had the sensitivity and paradoxical humility of a father-figure to hundreds of students and protégés to position them to finish what he started. I recall a few times when he would make a gruff rebuke to me. But I probably needed to hear it, as painful as it was. That's love. You needed to have some empathy for what he was going through with loss and health decline in his own life. But that just shows his humanity. He was not perfect. But he was relatable because he showed people every side of himself. A cheeseburger and three martini lunch. I love the many peculiar aspects of his personality. He had a lust for life, and he was a man of virtue.

—SEAN DAVID, Koop Institute colleague, now University of Chicago medical school faculty

I will always remember standing side by side with you and fighting the good fight. Now, all these years later, I remain deeply proud of the opportunity we had to work together.

—HILLARY CLINTON, 2010 letter to CEK

I covered science policy at the time for the Washington Post and I expected Koop to generate a lot of news. But neither I, nor anyone else, could have envisioned that by the time he left office eight years later, he would have managed to transform his job into the most electrifying bully pulpit in medicine. And he did it in the most unexpected way: by telling the truth. . . . In this era, during which progress, facts, and science are under unrelenting siege, it is thrilling to remember that even ideologues can love the truth. R.I.P. Dr. Koop.

—MICHAEL SPECTER, *New Yorker* obituary

In many ways *Dr. Koop* is an anachronism. Displaying the Schweitzer-like calm of a 19th century missionary, he will work imperturbably among the Tarascan Indians of Mexico or treat tribal chieftains in Africa, yet admits that helping the derelicts of Philadelphia's skid row has brought him "as close to despair as I have ever got—except when I was delivering babies in Harlem."

—*Roche Medical Image* interview

He suffers with the disease of AIDS and he suffers with the prospect of millions being affected. This is an agonizing situation for him, and it is very unsettling.

—Old friend, Harold O. J. Brown

Surgeon General C. Everett Koop has an opinion, which he will give you with great certainty at high speed.

—*Time* magazine

We were all scared out of our minds what he was going to report. . . . We're initially incredibly skeptical. OK, so he's pretending to be objective and scientific and wanting to learn. He turned out to be this incredibly engaging person, who, despite sort of his gruff manner was very sensitive. There were just so many incredible ironies. He became, you know, to all of us a major figure that made a difference.

—JEFFREY LEVI, now a professor at George Washington University, in the '80s led government relations for the National Gay and Lesbian Task Force, interview

He was a very able man, and a very nice guy. And a great personality, actually. He had a very fine sense of humor, and was a really, very, very good leader.

—EDWIN MEESE, President Reagan's attorney general, interview

When we're doing a PR campaign and we're looking for a national spokesman for an issue or a product, we recognize that you have Dr. Koop and you have everybody else. . . . He is absolutely unique in his ability to command attention.

—Washington public affairs firm, 1999

He had a huge ego. But we all have chinks in our armor and flaws in our character. And it has nothing to do with the good work that we do. All of us have feet of clay. And one thing I loved about Chick was that he had feet of clay. He had the walls of his office at Dartmouth covered with honorary degrees awarded from every prestigious university in the world. And yet, there he was sitting at his desk with his muddy L.L. Bean boots. And talking about where could we go to get some Korean chicken over waffles. Or I'd see a brilliant appetizer section on the menu. Dr. Koop would order all of the appetizers instead of ordering an entrée, and that would be his meal, and three double vodka martinis. He was a man's man, let me tell you.

—DAVID SERRA, an early director of the Koop Institute, interview

I came back to the house one afternoon to find him having trouble taking deep breaths. Drove him to the hospital, and he ended up in the ER. . . . Before admission, the young nurse came in to get his vitals and personal info. He was very rude (letting her know that all his information was already on file and she was wasting time) and she left in tears. In just a few minutes this petite female doctor came in, approached the bed and informed him that she knew who he was, his reputation, and what he had said to the nurse was not appropriate since she was only doing her job. She then told Dr. Koop that the girl would be back, and if he gave her any problems, he would end up with so many IV's and tubes that his head would spin! He gave her a snappy salute, and finally got admitted with pneumonia. The next day he had me bring a pair of earrings and a necklace so he could give them to the little nurse. That young nurse visited him several times each day. He did have a way with the ladies.

—LESTER GIBBS, personal aide, by email

Before evangelicals were pro-life, he sees the unborn child as a patient. He doesn't give a damn whether he goes down well at Wheaton. When he's a pro-life hero, and the right wing loves him, he pisses them off, because he doesn't give a damn whether they don't like gay people or not. These are patients we're talking about, and that's Chick. You know, I think his theology's crazy, but I think he was an admirable human being. And I would say the same thing with him

as I do with my own father. And that is both of these men were far
better human beings than their theology.

> —FRANK SCHAEFFER, son of theologian Francis Schaeffer,
> producer of *Whatever Happened to the Human Race?*—with
> a revised perspective on what he once believed; interview

Well, I think the Bible says we've all sinned and fallen short. I think
he didn't do a good job of controlling his own ego. To be a surgeon,
you've got to have an ego. It's necessary to do the job properly. So in
surgery, it served him well. In politics, not so much. He couldn't let
go. It's common here in Washington, you see people who have been
central to public events in a really important way. And now they're
retired and nobody cares what they think. And they just can't deal
with it. I think we saw that in Koop in retirement as well.

> —GREGG EASTERBROOK, author of *Surgeon Koop*, interview

It was almost impossible to even wish for him to go into retirement,
as he could not get away from the limelight of Chick Koop. . . . Chick
had a hard time dealing with becoming a has-been.

> —Family friend, from Philadelphia days, interview

He was a difficult man. But a lot of times, it takes a difficult man to
do difficult things.

> —PHILIP RYKEN, president of Wheaton College; the minister
> who married Koop and Cora Hogue, interview

With his Lincoln-style beard, military uniform and frequent television appearances, Koop raised the profile of the previously obscure
post of surgeon general to celebrity status.

> —MARK SCHOIFET, *Bloomberg* obituary

The Surgeon General's role all but ended with Dr. Koop because of
his extraordinary charisma and his impact. He became a dangerous
person to anybody that would want to wield any health related power.

> —DONALD SHOPLAND, tobacco control expert and Koop
> colleague, interview

There was when you met him a certain aura you know, an élan, which
you couldn't help. . . . The thing he taught me, that I've carried on
and taught other people is, you decide what the right thing to do
is. And you do it. He must have said that to me twenty times. And I
took it away is the biggest lesson I ever learned. . . . He would listen
to a bunch of people, but then he would decide. And then when he
decided that was it.

> —EDWARD MARTIN, friend, vice admiral, and chief of staff,
> interview

I introduced him to Jonas Salk. It was a really deep interaction. Jonas Salk's most important work was not the polio vaccine. But it was what happened after he set up the Salk Institute with the most amount of Nobel Prize winners in the life sciences. And then he was thinking beyond that to a phase two of the future evolution of humanity. And I think some of Chick's work after being Surgeon General was also really important. It wasn't really quite the same as Jonas's phase two, because Jonas was more of a sage and Koop kind of led the life of a hero.

—MICHAEL MCDONALD, colleague and friend, interview

He became the only memorable surgeon general. Koop turned his notoriety into influence, undertaking public health campaigns against smoking, domestic violence and preventable accidents. But his main contribution concerned HIV/AIDS. In the early days of the crisis, which coincided with the beginning of the Reagan administration, fear and uncertainty produced various proposals for mandatory testing, tattooing and isolation in camps. Koop was initially ordered by a superior to keep any views on the topic to himself. But Koop maneuvered to produce the "Surgeon General's Report on Acquired Immune Deficiency Syndrome," explicitly detailing the modes of HIV transmission, making clear it could not be spread by casual contact, and affirming that "We are fighting a disease, not people."

—MICHAEL GERSON, chief speechwriter to President George W. Bush, *Washington Post*

Koop's career bears a striking resemblance to that of Thomas à Becket, archbishop of Canterbury in the twelfth century. . . . The king appointed Thomas archbishop in hopes of using his buddy to gain more state control over the church. C. Everett Koop was the darling of the Christian right, appointed by the President in hopes of exerting more church influence over the state. Becket, however, was transformed by the responsibilities of his office. . . . Koop, too, chose the integrity of his office over the hidden agenda of his ruler. One man was a secular appointee to a religious position, the other a religious appointee to a secular position. But in both cases they chose to fulfill the high calling of their office rather than the political demands of their friends. And both of them will long be remembered as outstanding examples of Christians who had a job to do, and did it well.

—ALAN GOLD, *MarketPlace Networks* newsletter

To millions . . . C. Everett Koop is a folk hero, a real-life Dr. Welby swelled to stately proportions, steering America's course through the perils of modern illness. His stern face glares nightly from TV newscasts. Strangers pursue him for autographs. Here he is at a Hollywood gala, chatting with Bob Hope. Now he's lunching at New York's posh 21 restaurant, with fans lined up at his table. People magazine? "Good morning America"? He's practically a regular. "General, general," shouts a man racing after him on a New York street.

—*US News and World Report*

I had a two year old cousin named David who was dying of cancer.... Dr. Koop wrote a short story in Reader's Digest about my aunt and uncle and David.... My brother Ari had an infected toe when he was one year old. My mother wanted the best doctor in the city to see my brother. Since Dr. Koop had just successfully separated Siamese twins...he was the best person to call.... When my mother took Ari to see Dr. Koop he explained it was just an ingrowing toenail. Since he was so kind he didn't make my mom look like a fool, but instead said she had done the right thing.

—GREGG, in a high school report, December 10, 1987

I organized an event that incorporated the Surgeon General's annual dinner dance and a visit to the NIH Clinical Center. Everyone who attended the dance was asked to bring a stuffed animal toy to the party to be collected for distribution later.... I accompanied Dr. Koop and a few others to distribute the toys to any child that was in the hospital for treatment during the holiday season. Dr. Koop was a master at entering each child's room, speaking with the child and parents for a very brief, intense time, and leaving the toy with the child. I would stand outside the room and try to keep my composure, while he ... talked, and consoled, gave hope, but mainly gave his complete attention to the patient and family. One room he visited had a pair of red high-heeled shoes at the end of the bed, for the little girl's "journey" into the unknown. I lost my composure outside that room.

—SANDY ROBERTS, president of the US Public Health Service Wives' Club, by email

Chick Koop was able to spend, literally, maybe five minutes with a family and the family leaves the room feeling they have spent two days with the world's most famous pediatric surgeon.... [He could] concentrate an enormous amount of pathos in a short period of time.

—HARRY BISHOP, Koop's longtime surgical partner, to Victor Garcia

I think they didn't appreciate that, even though he was a right-to-life person that was very conservative, they didn't know about his character.... His record was fighting for the lives of children, even with very advanced, difficult diseases ... they never really understood his character. And his character was to do the right thing.

—ANTHONY FAUCI, interview

———

Maverick. An unorthodox or independent-minded person; a person who refuses to conform to the views of a particular group or party; an individualist.

—*Oxford English Dictionary*

The Passage of a Man

In his classic lectures on *The Art of Biography*, Paul Murray Kendall writes that the biographer's task is "to perpetuate a man as he was in the days he lived—a spring task of bringing to life again."[1] It is "to mark, to keep alive, the passage of a man by recapturing the life of that man."[2] i

Looking back after his death, two of Koop's final trainees, Michael W. L. Gauderer and Moritz M. Ziegler, recall the "towering figure . . . whose life's work as a pioneering pediatric surgeon, an extraordinarily effective public servant, and a thoughtful and dedicated educator, has had an immeasurable impact that has ranged from the survival of a single newborn with a major congenital abnormality to the health of an entire nation."[3] On smoking, he "totally changed the landscape," according to tobacco control expert Michael Fiore, who became a close friend.[4] On AIDS, Jeffrey Levi, Washington health professor who in the 1980s met with Koop on behalf of the National Gay and Lesbian Task Force, remarked: "He was as transformative as all the obits are saying."[5] Koop's AIDS report, according to President George W. Bush's chief speechwriter, Michael Gerson, was "one of the most important public health documents of the past century."[6] It also proved the key precursor to Bush's President's Emergency Plan for AIDS Relief (PEPFAR) program, that has been estimated to have saved the lives of twenty-five million Africans; "the single best policy

---

i   An earlier draft of this chapter was shared with half a dozen of those who knew Koop best, though not with members of his family. The consensus among them was that it offers a good likeness of their old friend.

of any president in my lifetime," according to the *New York Times*' liberal columnist Nicholas Kristof.[7]

Few among us have been called on to play so many different parts, and very few with the energy, resolution, and exacting execution, of the boy delivered by his eccentric Uncle Henry on October 14, 1916, at 216, Fourteenth Street, Brooklyn.

Some things are clear about this extraordinary life. Koop started out with a powerful physique (a rising star footballer until injury threatened his medical career plans, who continued to ski through a series of serious accidents), an effortless self-confidence (the only child of doting parents and grandparents), a brilliant mind (Dartmouth, Cornell, Penn), and a commanding presence. His confidence in himself was further honed when at twenty-nine he was offered the post of surgeon-in-chief of the nation's oldest children's hospital and was soon established as the pioneer of his emerging specialty. In tandem, he arrived at a place of distinctive religious faith—shifting from nominal Baptist origins into deeply-held conservative Presbyterian conviction, which offered a clear moral basis for his decisions and an equally clear sense of "call" in his many endeavors.

Koop's faith, and also his character, were influenced profoundly by his friendship with Donald Grey Barnhouse, a dominant figure in midcentury American Protestantism, with whom he worked closely during the 1950s. One Philadelphia friend shared that Barnhouse was "imprinted" on Koop's life.[8] Historian and friend Michael Horton commented on the "largeness, the ego, but also the playfulness—that combination" that Koop and Barnhouse shared.[9]

Koop's innate self-assurance, bolstered by decades of surgical deference, cohabited with a warm spirit and a gentle personal touch, as colleagues became lifelong friends, and as he spent decades saving the lives of babies, sometimes losing them, and comforting their parents. When challenged, he could sometimes be gruff, overbearing, and bad-tempered. Yet he was a man of great generosity, with his time as well as his money—spending Sundays for years on Philadelphia's skid row, helping his cousin with four children escape their one-bedroom apartment, steering or starting a slew of nonprofits, and in his later years quietly putting young people through college and seminary and medical school. It was, perhaps, because of his self-confidence that he was comfortable through it all with his college nickname Chick. And, as one writer noted of his time in Washington, in a city of designer briefcases he carried a tote bag.[10]

Koop's "elevation" of the office of Surgeon General was a remarkable achievement, as David Kessler noted, and also two of his severest critics, James T. Bennett and Thomas J. DiLorenzo.[11] Alongside the hard work and the politics involved, Koop developed a way of speaking about his office and himself in almost numinous terms, at once bizarre and extraordinarily potent. He famously declared, "I am the surgeon general of the heterosexuals and the homosexuals, of the young and the old, of the moral or the immoral, the married and the unmarried. I don't have the luxury of deciding which side I want to be on. So I can tell you how to keep yourself alive no matter what you are. That's my job."[12] His language suggests a personal relationship between the holder of the office and every individual American. For example, of the Baby Doe case: "I was the Surgeon General of all the people. That meant that I was the Surgeon General to Baby Doe. . . . I thought he had badly confused, and extraordinarily badly advised, parents, but I was also the Surgeon General to them. I thought that the people who gave that advice were crass . . . and I realized that I was the Surgeon General for those people as well."[13]

We have tracked Koop's meteoric career as a pioneer of pediatric surgery, leader in the agonizing process of specialty recognition, and architect at the Children's Hospital of the specialty's professional structure. We have observed his dramatic intervention in America's emerging debate over abortion, as he galvanized his fellow evangelical Christians to conviction and action, and stepped aside from the final years of his surgical career to warn America of where he believed legalized abortion would lead. We have seen how his crusade caught the attention of the incoming Reagan administration, who sought to please their social conservative supporters by appointing this campaigner MD to the largely symbolic office of Surgeon General, on the assumption that he would use it as a platform to continue his pro-life speech-making. And we have seen how Koop astonished everyone by deciding to do something altogether different—to set abortion to the side and become America's greatest ever leader in public health.

Koop never seems actually to have understood the political logic of his appointment, and that may have been a good thing. He saw the job as a professional step, the start of a new career, and turned his ferocious energies, beginning every day at 4:30 a.m. with coffee and prayer, to becoming "America's doctor."

Koop's adopting this defiantly apolitical persona mattered little at the outset of his appointment, even though it disappointed his pro-life supporters. But it mattered a good deal later, when he was called on to write two potentially momentous reports, on AIDS and abortion, and in both cases made conscientious choices that cut across the expectations of the administration (and everyone else). On AIDS, he decided to set aside the lifestyle issues that were closely related to HIV infection and that colored much conservative thinking, and to fall back on his fundamental "pro-life" commitment: To save lives at all costs.[14] To that end, he listened to many people, but especially to the gay community, tens of thousands of whom were wasting away and dying. On abortion, his skepticism of political motivation, and resentment that the issue he had set aside had finally caught up with him, led to a curious and un-Koop-like indecision, between a comprehensive report that sought to limit abortion, through such means as contraception and aid for mothers, and a technical conclusion that the jury was out on the matter of psychological sequelae. By opting for the latter and delaying submission until Reagan was days from leaving office, he sowed surprise, disappointment, and misrepresentation, as well as revealing his deep indifference to the dynamics of American politics.

Meanwhile, his hope that incoming President Bush would make him secretary of health and human services offered a further illustration, were it needed, that this celebrated Washington figure remained to the end a political novice. He genuinely believed something that friend and colleague Edward Martin told him no one else in Washington believed, that after eight years as Surgeon General, having "understudied" the role of secretary, he would get a promotion. Not only so. He believed this despite having made it clear that he had no plans to become a team player. Even in his final years, he remained convinced that his mistake had been not to press his case harder.

Once the visionary slipped the constraints of public office and stepped into the life of Citizen Koop, the scope of his activities was remarkable—symbolized in the November 1996 note to a correspondent that, at the age of eighty, "I've reached the insanity in my life where I have five offices in three states."[15] One journalist glimpsed an org chart on his office wall with twenty-nine nodes.

We noted the enthusiasm he felt for new possibilities as he stepped down as Surgeon General. We noted also that after his two previous careers, in medicine and in government, this man with seemingly limitless energy was suddenly free to carry forward his flood of ideas with neither guardrails nor the need for counsel. Some of these efforts saw great success. Some led to failure and embarrassment.

The Clinton administration shrewdly recruited Koop as a key advocate of their healthcare reform plan, and Koop in return recruited Hillary Clinton to help him launch Shape Up America!, the nonprofit diet effort he called his "last crusade." Much less well-known are the projects he led on bioinformatics, which overlapped both with the Clinton healthcare reform effort and also with Vice President Gore's internet initiatives. While his hope to use the medical school at Dartmouth as a test bed for the reform of doctors' training went awry, his determination to press his vision for the future of medicine was unaffected. He urged a twin focus on technology, which needed to begin with computer literacy among medical students and would end up transforming healthcare delivery, and the human dimension. The relation of doctors and patients should be as it had been when he was a child. As he put it, back then patients loved their doctors, even if there was often little they could do. Now they can do a great deal, but patients distrust and even hate them.

As controversy swirled around the AIDS report in the late 1980s, and the press lionized Koop as never before, this rather self-confident man discovered that he had become a celebrity. Celebrity can be a hard thing to slough off. It was during the glory days of the AIDS report and soon after that he "became Koop," the "most-trusted physician in America," a "folk hero," an "icon"—terms others had coined but that he liked to use of himself. It all super-charged his ego; celebrity went to his head. We reviewed his response to *Nova*'s Paula Apsel explaining that awarding Surgeon General medals to her staff would breach journalistic ethics. Koop was furious and insulted. He believed his reputation for integrity set him above such norms. As someone who counsels celebrities in trouble told me, "I think if you find yourself walking into a room for decades and people are bowing and scraping it cannot not affect you." The tragedy of celebrity is "to think you can maintain icon status forever."[16]

Yet in his later years, friends would speak of his desire to remain "Koop"—Koop, larger than life, the figure of authority who commanded vast respect; Koop, the man who was once told by Gallup that his was the most trusted name in America. Yet, as one candid friend told him in his old age, "I can't bring back the 1980s."[17] He learned hard the lesson articulated in the lapidary dictum of celebrated British politician Enoch Powell, that "all political lives . . . end in failure."[18]

Koop is the host of many seeming contradictions. Perhaps most striking is the contrast between what looks like a flint-faced lack of interest in what others think of him, and his thin-skinned sensitivity. He wrote about how hurt he was by criticism during the confirmation process—not simply annoyed, but hurt; generally speaking, controversialists don't get "hurt." Koop was specially hurt, in succeeding years, by the failure of friends and allies in pro-life or religious circles to stand by him, when they denounced him first over his AIDS report, and then his abortion non-report. "He needed his ego stroked," said a candid colleague at the HHS. Close up, his skin can look a lot thinner. We know he was deeply depressed for a period before his death, and we also know that way back in the mid-1950s a discouraging incident triggered a depression that led him to doubt his work as a pediatric surgeon and consider a change in career. The bold face he put on to the world at large masked a sensitive individual, who could over-react to slights and also to setbacks.

There were circumstances in which Koop's ego helped, but it could also lead him astray. Joshua Nelson, who as a young man worked with him at the Koop Institute, captures this well: "He was a brilliant man, but he couldn't do everything. And he tended to think he could do everything. And because he'd been really very lucky, or surprisingly skilled, at things like public relations and so on . . . well, he tended to think he could always out-guess the experts, he knew all the answers. I didn't blame him for the Time Life thing. I know, people warned him, Time Life is doing this arm's-length thing, because they regarded it as a risk and so on. And then DrKoop.com. I mean, he had good friends who said do not do this."[19] But he did it, he did them both, because he thought he knew better. And also because at heart he was still that young man who had more than once cheated death on a ski jump.

The sad result was that the author of gargantuan achievements ended up feeling a failure. As one friend said, "He was uncomprehending of his growing irrelevance, there was no maturation or evolution. It was binary. He had to be either Koop or not."[20] And when the limelight faded, instead of kicking back, relaxing, rejoicing in all that had been achieved, maybe writing the medical mystery he had told Henry Waxman that he had always wanted to, "he felt lost, adrift, in a sadness made worse by his consciousness of the fading of his celebrity."[21]

We have seen him criticized for his role in defending latex gloves and phthalates, products that environmentalists deemed risky, and failing to declare potential conflicts of interest in the process. Meanwhile, DrKoop.com was just getting off the ground. The earlier controversies had primed critics in the press to go after Koop as soon as problems developed with this far more prominent effort. His reputation as the straight-shooter doc suddenly collided in the public mind with the prospect of Koop the internet millionaire. This was no easy time.

Koop made things much worse by the way he chose to defend himself. Forgetting that the Book of Proverbs and image consultants both advise that "a soft answer turneth away wrath," he announced to the press: "I have never been bought. I cannot be bought. I am an icon, and I have a reputation for honesty and integrity, and let the chips fall where they may."[22] Many editorials, much heart-searching, and three months later, chips had been falling. When a journalist asked him about the "icon" remark he covered his face with his hands. But damage had been done. As the *Boston Globe* observed in its pithy reviews at the close of 1999, Koop had "dropped out of the sainthood sweepstakes."[23] The *Washington Post* quoted a source who had worked with him for years: "Those of us who know him reasonably well are convinced he's not corrupt—but that doesn't make it right."[24]

"In good, successful people," someone who counsels celebrities in trouble told me, "there is an ego, and an element of self-hypnosis, that what I do will be embraced as good because it is. And that's not what happens." He continued: "When you're dealing with ego, and that icon status doesn't continue, it's very, very hard for people. . . . That's the curse of celebrity, and it doesn't register." And the result can be described only as an existential crisis. But, he added, "I really adored this guy."[25] His friends' take is reminiscent of something Koop himself had said, more than half a century before, of his friend and mentor Donald Grey Barnhouse. "This man is one of the most remarkable I have ever known. . . . To know him as I do is to love him although at times I do not necessarily like what he does."[26]

"People wanted to benefit and profit from his celebrity," his close friend Woodie Kessel shared with me, "and he was not sophisticated enough, and they would draw him in and launch all these things. They would play to his ego to make him feel good about all of that stuff."[27] Edward Martin noted simply that "he was easy to con."[28] Another friend and colleague shared that "he had a child-like enthusiasm. It was quite innocent. I don't think he was malicious, I don't think there was avarice . . . he would sit and evangelize with you about these things [business projects] without an understanding that there were motivated adversaries out there."[29] Koop Institute director David Serra recalled: "My job really, as I see it, was to protect Dr. Koop from all of the people who came here with ideas wanting to use him or his name for their project."[30]

When DrKoop.com got in trouble for blurring the line between ads and editorial, he was targeted by some particularly acerbic journalists. It's actually harder to find Koop at fault in this case than in his missteps over gloves and chemicals when he failed to declare conflicts of interest.[31] The commercial internet was very young. Standards had yet to emerge to determine what was ethical and what was not, and in particular how editorial and advertising should be distinguished. Koop's response was smart and strategic, to pull leading sites together in the "HI-ethics" group that would set industry standards. But by then damage had been done.

As these controversies came to a head, Koop decided to make a major effort to explain himself, addressing a meeting of some fifty New England newspaper editors. He began on the defensive, making his case. Then, suddenly, his mind took him back thirty years, and he began to talk about his lost son. He shared with the editors that, shortly before David's death, he had been invited to address a prayer breakfast, and had prepared his remarks. A few days later, he duly attended the breakfast, and was reading the speech as prepared. Then he had to break off, to tell his audience that his son was dead. "Standing before the editors," reports the *Washington Post*, "Koop went on: 'Now I find myself in the same position.'"[32]

For such an outwardly self-assured public figure, he remained a surprisingly private man. He wrote and spoke voluminously, but rarely about his personal life, his inner life. His memoir, written with the aid of historian son Allen, is well-crafted and informative—a cut above the usual after-office ghost-written Washington money-spinner (which may explain why sales were disappointing), but we finish it without learning much about what makes him tick.

"What did Chick most like to do?" I asked his longtime friend Tony Fauci. "Chick liked to eat," he replied, "and he liked his martinis." In spring of 1989 *Washington Post* columnist George Will wrote of a memorable lunch: "Our little group . . . would chow down on tuna melts, french fries, and other things not recommended by the American Heart Association. One guest, Surgeon General C. Everett

Koop, the nation's doctor, washed down a cheeseburger and fries with two martinis, bless his heart."[33] Another time, a colleague pled with him not to pile his plate so high with bacon at a buffet, as he was in public.[34] "The guy is a bit peculiar," wrote *US News and World Report*. "He is just gobbling double handfuls of shrimp and deviled eggs at a Boston buffet in his honor. . . . He drinks two dry martinis at lunch. He's overweight. He doesn't exercise much. He has an answer, of course. 'If you look and feel as well as I do at 71, call me.'"[35] Lunching with a group of medical school faculty, he was quizzed after asking someone to pass the butter. "I'm paid to give the American people advice on their health," he quipped. "I'm not paid to set them an example!"[36]

He liked to cook as well as eat, and friend and colleague Woodie Kessel recalled the many occasions when the Surgeon General would propose in his commanding voice an omelet at 5:30 the next morning.[37] Yet as Koop cooked and ate and drank and greatly enjoyed raising eyebrows, he proved surprisingly successful at keeping his weight under control. For some years he was around 210 pounds, "overweight" in BMI terms but not much. He then dropped to 190 —thanks to Fauci's encouragement and the pressure of a planned but ultimately unnecessary knee replacement. Fun food and double vodka martinis notwithstanding, he maintained that weight for years, showing remarkable self-control alongside the braggadocio.

We know he loved—over many years—to sail with friends and colleagues, and to cruise across the Atlantic with his wife. We know he loved a good mystery (he was a particular fan of the psychologically twisted novels of Patricia Highsmith) and had toyed with writing one of his own.[38] We know about his disciplined early-morning routine over many decades, his habit back at the Children's Hospital of slipping tomorrow's schedule into his socks, so he would be reminded as he went to bed. We've seen him railing in conventionally conservative, old guy, terms, against a young man with a mohawk, the evils of video games, and television that takes kids way from their grandparents. While in advancing years he felt bad about how little he had seen of his children when they were small, he seems never to have grasped how profoundly different their family experience was from his own—the hands-on parenting and grandparenting he knew in Brooklyn, as day by day his father would spend lunch-hours in the New York Public Library looking up the answers to his precocious son's latest questions, as he became his lifelong best friend.

We have seen a teenage boy who loved to collect things—in later life plastering his home with honorary degrees and Koop cartoons, and making it a repository for orchids, and bowties, and canes, one of which concealed a Jameson flask.

And we have also seen a remarkable young man—hardly a typical "social conservative" of the 1940s and 1950s—fighting racism and anti-semitism and ableism, taking on a succession of women trainees, and spending what little free time he had, year on year, helping the homeless on Philadelphia's skid row.

"I have always had what might be called a passion for healing and I would give all I had to be in the position where I might help my fellow man," wrote seventeen-year-old Charles Everett Koop; and over the next eight decades he did just that.[39] "My whole career has been dedicated to prolonging lives," he said, looking back from his 90s, "especially the lives of people who are weak and powerless, the disenfranchised who needed an advocate: newborns who needed surgery, handicapped children, unborn children, people with AIDS."[40]

ACKNOWLEDGMENTS

From Koop's days at the Children's Hospital, Moritz Ziegler kindly introduced me to former trainees, including Howard Filston, Victor Garcia, Michael Gauderer, and Martin Eichelberger, who have been generous with their time and their memories. Matthew Hornick, now at Yale, and Clyde Barker, former chair of surgery in the Hospital of the University of Pennsylvania and more recently president of the American Philosophical Society, helped broaden my understanding of major figures from the Koop years. Among patients and their families, Paul Sweeney, Carl Lingle, Robert Douglass, and Joe and Joyce Stein, have kindly added their testimony.

Among former Koop colleagues at the Department of Health and Human Services, and key advisers, I've been much helped by Edward Martin, Samuel "Woodie" Kessel, Peter Hartsock, Anthony Fauci, Jack Henningfield, Donald Shopland, Charles "Mac" Haddow, Robert Mecklenburg, Thomas Novotny, Michael Fiore, Alan Blum, John Svahn, and Jeffrey Nesbit, among others. Since Koop was a leader in making friends out of colleagues, these mostly stayed in touch, and some became very close. Another special friendship hatched in Washington was with NBC's "Dr. Tim" Timothy Johnson, who has been most kind and helpful. Other close Koop friends who have been gracious in sharing reflections, especially on Koop's latter years, include Kenneth and Evelyn Larter, and Michael DellaVecchia.

Others from the Washington community, Koop interlocutors from the 1980s Henry Waxman, James Baker III, and Edwin Meese have all been responsive to my inquiries, as has Surgeon General Richard Carmona, who helped me understand the office post-Koop. (The current Surgeon General declared himself too busy.) Karen Tumulty, biographer of Nancy Reagan, graciously introduced me to Reagan's son Ron Reagan, Jr., and Landon Parvin, Nancy's speechwriter who crafted the celebrated Reagan AIDS speech. Charles (Chuck) Donovan (a Reagan appointee), Edward Grant, and Richard Doerflinger are among the most thoughtful of pro-life leaders.

From Dartmouth, former colleagues in and around the Koop Institute who have shared their memories include Joseph O'Donnell, David Serra, Sean David, Virginia Reed, Christopher Jernstedt, Joseph Walsh, Joshua Nelson, Joseph Henderson, Peter Culp, and longtime hospital president James Varnum. Others include Koop's aide, Lester Gibbs, and Matthew Wetherell. And I am also much in debt to Dartmouth historian Randall Balmer for counsel and encouragement.

For perspective, Alyssa Burgart from Stanford and the *American Journal of Bioethics* discussed with me the significance of Baby Doe, and Stephanie Meredith and Joni Eareckson Tada Koop's importance for disability rights. Douglas John is among those who have helped me think through Koop's activities after he stepped down. Jan Strode helped me understand Shape Up America! Donald Hackett helped with DrKoop.com.

Other witnesses have included Michael Gottlieb, who first identified the AIDS virus; Jeffrey Levi and Gil Gerald, key interlocutors on behalf of the gay community as Koop wrote his AIDS report; George Lundberg, former editor of the *Journal of the American Medical Association*; Alan Goldberg, former president of the American College of Chest Physicians; Frank Schaeffer, who worked with his famous father and Koop on the *Whatever Happened to the Human Race?* movie series; and Timothy Westmoreland, who worked on Capitol Hill as well as at HHS and with the Clinton transition.

It's a truism that the *families of biographical subjects* tend to be uneasy. I am grateful to the Koop family for gracious responses to my inquiries, in particular to his oldest son, Allen, also a Dartmouth historian; to Anne, widow of his second son Norman; to Anne and

Norman's daughter Christina (Tina) Bazala; to his cousin's daughter, Dale Alekel; and to his widow, Cora Hogue Koop.

For many years, the Koops' lives were centered around *Tenth Presbyterian Church in Philadelphia*. Former ministers Liam Goligher and Carroll Wynne kindly made introductions, in particular to Linda Boice, widow of James Montgomery Boice who was minister at Tenth from 1968 until his untimely death in 2000. Linda has been a steady source of counsel, and in turn offered introductions to old friends of the Koop family. Philip Ryken, now president of Wheaton College, was minister at Tenth when Koop married Cora Hogue.

Robert Case, Melinda Delahoyde, Curtis Young, and Matthew Miller have shared *memories of Koop's efforts on abortion, and the Christian Action Council he helped establish.* John Freeman spoke with me of the AIDS ministry that Koop supported and in which Erna Goulding later got much involved. Michael Horton knew Koop then and also later. Others who have helped include Peter and Judi Mollenkof.

Thomas Getman also knew the Koop family in Philadelphia, and then met Koop again when he was on the staff of Senator Hatfield. Medical journalist Mona Khanna was a young Hill staffer who met Koop when she was working with Senator Kennedy.

And thanks also to those who have preferred to share their witness in private.

My friend Matt James of BioCenter in London has kindly assisted with various research tasks, as has David Caprio in Washington, DC.

More than a handful of those I have interviewed, named and unnamed, also kindly agreed to review parts, or in some cases all, of the manuscript in draft, as did my old friend C. Ben Mitchell (who way back worked on ethics for the Southern Baptist Convention). This has been of special importance in light of the extraordinary range of Koop's activities, and if the text shows evidence of sure-footedness across these several fields they deserve much credit.

NOTES

Introduction

1 *Boston Globe* obituary, February 26, 2013.

2 Philip Yancey, *Sole Survivor* (New York: Penguin Random House, 2003), 187.

3 Margaret Carlson, "A Doctor Prescribes Hard Truth," *Time*, April 24, 1989.

4 IMDB blithely defines him as an actor. https://www.imdb.com/name/nm0465
601/?ref_=tt_cl_t_9.

5 Zappa lyrics for "Promiscuous" at https://mojim.com/usy102840x7x8.htm.

6 Mullan/Martin, 37.

7 "In a memo to the Senate last month, officials of the Department of Health and
Human Services sharply limited the duties of the office, making Koop subordinate
in nearly all matters to the assistant health secretary." *The Bulletin* (Philadelphia),
November 17, 1981.

8 Richard Kluger, *Ashes to Ashes* (New York: Knopf, 1996), 537.

9 Memorandum to Agency Heads et al., April 8, 1982. MSC 489 Box 143 F12 Cor.

10 James T. Bennett and Thomas J. DiLorenzo, *Public Health Profiteering* (New York:
Routledge, 2001), 8.

11 Available at https://profiles.nlm.nih.gov/spotlight/qq/catalog/nlm:nlmuid-1015
84930X779-doc.

12 *Mademoiselle*, May 1989, 126.

13 "God's Plan for a Surgeon," *The Presbyterian*, January 1987. ACC Box 10.

14 "God's Plan for a Surgeon," *The Presbyterian*.

15 *Whatever Happened to the Human Race?* was issued as a five-part documentary
series by Gospel Films in 1979. It is available here: https://www.youtube.com/watch?v
=pyo2pQTyeTE.

16 Yancey/Koop.

17 But he noted that while annual deaths from smoking stood at 380,000, the number
of "unborn children then aborted each year" stood at "well over 1,000,000." Koop
memoir, 270.

18 Stridency: E.g., Koop memoir, 271. That stridency helped lead to a series of violent
attacks on abortion providers, mostly after Koop stood down. See Liam Stack, "A
Brief History of Deadly Attacks on Abortion Providers," *New York Times*, November 29, 2015. Moral question: CACE Forum, "Ethics of Activism, Protest, and Dissent," Dr. C. Everett Koop's Remarks. Undated, early 1990s, CACE Wheaton College
archive. Shortly before he stood down, he had raised questions about the value of

overturning Roe, since that would mean we would have "50 problems instead of one." "Koop Foresees 50 Different Laws if Abortion Ruling Is Overturned," *New York Times*, January 20, 1989. This prescient observation does not imply that he would oppose such a ruling, but that the pro-life movement's focus on overturning Roe had been excessive.

19 In discussing abortion protagonists, I simply use the terminology they apply to themselves, pro-choice and pro-life. I am well aware that each of these terms comes laden with values and history, and that many who are "pro-choice" dispute the term "pro-life," and vice versa. Only for special reasons will I use quotation marks around these words. The narrative is intended to be respectful of both these strongly held, conflicting, moral visions.

20 C. Everett Koop, *Koop. The Memoirs of America's Family Doctor* (New York: Random House, 1991; a paperback edition was published in 1993, under the joint imprint of HarperCollins and the evangelical publishing house Zondervan). Koop explained to Philip Yancey shortly before he stepped down that he had kept a journal of his time in Washington, and passed it, plus hours of dictation "on my pre-Washington life," to his son Allen. Allen, a history professor at Dartmouth "and a good writer," had taken a year off teaching to work on the book. He shares the copyright. Yancey/Koop.

21 Gregg Easterbrook, *Surgeon Koop: Medicine and the Politics of Change* (N.l.: Whittle Books, 1991). *Surgeon Koop* is one of a curious series of brief books filled with drug advertisements, intended to be placed in physicians' waiting rooms. Anne Bianchi, *C. Everett Koop: The Health of the Nation* (Brookfield, CT: Milbrook Press, 1992).

22 Bennett and DiLorenzo, *Public Health Profiteering.*

23 I'm grateful to Bennett and DiLorenzo for collating every conceivable criticism of Koop, and also for serious research including FOIA requests. Their cartoonist approach to biography can be amusing, though the humor quickly wears thin.

24 In Terry L. Cooper and N. Dale Wright, ed. *Exemplary Public Administrators* (San Francisco: Jossey-Bass, 1992).

25 Philip Yancey, "The Embattled Career of Dr. Koop," *Christianity Today*, October 20 and November 3, 1989.

26 Letter and draft proposal to Koop, May 11, 1988. AC 2014–016 Box 26/33.

27 Koop also told a correspondent that the book contained "many inaccuracies," though it is not clear what he was referring to. Koop to Will Devlin, November 25, 1991. DA-698 Box 1964.

28 After recent controversy over a projected life of exuberant journalist Christopher Hitchens, the editor-in-chief at W. W. Norton declared he couldn't remember a single estate that actually approved one of theirs. John A. Glusman, quoted by Elizabeth A. Harris, "Hitchens Biography Proceeds, against His Widow's Wishes," *New York Times*, February 4, 2021.

29 Romans 3:23.

30 Robert A. Caro, *Working. Researching, Interviewing, Writing* (New York: Knopf, 2019), 3, cited in Melanie Nolan, "The Great Individual in History: Historicising Historians' Biographical Practice," in Hans Renders and David Veltman, ed., *Fear of Theory. Toward a New Theoretical Justification of Biography* (Leiden: Brill, 2021).

31 Sean David interview.

Prologue: A Party in Washington

1 *Dartmouth Medicine*, Winter 2006.
2 *American Journal of Public Health* 96 (December 2006).
3 Michael Fiore interview.

Part I: FAMILY AND FAITH

1 Carl F. H. Henry, *The Uneasy Conscience of Modern Fundamentalism* (Grand Rapids: Eerdmans, 1947).
2 Founded in 1956, *Christianity Today* retains that role. See christianitytoday.com.
3 Richard J. Mouw, foreword to 2003 repr. of Henry, *Uneasy Conscience of Modern Fundamentalism*, ix, x.
4 Jon Meacham looks back thirty years on. See "The Editor's Desk," *Newsweek*, November 12, 2006. The entire issue offers a series of fascinating reflections.
5 Christian Smith, *American Evangelicalism: Embattled and Thriving* (Chicago: University of Chicago Press, 1998), 13. See also: Steven P. Miller, *The Age of Evangelicalism* (New York: Oxford University Press, 2014) and George M. Marsden, *Fundamentalism and American Culture* (New York: Oxford University Press, 2006).
6 Graham's archives were held for many years at Wheaton College's Graham Center in Wheaton, IL. In 2018, a year after Graham's death, they were controversially moved to an evolving museum/library/exhibition complex in Charlotte, North Carolina, that includes Graham's childhood home. See https://religionnews.com/2022/11/07/a-new-billy-graham-archive-opens-on-the-late-evangelists-birthday/. See also: https://thewheatonrecord.com/2019/04/04/billy-graham-archives-moving-out-of-bgc/.
7 Dartmouth went co-ed in 1972.
8 See Koop memoir, chapter 2, for various details.
9 She was known as Betty, but "I call her Liz; nobody else does," he told Marlene Cimons of the *Los Angeles Times Magazine*, September 14, 1986, 19.
10 Vassar commencement speech, May 28, 1990. https://digirepo.nlm.nih.gov/ext/document/101584930X972/PDF/101584930X972.pdf. The hurricane that struck New England a couple of days later was "one of the most powerful in recorded history." https://www.weather.gov/okx/1938HurricaneHome.

CHAPTER 1: The Koops

1 Census 1920, 1930, accessible at Ancestry.com.
2 Undated memorandum. ACC 2017–018 Box 1/3. "Anabaptists" were a collection of religious groups that arose during the Protestant Reformation of the sixteenth century, but refused to join with either Lutherans or Calvinists because they opposed the baptism of infants. They were opposed and sometimes severely persecuted by both Catholics and other Protestants. Today, their descendants include both the Baptist churches and groups such as Mennonites. See, for example, the *Catholic Encyclopedia*: https://www.newadvent.org/cathen/01445b.htm.
3 See *New York Times* obituary, February 25, 2013. His birth was preceded, five years

before, by that of a stillborn brother. Koop memoir, 11. It is interesting to mull how different Koop might have been had he grown up as a younger brother.

4 Marlene Cimons, *Los Angeles Times Magazine*, September 14, 1986, 19. Apel had been born in Germany, and immigrated as a child.

5 Koop, Summer I was 12, going on 13. ACC 2015–011 Koop Papers 1942–2009 Box 1. This is one of Koop's several efforts at writing an autobiography. They all petered out.

6 Margaret Carlson, "A Doctor Prescribes Hard Truth. . . . America's Surgeon General, has an opinion on everything healthful, but he nonetheless enjoys meat and martinis," *Time*, April 24, 1989.

7 Koop, Summer I was 12.

8 Koop to Hudson T. Armerding, January 15, 1976. Armerding replied: "there is a good possibility that she will be accepted." Armerding to Koop, January 22, 1976. ACC 2014–016 Box 24/33.

9 Dale Alekel interview.

10 Koop, Summer I was 12.

11 Ziegler/Koop, 1–2.

12 Ziegler/Koop, 2.

13 George Hoyt Whipple, George Richards Minot, and William Parry Murphy were awarded the Nobel Prize in Physiology or Medicine in 1934, "for their discoveries concerning liver therapy in cases of anaemia." https://www.nobelprize.org/prizes/medicine/1934/summary/.

14 Ziegler/Koop, 2.

15 Ziegler/Koop, 4.

16 Maurice J. Stack to Koop, March 18, 1993; Koop to Stack, March 25, 1993. DA-698 Jan-Jly 1993 KI Cor.

17 "Then I have some other relatives here. These are the ones that really call me good old Ev," said Koop at his retirement dinner. Transcript courtesy of Scott Adzick, MD, Children's Hospital of Philadelphia.

18 Koop to Frederick W. Platt, March 5, 1993. DA-698 Box 1965. Koop had planned to drop "Chick" when he moved on from college to medical school, but shortly after term began an old friend spied him across a room and yelled "Chick Koop!" He knew it was all over. Personal conversation.

19 He noted that one year his expenses, from tuition to travel, added up to $999; that equates to around $23,000 today. https://www.dollartimes.com/inflation/inflation.php?amount=999&year=1933. Student jobs included running a laundry and a dishwashing business and selling saddleshoes. Notes on biography. ACC 2014–016 Koop papers Box 26/33.

20 Koop memoir, chapter 2, for details.

21 Koop memoir, chapter 2, for details.

22 Koop memoir, 42.

23 Koop memoir, 53.

24 Ziegler/Koop, 1.

25 Koop, Autobiographical sketch.

26 Koop, Autobiographical sketch.

27 Koop, Autobiographical sketch.

28 *US News and World Report*, May 30, 1988, 57.

29 Koop memoir, 88.

30 Koop to Maurice J. Stack, March 25, 1993. DA-698, Jan-Jly 1993 KI Cor.

31 Anne Koop interview.

32 There were four Koop children: Allen (1944), Norman (1946), David (1947), and Elizabeth (Betsy) (1951).

33 ACC 2014–016 Box 26/33. The house is on Three Mile Road, Etna, just outside Hanover, and remains in the family.

34 Koop, Summer in New Hampshire. ACC 2015–011 Koop Papers 1942–2009 Box 1.

35 Koop file note Insert re David #1. ACC 2014–016 Koop Papers.

36 Ziegler/Koop, 62.

37 Ziegler/Koop, 62.

38 Granddaughter Christina (Tina) Bazala interview. Tina became a photographer, but in mid-life has retrained as a pediatric nurse.

39 Ziegler/Koop, 62.

40 Confidential interview.

41 Confidential interview.

42 Confidential interview.

43 Confidential interview.

44 Confidential interview.

45 Anne Koop interview.

46 Christina Bazala interview.

47 Christina Bazala interview.

48 Tina Bazala loves to tell the story. "I mean, doesn't Hillary Clinton call your house on Thanksgiving and interrupt your dinner?" Christina Bazala interview.

49 "What I Tell the Parents of a Dying Child," *Reader's Digest*, February 1968.

50 Marlene Cimons, *Los Angeles Times Magazine*, September 14, 1986, 19.

51 Gregg Easterbrook, *Surgeon Koop* (N.l.: Whittle, 2001), 18.

52 David was plainly expert, and not without a sense of humor. His father recalled the time he rappelled from his fourth-floor dorm window to the floor below to ask his neighbor to turn down his stereo. Biographical notes. ACC 2014–016 Koop papers Box 26/33.

53 *Nashua Telegraph*, Nashua, New Hampshire, April 29, 1968.

54 Easterbrook, *Surgeon Koop*, 18.

55 *Nashua Telegraph*, April 29, 1968.

56 Anne Koop interview.

57 Anne's relationship with the Koop family was especially close. She and Norman had met in their teens, when like the other Koop kids he had a summer job on the celebrated Cog Railway on Mount Washington, New Hampshire, which was owned and operated by her parents. When her father shot himself on August 4, 1967, her mother took over the management of the railway, a story she tells in her engaging memoir *I Conquered My Mountain* (Canaan, NH: Phoenix Publishing, 1982). Her mother wrote, "Anne was just numb, she was so attached to her father." 105, 106.

58 December 28, 1968. In addition to a maid of honor (her sister), she was attended by a flower girl and ten bridesmaids. The *Philadelphia Inquirer* (December 29, 1968) describes her as "a debutante of the 1968 season." She was given away by her godfather.

59 Joe and Joyce Stein interview.

60 "It was so nice to hear from you on my birthday and to get the pictures of your adorable children." Koop to Dr. and Mrs. Warren (and Lark) Lambard, October 30, 1978. ACC 2014-016 Box 25/33.

61 His call followed the departure the previous year of Barnhouse's immediate successor, Canadian Mariano di Gangi (1923-2008), who served at Tenth 1960-67. Boice, like Barnhouse, was an intellectually gifted man of great energy.

62 Email from Carroll Wynne, April 15, 2021.

63 Linda Boice interview.

64 Paul Brand interview with Philip Yancey, July 27, 1989; notes in my possession courtesy of Yancey.

65 Donald C. Drake, "Zealot for life," *Philadelphia Inquirer*, September 2, 1979.

66 Koop to Frank E. Gaebelein, September 19, 1968. Wheaton Koop Box B.

67 Koop to Joseph Bayly, Cook Publishing Company, November 17, 1969. Wheaton Koop Box B.

68 C. Everett and Elizabeth Koop, *Sometimes Mountains Move* (Wheaton, IL: Tyndale House, 1979), 7.

69 Koop, *Sometimes Mountains Move*, 10.

70 Koop, *Sometimes Mountains Move*, 17.

71 Koop, *Sometimes Mountains Move*, 25. A coda to *Sometimes Mountains Move* lies in another small book about the death of a son, by another deeply religious father in the evangelical and reformed tradition of the Christian faith. Philosopher and theologian Nicholas Wolterstorff tells in *Lament for a Son* how after Eric's death, in 1983 and at the age of twenty-five, someone gave him a copy of the Koops' book. It made him angry. "His son's foot had not slipped. *God* had shaken the mountain. God had decided that it was time for him to come home." He goes on: "I find this pious attitude deaf to the message of the Christian gospel. Death is here understood as a normal instrument of God's dealing with us. 'You there have lived out the years I've planned for you, so I'll just shake the mountain a bit. All of you there, I'll send some starlings into the engine of your plane. And as for you there, a stroke when running will do nicely.'" For Christians, Wolterstorff pleads, death can never be "normal;" "God is appalled by death." His own explanation? "I have no explanation. I can do nothing else than endure in the face of this deepest and most painful of mysteries." Wolterstorff, *Lament for a Son* (Grand Rapids: Eerdmans, 1987), 66-67. Wolterstorff, oddly, does not refer to the Koops or the book by name, and it's not clear if Koop ever read the book. A gentler gloss was shared with me by Koop's friend and trainee Howard Filston. "That certainly describes his faith, and how he believes that God engineered every bit of that whole thing. David's death. And . . . be able to see God's hand in all this. You know, I read the book after [my son] Scott died. And it really didn't help me very much because I find it hard to see God's hand in some drunk coming out of a bar and killing my kid. I'm a Presbyterian and a Stephen Minister [a kind of lay ministry] and I've dealt with a lot of grief in folks. I've never recommended this to anybody except some very few people that had very, very similar experiences, because it doesn't leave much room for happenstance or evil people. It didn't work for me." Howard Filston interview. Koop himself shared with Philip Yancey that he and Schaeffer had a related disagreement when Schaeffer was in the Mayo Clinic with cancer. Schaeffer said it was a "terrible heresy" to say that God had

given him the cancer. Koop told him God had planned it "before the foundation of the world." Yancey/Koop.

72 Comments of Norman Koop, memorial service for C. Everett Koop, First Congregational Church of Woodstock, Vermont, March 9, 2013 (notes in Mike Stobbe's possession); Norman Koop, interview with Stobbe, March 11, 2013. Mike Stobbe, *Surgeon General's Warning* (Oakland: University of California Press, 2014), 329–330, 173.

73 Koop, *Sometimes Mountains Move*, 29–31.

74 Koop, *Sometimes Mountains Move*, 32.

75 The Steins shared the "memorial service of thanksgiving for the life of our son" and it was "adapted for David's memorial service." Retirement dinner transcript, courtesy of Scott Adzick, MD, Children's Hospital of Philadelphia.

76 Koop, *Sometimes Mountains Move*, 41.

77 Easterbrook, *Surgeon Koop*, 17–18.

78 Marlene Cimons, *Los Angeles Times Magazine*, September 14, 1986, 19, 20.

79 Kenneth Larter interview.

80 Michael DellaVecchia interview.

81 Marlene Cimons, *Los Angeles Times Magazine*, 19.

82 Koop's will is available from Haverhill Probate Division, NH, case 315-2013 -ET-00182.

83 Allen Koop email, September 23, 2021. "My father would have accomplished nothing without the advice and direction provided by my mother, who was the person who made sure he took advantage of opportunities and avoided pitfalls."

84 She would refuse to permit her husband to buy new shoes unless first he discarded an old pair! Christina Bazala interview.

85 As *Bloomberg News* summed up its Koop obituary, "Though he was raised by a church-going family, Koop wasn't especially devout until he joined the Tenth Presbyterian Church of Philadelphia in 1948. He had a spiritual awakening." https://www .bloomberg.com/news/articles/2013-02-25/c-everett-koop-surgeon-general-who -took-on-tobacco-dies-at-96?leadSource=uverify%20wall. (The Koops did not actually become formal members of the church until 1952.)

86 Gallup first measured church membership in 1937. It was then at 73 percent. https://news .gallup.com/poll/341963/church-membership-falls-below-majority-first-time.aspx.

87 Koop, Notes for a biography. ACC 2015–016 Koop Papers 1942–2009 Box 1.

88 Foreword to Margaret N. Barnhouse, *That Man Barnhouse* (Wheaton, IL: Tyndale House, 1983).

89 Bernard R. DeRemer, in *Disciple* magazine, quoting *Pulpit Helps*, February 2003. The Barnhouses lived on a farm outside the city in Doylestown, Pennsylvania— Barchdale, on Route 3. F. F. Bruce to Barnhouse, September 11, 1955. PHS Barnhouse Biographical Files.

90 C. Allyn Russell, "Donald Grey Barnhouse: Fundamentalist Who Changed," *Journal of Presbyterian History* 59, no. 1, 33.

91 Koop to Peter Paul Rickham, October 9, 1979. ACC 2014–016 Box 26/33.

92 Barnhouse in 1954; Koop in 1980. For Barnhouse, Margaret N. Barnhouse, *That Man Barnhouse*, 171. For Koop, see chapter 5. The awards were at the "Chevalier" (entry-level) grade. As we note later, Michel Carcassonne's efforts to boost Koop's grade were unsuccessful.

93 In his memoir, 85, Koop refers to "grand rounds" that morning, a term used for a hospital case conference; this is most unlikely.

94 Koop, Notes for a biography, c. 1990. This outline was drafted soon after the 1974 twin separation, and with an evangelical publisher in mind. ACC 2014–016 Koop Papers Box 26/33.

95 Koop, Notes for a biography.

96 Koop, Notes for a biography. His reference to his sons as "*her* toddling boys" (my emphasis) is telling; as more broadly the assumption that since they have small children only the husband may attend church.

97 Koop, Notes. The AMA meeting was actually in June. Perhaps they were in Atlantic City for this decisive conversation at another time that year. Elsewhere, he confirms that it took place seven months after he began attending Tenth Church. "God's Plan for a Surgeon," *The Presbyterian*, January 1987. ACC Box 10.

98 Donald C. Drake, "Zealot for life," *Philadelphia Inquirer*, September 2, 1979.

99 Koop, Notes for a biography.

CHAPTER 2: At Tenth Church

1 Koop, Notes for a biography. ACC 2015–016 Koop Papers 1942–2009 Box 1.

2 Oddly, despite his evident importance for the Koops in their early days of evangelical faith, "Cornie" is not referenced in the Koop memoir. Koop, Notes for a biography.

3 Koop, Notes for a biography.

4 Colleague and friend Erna Goulding, who had urged the Koops to attend Tenth, joined at the same time as the Koops. PHS, Tenth Presbyterian Church Session Minutes, May 28, 1952.

5 Koop, Notes for a biography.

6 PHS, Tenth Presbyterian Church Session Minutes, October 26, 1952. Koop was a member of the Foundation board of directors from at the latest November 1952. Herron to Hopkins, December 1, 1952. PHS Evangelical Foundation files.

7 Koop, Notes for a biography.

8 This was apparently toward the end of 1948.

9 Koop, Notes for a biography. See also William Edgar, *Schaeffer on the Christian Life: Countercultural Spirituality* (Wheaton, IL: Crossway Books, 2013), 58.

10 See Chapter 6 for further discussion of Schaeffer. In 1979 Koop would nominate him (unsuccessfully) for the Templeton Prize in Religion. Koop to Wilbert Forker, June 20, 1979. NLM 205–011 Box 2 Cor.

11 Koop, Notes for a biography. The town is properly Champéry.

12 Koop, Notes for a biography.

13 Missions: Koop to Calvert N. Ellis, December 12, 1967. ACC 2016–016 Box 18/33. Contributing: For example, a Mrs. Philip Ward. Koop to Ward, October 15, 1957. ACC 2014–016 Box 25/33.

14 Thomas Getman interview.

15 Re-founded as *Eternity* from 1950. C. Allyn Russell, "Donald Grey Barnhouse: Fundamentalist Who Changed," *Journal of Presbyterian History* 59, no. 1, 37. Barnhouse's magazine, the heart of the work of the Evangelical Foundation, was published from 1931 under its original title, *Revelation*. In 1949 a crisis developed

after two of the key staff members, one of whom was then married, began an affair which ended in a divorce and their subsequent marriage. Barnhouse regarded this as improper and sought their resignation or dismissal. However, Barnhouse himself did not control the board of the company, and he was outvoted. As he wrote in a lengthy statement, evidently circulated to various evangelical leaders "in order to reestablish my written ministry," a Mr. J. G. Becker, evidently leading for the board, refused to "give the magazine back to me." So Barnhouse resigned as editor of *Revelation*, and persuaded other writers to pull out. As a result, *Revelation* folded. In 1950, Barnhouse began its successor, *Eternity*. Undated (mid-1949) Barnhouse memorandum, apparently personally typed. PHS RG 480-15-32. In a letter to Russell, former Foundation staffer Paul Hopkins explained: "Two of us spent until 2 a.m. at his farm trying to convince him to start what turned out to be *Eternity*. Once we did, *Revelation* quickly faded and we took over its assets and liabilities about the time the first issues of *Eternity* came off the press." Hopkins to Russell, October 7, 1981. PHS RG 480-15-21. Hopkins broadly approved Russell's Barnhouse analysis, though "he eschewed (especially in his Foundation years) a fundamentalist tag, seeking rather to be called . . . evangelical." Hopkins to Russell, July 29, 1981. PHS RG 480-14-19.

16 Russell, "Donald Grey Barnhouse," 37.

17 See Vern J. Wirka, "Religious Broadcasting Influence on Presbyterians," (MA diss., University of Omaha, 1997); Mark Ward, Sr., A*ir of Salvation: The Story of Christian Broadcasting* (Grand Rapids: Baker, 1994), 210; Russell, Donald Grey "Barnhouse," 37. $40,000 in 1928 equates to around $700,000 today. Ward notes that in 1927, when the church broadcast locally, at year's end Barnhouse had 11 cents in the radio account.

18 Russell, "Donald Grey Barnhouse," 53.

19 Russell, "Donald Grey Barnhouse," 38.

20 Russell, "Donald Grey Barnhouse," 48. "Lonely" is a curious term for the famously gregarious Barnhouse. But he was certainly a loner.

21 W. L. Taitte, "The Lady is a Priest . . . and a Psychiatrist, a Professor, a Peace Activist, a Mother of Seven . . . ," *D Magazine*, June, 1983.

22 Karen Maroda, "Sylvia and Ruth," *Salon*, November 29, 2004. The Barnhouse children all kept the faith, though sometimes not quite as their father had hoped. The eldest, Ruth, became one of the first women episcopal priests, and the psychiatrist who treated, and befriended, poet Sylvia Plath for the decade before her death. I am presently working on her biography.

23 Dorothy Barnhouse to Koop, NLM Box 86 Cor.

24 Yancey/Koop. See Russell, "Donald Grey Barnhouse." There were at least six potential writers of a Barnhouse biography! Sadly, all came to nothing. Barnhouse's second wife Margaret Barnhouse's lively book, *That Man Barnhouse* (Wheaton, IL: Tyndale House, 1983) is a personal memoir, focused largely on the period after their marriage in 1954.

25 The Foundation was established in 1950 to host the new magazine, *Eternity*, and several other Barnhouse projects. Koop states at various places that he was president of the Foundation from 1951, but the record states that he joined the board in 1952, when Barnhouse was president. PHS RG 480-5-8. In 1958 Koop, then board chair, complained that board members were insufficiently engaged.

"As a Board, do we feel that this is Barnhouse's show and we are here to rubber stamp activities unless they are way out of line?" He added: "My position is an anomalous one in being chairman of the meeting while the president sits in the chair.... The effort of trying to keep to the agenda ... becomes so enervating that I have all but ceased to make efforts in this direction." Memorandum from Koop to Board of Directors, October 15, 1958. PHS RG 6480 Evangelical Foundation Cor. This was no new situation. Back in 1953 another board member, F. Leon Herron, had resigned, writing to Barnhouse in a candid letter: "If you insist on going, 'your own way,' then I think you should pause and weigh the consequences." Herron to Barnhouse, February 19, 1953. PHS Barnhouse Biographical Files. The Foundation continues under the name the Alliance of Confessing Evangelicals; historical Barnhouse radio broadcasts continue as "Dr. Barnhouse and the Bible." See alliancenet.org. Koop rejoined the board some years after stepping down as Surgeon General. Michael Horton interview. See also, Undated memorandum. ACC 2014–016 Box 18 Misc.

26 Russell, Allyn C., "Donald Gray Barnhouse," 37.

27 It is telling that in the formal "Questionnaire," required by the government of France in advance of his award of the *Légion d'honneur,* Barnhouse made no mention whatever of his role at Tenth Church. June 30, 1954. PHS DG 1180-14-29.

28 Koop to James E. Eckenhoff, February 8, 1956. ACC 2014–016 Box 24/33.

29 The vote was 372–7. Linda Boice interview.

30 Evan Todd Fisher, "Strengthen What Remains: The rhetorical situation of James Montgomery Boice" (PhD dissertation, Southwestern Baptist Theological Seminary, 2018), 246–47.

31 Koop to Schaeffer, July 1, 1980. 2015–11 NLM Box 2 Cor.

32 Linda Boice interview.

33 Linda Boice interview.

34 See Chapter 18.

Part II: SURGEON

1 Ziegler/Koop, 5.

2 The originally British term "anaesthetist," spelled "anesthetist," was commonly used back then in the United States, where "anesthesiologist" and cognates are now universal. But the issue is a little more complicated. See Wei-Zen Sun and James L. Reynolds, "Anesthesiologist, Anaesthetist, Anesthetist, Et Cetera: A Summary of English Names for Anesthesia Professionals in Several Regions," *Asian Journal of Anesthesiology,* 56:2, 43–44.

3 *Pennsylvania Medicine* 28 (December 1985).

4 Willis J. Potts, "Pediatric Surgery," *Journal of the American Medical Association* 157 (1955), 629. Quoted by Catherine Musemeche in *Small: Life and Death on the Front Lines of Pediatric Surgery* (Hanover, NH: Dartmouth University Press, 2014), 23.

5 Ziegler/Koop, 1. Moritz Ziegler, one of Koop's final trainees at the Children's Hospital, interviewed him in Hanover on May 8, 2006, as part of the Oral History Project of the American Academy of Pediatrics. Ziegler shared with me that when he was a medical student, living at home, one Saturday he picked up a copy of the *Reader's Digest.* It happened to include an article titled "What I tell the parents of dying children," by "a certain C. Everett Koop, a name I did not recognize." Ziegler

continued: "I read the piece and I was immediately smitten, saying to myself 'That is what I want to do one day!'" Moritz Ziegler interview.

6 Ziegler/Koop, 1.

7 *Washington Post* obituary, February 25, 2013.

8 *New York Times Good Health Magazine*, October 9, 1988, 32.

9 Ziegler/Koop, 5.

10 *Good Health Magazine*, 32.

11 Ziegler/Koop, 5.

12 Koop retirement dinner transcript, April 27, 1981. Should readers find Koop's account of his teen surgeries implausible, these comments from Rhoads offer confirmation, in light of his close relationship with Koop's mother.

13 *New York Times* obituary, February 26, 2013.

CHAPTER 3: The Making of a Surgeon

1 Ziegler/Koop, 6, 7.

2 Ziegler/Koop, 10.

3 Ziegler/Koop, 8, 9.

4 Ziegler/Koop, 10.

5 Ziegler/Koop, 10, 11.

6 Ziegler/Koop, 11, 12.

7 Koop later described Ravdin in the decade after the end of the Second World War as "perhaps the most important figure in American surgery." Heskel/Koop, 2.

8 I.S. Ravdin to Koop, October 31, 1956. Penn 21.

9 Though he need not have worried. Some years later Koop realized that, unusually for the time, Ravdin had no difficulties with married staff: "He had a habit of making rounds just before dinner, and we'd go tearing through the hospital and see all the patients, and then he'd look at his watch and he'd say, 'Those of us who have wives ought to get home for dinner. The rest of you can finish up here.'" Ziegler/Koop, 12.

10 In his memoir, Koop's memory is somewhat altered. Ravdin directs him to seek the internship at the Pennsylvania Hospital, and threatens only two years in the dog lab, not four. Koop memoir, 60. It used to be standard for medical schools to train students and residents in surgery using dogs and pigs and other animals. The last north American medical school only just ended the practice. Of course, as we have seen, Koop had had his own surgical practice on small animals as a boy—at home, with the help of his mother! See "Last U.S. Medical School Still Killed Animals to Teach Surgery but No More," *Washington Post*, June 30, 2016.

11 Ziegler/Koop, 12.

12 "The reminiscences of Isadore Ravdin, 1894–1972," 221. Even here in the title Ravdin's given name is mis-spelled! The Penn archives recommend Isidor, though their own usage varies. https://archives.upenn.edu/collections/finding-aid/upt50r252/. He went by I.S. or Rav. Ravdin spent forty years in the U.S. military, retiring in 1956 as a Major General, the first officer on non-active military service to achieve that rank.

13 Ravdin to Rhoads, October 6, 1940. Penn Box 23.

14 Ziegler/Koop, 11, 12.

15 His early publications included a paper on gelatin as a plasma substitute, co-written with Louisa Bullitt, for the *American Journal of the Medical Sciences*, January 1945.

16 *US News and World Report*, May 30, 1988, 56.

17 Koop to Rhoads, undated [June, 1945]; Koop to Bender, June 28 and July 11, 1945; Koop to Pipes, July 11, 1945. ACC 2014–016 Box 26/33.

18 *Washington Post* obituary, February 25, 2013.

19 Ziegler/Koop, 11–14.

20 I.S. Ravdin to Koop. Penn Box 22 F 23.

21 Ziegler in Ziegler/Koop, 16.

22 *Washington Post* obituary, February 25, 2013.

23 Ziegler/Koop, 19.

24 Elsewhere, he recalls responding with news of the position he had discussed with Memorial Hospital in New York City and Cornell. Either way, he was overruled! Children's Hospital History Project, interview November 22, 2002. ACC 2015–011 Koop Papers 1942–2009 Box 2/4, 2.

25 Children's Hospital History Project, interview November 22, 2002. ACC 2015–011 Koop Papers 1942–2009 Box 2/4, 10.

26 The system seems to have been for a roster of "consultants" to work with Koop for six-month stints. Koop discusses this in a letter to Rhoads of August 11, 1947. ACC 2014–016 Box 26/33. Koop, untitled reminiscence. ACC 2015–011 Koop Papers 1945–2009 Box 1.

27 Eugene Betts, National Memorial Service, at 1h15m. https://www.youtube.com /watch?v=FBm6xZSmgro.

28 Ziegler/Koop, 20.

29 Ziegler/Koop, 20.

30 Ziegler/Koop, 20.

31 Ziegler/Koop, 18–20.

32 Gregg Easterbrook, *Surgeon Koop* (N.l: Whittle, 2001), 7.

33 Don K. Nakayama, "Vignettes from the History of Pediatric Surgery," *Journal of Pediatric Surgery*, 2019, S5.

34 Ziegler/Koop, 18. One of the part-time surgeons did not respond to a call, and a child with an intussusception (an obstruction of the intestine, where one segment slips into another) died as a result.

35 Koop, untitled reminiscence.

36 *New York Times* obituary, February 26, 2013.

37 Catherine Musemeche, *Small: Life and Death on the Frontlines of Pediatric Surgery* (Hanover, NH: Dartmouth College Press, 2014), 27.

38 Discussed in Briana Ralston, "'We Were the Eyes and Ears . . .': Nursing and the Development of Neonatal intensive Care Units in the United States, 1955–1982." (PhD diss., University of Pennsylvania, 2015.)

39 Koop memoir, 79.

40 Kristin A. Zeller, et al., "History of Pediatric Surgery," www.pedsurglibrary.com/apsa.

41 Peter J. Safar, *An Autobiographical Memoir* (Park Ridge, IL: Wood Library Museum of Anesthesiology, 2000), 74.

42 Koop memoir, 75 and 79.

43 Ehrhart/Bishop, 2.

44 Koop to Ravdin, May 2, 1946. Penn Box 23.

45 Koop to Ravdin, May 9, 1946. Penn Box 23.

46 Heskel/Koop, 16,17. It was at either 15 or 17 Adams Street; Koop gives both numbers in different interviews.

47 Heskel/Koop, 18. The housing situation must have been extraordinarily difficult for Betty, with a two-year-old and a newborn to care for.

48 It's interesting to note Koop's use of "pediatric surgery" here, which anticipates his later decision to make it his preferred term for the discipline. His departmental letterhead at the Children's Hospital through the end of the 1940s continued to read, "Surgery of Infancy and Childhood."

49 Ravdin to Koop, May 12, 1946. Penn Box 23. The Boston Children's Hospital had (and has) a similar relationship with Harvard as do their equivalents in Philadelphia. In his c.v. Koop records a fellowship at the hospital, though the Harvard archives have no record of his visit. Email from Stephanie Krauss of the Countway Library, October 24, 2022. C.v. at Ziegler/Koop, 73.

50 Untitled memo. ACC 2015 Koop Papers 1942 Box 1. At another place Koop states it as $1,000 and adds that he got a further $1,000 from Knox Gelatin Co. for his work in assisting their development of gelatin as a plasma substitute. Biographical notes. ACC 2014–016 Koop papers Box 26/33.

51 Ravdin to Koop, August 15. Penn 23. Koop notes that this is the first time his chief has signed off with his nickname, Rav, doubtless to cushion the blow. Koop's memoir records that he fired off a furiously impertinent response: "Dear Rav, I wouldn't worry about $50.00 if I were you," signed "Chick." He remarks, "I don't know what he thought about my reply; no additional money came my way."

   Koop's memory is unreliable. The sum involved was actually $15, not $50, and his response to his chief was a good deal more polite. On August 11 he reminds him that hitherto he has received a raise of $115 each year, to begin with the July check. This year there has been none, so the financial news has been bad on two scores. His final paragraph: "Sorry to write you about the . . . money question, but a hundred fifteen dollars still seems like a lot of money to me." Koop to Ravdin August 11, 1946. Penn Box 23.

52 Ravdin to Koop, June 11, 1948. Penn Box 23.

53 Koop to Ravdin, August 8; Ravdin to Koop, August 15. Penn Box 23.

54 Children's Hospital History Project, interview November 22, 2002. ACC 2015–011 Koop Papers 1942–2009 Box 2/4, 5,6.

55 Nakayama, "Vignettes," S36.

56 Judson Randolph, "The First of the Best," *Journal of Pediatric Surgery*, 20 no. 6 (1985), 580.

57 Randolph, "First of the Best," 580.

58 Koop to Rhoads, July 31, 1948. ACC 2014–016 Box 26/33.

59 "Did you know? Surgical pioneer defied authority to conduct landmark operation," *AAP News*, December 17, 2015. See also Children's Hospital History Project, interview November 22, 2002. ACC 2015–011 Koop Papers 1942–2009 Box 2/4, 5–7.

60 Heskel/Koop, 19. They got a car soon after.

61 Koop to Gross, December 5, 1946. ACC 2014–16 Box 25/33.

62 Koop's trainee Moritz Ziegler would later occupy the chair named for Gross.

63 Ziegler/Koop, 24–27.

64 Koop memoir, 102. The American Pediatric Surgical Association (wrongly) names Koop's later trainee Rowena Spencer as the first woman to be trained in pediatric surgery in the United States, perhaps because Bender did not go on to practice in the specialty, whereas Spencer became a celebrated pediatric surgeon. See Don

Nakayama, David Powell, Mary Fallat, George W. Holcomb III, *Saving Lifetimes. Celebrating the 50th Anniversary of the American Pediatric Surgical Association* (N.l.: American Pediatric Surgical Association, 2019). Available at: *https://www. pedsurglibrary.com/library/Saving_Lifetimes_2019.pdf*.

65 Rhoads to Koop, December 31, 1945. ACC 2014–016 Box 26/33. Rhoads' tone suggests this is a personal gift.

66 Memo to self, undated, mid-1950s. ACC 2014-016 Box 26/33.

CHAPTER 4: Shaping a Specialty

1 AAP Tumor Registry Committee minutes, June 24, 1951.

2 AAP Board minutes, March 31, 1955.

3 AAP Committee on Accident Prevention minutes, October 2, 1955.

4 AAP Committee on Accident Prevention minutes, October 2, 1955.

5 AAP Committee of Section on Surgery minutes, April 4, 1953.

6 C. Everett Koop, "Pediatric Surgery: The Long Road to Recognition," *Pediatrics* 92 no. 4 (1993), 620–21.

7 It's not entirely clear whether he was the fourth full-time pediatric surgeon. In one interview he states that he was the sixth, though at the same time actually the first to refuse *any* adult surgery. "Even Robert E. Gross did occasional gallbladders." Heskel/Koop, 20. Another time he says he was sixth or seventh. "Pediatric Surgery—Reflections on the First Quarter Century," speech at the Children's Hospital, February 9, 1971. HML CHOP records Box 63.

8 Don K. Nakayama, "Vignettes from the History of Pediatric Surgery," *Journal of Pediatric Surgery* (2019), S3, S4.

9 Judson Randolph, "The First of the Best," *Journal of Pediatric Surgery* 20, no.6 (1985), 580–81.

10 Ziegler/Koop, 20–21.

11 Kristen A. Zeller, et al., "History of Pediatric Surgery," www.pedsurglibrary.com/ apsa. 1/18 actually gives both 1930 and 1936 as cut-off dates for his general practice on the same page! He has written that it was "As soon as it became feasible after the first world war." Ladd later clarified: "As far as the effect [Halifax] . . . had on my selection of a specialty I would say nil."

12 Nakayama, "Vignettes," S3.

13 Zeller, "History of Pediatric Surgery," 1/18.

14 Zeller, "History of Pediatric Surgery," 2/18. These early leaders were strong personalities. For all their shared commitment to children's surgery, they could be very difficult people, and there had been a falling out between Ladd and Gross. Discussed in Chapter 3.

15 Dale G. Johnson, "Excellence in Search of Recognition," *Journal of Pediatric Surgery* 21 (1986), 1019.

16 Zeller, "History of Pediatric Surgery," 2/18.

17 Nakayama, "Vignettes," S6, S7.

18 Zeller, "History of Pediatric Surgery," 33, 34

19 Nakayama, "Vignettes," S34.

20 Koop, "Pediatric Surgery," 619.

21 Ziegler/Koop, 29; Nakayama, "Vignettes," S28.

22 Nakayama, "Vignettes," S28.

23 Zeller, "History of Pediatric Surgery," 2/18.

24 Zeller, "History of Pediatric Surgery," 2/18.

25 For a brief history of the journal, see Jay L. Grosfeld, "The *Journal of Pediatric Surgery*—Celebrates its 50th Anniversary," *Journal of Pediatric Surgery* 50 (2015), 1–4.

26 Quoting Johnson in Zeller, "History of Pediatric Surgery," 2/18.

27 Willis Potts wrote to congratulate Koop on the first issue of the new journal in a letter Koop likely found slightly uncomfortable, since amidst his congratulations he notes that Koop's appointment as editor had actually been Potts' idea! Potts to Koop, ACC 2014–16 Box 26/33.

28 Zeller, "History of Pediatric Surgery," 3/18.

29 Quoted in Grosfeld, "The *Journal of Pediatric Surgery*," 1.

30 Koop, "Pediatric Surgery," 621.

31 Zeller, "History of Pediatric Surgery," 4/18.

32 Dale G. Johnson, "Excellence," 1027–28.

33 Koop to Rhoads, February 14, 1968. ACC 2014–016 Box 26/33.

34 Holcomb/O'Neill, 42.

35 C. E. Koop, "A Perspective on the Early Days of Pediatric Surgery," *Journal of Pediatric Surgery* 38, no. 5, S1, 38.

36 Holcomb/O'Neill, 42–43.

37 Grosfield/Beardmore, 34, 26–7.

38 John Foster Cooper, *The Surgical Diseases of Children* (London: Parker, 1860; repr. Miami, FL: Hardpress, 2017).

39 Nakayama, "Vignettes," S10.

40 Children's Hospital History Project, interview November 22, 2002. ACC 2015–011 Koop Papers 1942–2009. Box 2/4, 19.

41 Nakayama, "Vignettes," S8.

42 *The Bulletin* [Philadelphia], April 29, 1981, B4.

43 C. Everett Koop, "A Glimpse at the Early BAPS," *Journal of Pediatric Surgery* 38, no. 7 (2003), 23.

44 Koop to Ravdin and his wife, September 5, 1963. His visitors were Peter Paul Rickham, Robert Zachary, and David Waterston, the first two accompanied by their wives. Penn Box 19.

45 Koop to Ravdin, October 22, 1963; reply November 15, 1963. Koop in turn solicits ideas from the British surgeons, and forwards Rickham's response to Ravdin on December 17, 1963. Penn Box 19.

46 C. Everett Koop, "A Glimpse at the Early BAPS," *Journal of Pediatric Surgery* 38, no. 7 (2003), 23.

47 Dartmouth College website bio.

48 Author of *Neonatal Surgery*, "for many years the standard text," per his London *Times* obituary, January 12, 2003.

49 Peter-Paul Reichenheim, born at Wannsee in Germany, was processed as an enemy alien but granted refugee status November 21, 1939. See Ancestry.com.

50 George W. Holcomb, III, "The Journal of Pediatric Surgery: its First 50 Years, *Journal of Pediatric Surgery* 53 (2018).

51 See Lewis Spitz, "Robert Bransby Zachary," *British Medical Journal*, April 17, 1999.

52 Koop to Margaret Barnhouse, June 25, 1966. ACC 2014–016 Box 24/33. Carcassonne was keen to have their daughter study at Bryn Mawr, though apparently his wife was less enthusiastic. Koop was encouraging, and assured his friend he will help out if she is admitted. Koop to Carcassonne, March 1, 1967. ACC 2014–016 Box 26/33. Per the office of the president of Bryn Mawr, Cathy did not matriculate. Email, May 18, 2023.
53 Holcomb, "The Journal of Pediatric Surgery."
54 Biographical notes, ACC 2014–016 Koop papers Box 26/33.
55 American Board of Medical Specialties. ABMS.org. See Koop, "Pediatric Surgery," 621.

CHAPTER 5: At the Children's Hospital

1 Ravdin to Koop, October 31, 1956. Penn Box 21.
2 Kristen A. Zeller, et al., "History of Pediatric Surgery," www.pedsurlibrary.com/apsa.
3 For a biographical sketch, see "I.S. Ravdin: Larger—and Smaller—than Life," *Penn Medicine News*, Summer 2015.
4 Ravdin built on the suggestion of his colleague Jonathan Rhoads. Transcript courtesy of Scott Adzick, MD, Children's Hospital of Philadelphia.
5 Dinner transcript courtesy of Scott Adzick, MD, Children's Hospital of Philadelphia.
6 Koop memoir, 68.
7 Moritz Ziegler, email March 25, 2023.
8 Ravdin to Koop, July 12, 1950. Penn Box 22.
9 Ravdin to Koop, May 8, 1952. Penn Box 21.
10 Koop to Ravdin, December 3, 1952. Penn Box 21.
11 Ravdin to Koop, March 9, 1955. Box Penn 21.
12 Ravdin to Koop, July 29, 1954. ACC 2014–016 Box 26/33.
13 Ravdin to Koop, April 28, 1954; Koop to Ravdin, April 29, 1954. ACC 2014–016 Box 26/33.
14 Ravdin to Koop, December 20, 1948. Penn Box 23.
15 Ravdin to Koop, February 12, 1955. Penn Box 21.
16 Koop memoir, 68.
17 Penn R252 Ravdin papers Box 22 F20.
18 Koop to Ravdin, April 21, 1961. Penn Box 19
19 Koop to Ravdin, June 11, 1962; Ravdin reply, June 16, 1962. ACC 2014–016 Box 26/33.
20 Koop to Ravdin, October 18, 1956; Ravdin reply, October 24. Penn Box 21.
21 Penn R252 Ravdin papers, Box 22 F20. No honorary degree was awarded to Ravdin; confirmed to me by Stefanie Diaz in the president's office, email March 1, 2023.
22 Ravdin to Koop, June 16, 1962. Penn Box 19.
23 Ravdin, *Reminiscences*. See also Columbia interviews of November 17, 1955; December 1, 1955; and December 15, 1955.
24 Ravdin, *Reminiscences*, 14–15. In the year before college, Ravdin worked with a printer/publisher setting up religious magazines.
25 Rhoads' remarkable life is well reviewed in this *New York Times* obituary, February 8, 2002. Clyde F. Barker summarizes his life in an introduction to a symposium convened in his honor following his death in 2002. *Proceedings of the American Philosophical Society* 147, no. 3 (September 2003). See also, Ravdin, *Reminiscences*, 221.

26 Barker, *Proceedings.*

27 Biographical notes. ACC 2014–016 Koop papers Box 26/33.

28 Koop to Rhoads, August 11, 1947; Rhoads to Koop, August 26, 1947. ACC 2014–016 Box 26/33.

29 Koop memoir, 75, 76.

30 Confidential interview.

31 Peter J. Safar, *An Autobiographical Memoir* (Park Ridge, IL: Wood Library-Museum of Anesthesiology, 2000), 71, 68.

32 Safar, *An Autobiographical Memoir,* 74.

33 Koop recalls approaching Ravdin about the need for action on anesthesia, thereby triggering Deming's move. ACC 201 Koop Papers 1942–2009 Box 1. The timing of her arrival makes this explanation implausible.

34 Safar, *An Autobiographical Memoir,* 82–83.

35 Selma Harrison Calmes, "The First Anesthesiologist at America's First Children's Hospital: Margo Deming, M.D.," *American Society of Anesthesiologists Newsletter,* October 1998, 22, 23. As we have noted, Koop actually returned to the hospital in October of the year. John J. Downes, later Anesthesiologist-in-Chief, in a 1992 oral history interview, oddly states that Deming did not begin her work full-time at the Children's Hospital until 1950. HML CHOP files.

36 Calmes, "The First Anesthesiologist," 22.

37 Calmes, "The First Anesthesiologist," 22.

38 Koop memoir, 99.

39 Gregg Easterbrook, *Surgeon Koop* (N.l.: Whittle, 2001), 10.

40 Koop memoir, 99.

41 See, for example, Christine L. Mai and Charles J. Coté, "A History of Pediatric Anesthesia: a Tale of Pioneers and Equipment," in *Pediatric Anesthesia,* 23 March, 2012.

42 Calmes, "The First Anesthesiologist," 24.

43 Koop to Ravdin, June 21, 1954. Penn Box 21.

44 Calmes, "The First Anesthesiologist," 23.

45 Easterbrook, *Surgeon Koop,* 10.

46 HUP refers to the Hospital of the University of Pennsylvania, where Koop and Deming were colleagues before their appointments to the Children's Hospital. Koop to Deming, January 23, 1992. DA-698 Box 1964.

47 Easterbrook, *Surgeon Koop,* 10–11.

48 Untitled, ACC 2015–011 Papers 1942–2009 Boxes 1, 11.

49 Untitled, ACC 2015–011 Papers 1942–2009 Boxes 1, 12–14.

50 Remarks to the Children's Hospital Alumni Organization, May 20, 1988. HML CHOP Box 79, 11–12.

51 I am indebted to Moritz Ziegler, who together with Ali Kaviani maintained over many years a contact list and organized get-togethers, the last of which was in association with Koop's funeral. Ziegler's list is of forty-three, to which I have added four more from other research. In addition there were occasional international trainees, for varying periods of time. Ziegler email, March 25, 2023.

52 Rowena Spencer was the first female surgical intern at Hopkins. See obituary, https://www.nola.com/entertainment_life/health_fitness/dr-rowena-spencer-trailblazing-pediatric-surgeon-dies-at-91/article_6e4da24c-2412-572d-982a-0983f6fac279.html.

When Spencer returned to Mississippi, she became the first woman surgeon in the state. Even the Association of Women Surgeons does not know how many women surgeons there were at the time. Email from Valerie Workman, February 21, 2024.

53 Bender: Doris Bender "held the fort" for Koop while he was in Boston. Heskel/Koop, 20. Later, in August 1948, she "supervised" Rowena Spencer and another trainee during his vacation. "Doris has a special knack for knowing a sick baby," he wrote to Rhoads, July 31, 1946. ACC 2014–016 Box 26/33. As noted above, the American Pediatric Surgical Association wrongly claims that his later trainee Rowena Spencer was the first American woman to be trained in pediatric surgery. Spencer: Ehrhart/Koop, 71. Jones: The precise dates of Jones' time with Koop are not clear, but apparently during 1951–52. In January 1953 we find him discussing whether she has improved her performance during her time at the Children's Hospital, for a professional reference; he notes that she spent one year there. Draft letter to James B. Flick, undated, enclosed with letter to Ravdin, January 7, 1953. Penn Box 21. Wagner: Ehrhart/Koop, 71. Schnaufer: Ehrhart/Koop, 71. Curiously, Schnaufer was the final woman trainee; the more than forty others would all be men. Koop's memory is a little different. He recalls six women out of thirty trainees. Koop to the editor, *Newsweek*, June 2, 1981. MSC 487 Box 68.

54 Koop to Ravdin, December 17, 1948; Ravdin to Koop, December 20, 1948. Penn Box 23.

55 Ehrhart/Taylor, 169–70. "I tried to know as much as I could about the wives of the residents whom I appointed on my service because I think they were responsible for the success of their husbands and the success of their marriage, and you can tell when you meet some wives that the battle is already lost; there's not much point in going on. I only had one female pediatric surgeon who came to me already married and others who did marry, so I'm not basing this on just gender, and I should say 'spouse.' I think in a surgical world, a spouse of a female surgeon has a tough road, because it is a tough life, and there are a lot of things that a man expects of his wife, even if she's got a job, that a female surgeon, who's busy, is not going to be able to satisfy. So I think that the right person in a marriage and the right of set of values of what it's all about are important." Ziegler/Koop, 63, 64.

56 Koop to Rhoads, July 31, 1948. ACC 2014–016 Box 26/33.

57 She would go on to endow a chair at Hopkins named for her surgeon father, the Lewis Cass Spencer Chair of Orthopaedic Surgery, in 1997.

58 "This Month in History: Dr. Rowena Spencer and Her Little Chickens," undated, at https://www.lsuhsc.edu/library/news/?p=7798. Blalock and Thomas would collaborate in developing a revolutionary treatment for "blue baby" syndrome, which became the theme of a PBS documentary. In 1976 Hopkins awarded Thomas an honorary doctorate. In the documentary, Spencer comments: "Many times in my career I was complimented on my surgical technique and I will admit that a good many people were shocked when I told them I learned my surgical technique from a black man who had only a high school education." The fascinating and generally unedifying story of Thomas and "academic larceny," which includes references to Rowena Spencer, is told in Don K. Nakayama, ed., *Black Surgeons and Surgery in America* (Chicago: American College of Surgeons, 2021).

59 *Hopkins Medicine*, Fall 2014.

60 Most of Koop's trainees kept in close touch with their mentor down the years.

Spencer's relationship with him may have been more distant because she credited Hopkins—and Thomas—with her key surgical training. She did not attend Koop's 1981 retirement dinner. Spencer's text: Rowena Spencer, *Conjoined Twins: Developmental Malformations and Clinical Implications* (Baltimore, MD: Johns Hopkins University Press, 2003).

61 Ziegler email, March 25, 2023.

62 Retirement dinner listing. ACC 2014–016 Post-APSA/BMP Phila. April 81.

63 "Dr. Rowena Spencer and Her Little Chickens."

64 Biographical summary in his obituary, *Philadelphia Inquirer*, May 14, 2009.

65 Obituary, *Philadelphia Inquirer*.

66 See https://www.philadelphia-reflections.com/blog/1748.htm.

67 Moritz Ziegler interview.

68 Ehrhart/Bishop, 15.

69 Ehrhart/Bishop, 10.

70 Moritz Ziegler interview.

71 Ehrhart/Koop, 88.

72 Ehrhart/O'Neill, 127.

73 Ehrhart/Bishop, 13.

74 Ehrhart/O'Neill, 120.

75 Penn Box 21.

76 Ehrhart/Koop, 72.

77 Ehrhart/Bishop, 13.

78 Ehrhart/Melhuish, 105.

79 Ehrhart/Koop, 87.

80 Moritz Ziegler interview.

81 Ehrhart/Taylor, 167.

82 Kristen A. Zeller, et al., "History of Pediatric Surgery," www.pedsurglibrary .com/apsa. Several Koop dates in this article are inaccurate, and Deming's name is misspelled.

83 Michael Gauderer and Moritz Ziegler, "Charles Everett Koop MD, DSc October 16, 1916–February 25, 2013," *Journal of Pediatric Surgery* 48, no. 6 (2013).

84 Judson Randolph, "The First of the Best," *Journal of Pediatric Surgery* 20, no. 6 (1985), 586.

85 Ehrhart/Koop, 81.

86 Bio notes. ACC 2014–016 Koop papers Box 26/33.

87 From undated notes for a book on leadership. ACC Box 21.

88 Briana Ralston, "'We Were the Eyes and Ears . . .': Nursing and the Development of Neonatal intensive Care Units in the United States, 1955–1982" (PhD diss., University of Pennsylvania, 2015), 275.

89 David G. Nichols, *Roger's Textbook of Pediatric Intensive Care* (Philadelphia: Lippincott, Williams and Wilkins), 4th edition, 2008, 97. It runs to 5,168 pages.

90 Confidential interview. See Chapter 5 on Erna Goulding's role at the Children's Hospital.

91 Koop memoir, 102.

92 Goulding memorial service at Tenth, December 18, 2012.

93 John B. Freeman interview. Freeman had first met Koop around 1990, and been surprised to find that he knew all about the organization; Koop handed Freeman

a check for $25,000 he had just received as an award. Erna Goulding, now retired from the Children's Hospital, was at this point a board member of Harvest. Freeman recalls the time he "questioned her about something I asked her to do in the office. She said, 'John, I was in charge of nine hundred nurses every day. I think I can do this.' Yes. She was a character!" For reasons that are unclear, she seems to have played no part in the Koop retirement dinner.

94 See Chapter 5.

95 Untitled memo. ACC 2–15 Koop Papers Box 1. The comment was relayed to Koop by his trainee, Dorothy Bender.

96 Koop to Erna Goulding, January 31, 1947. Penn 23.

97 Koop to Ravdin, with Koop's addendum and Ravdin's reply at the foot. Penn Box 23. This rather curious document resembles an email exchange! Koop's December 13 recruitment letter to Goulding had fortunately begun by stating that he had heard of her plan to leave the University Hospital. The following year a similar misunderstanding would strain the relationship, this time over a part-time affiliation with the Children's Hospital of a University Hospital anesthesiologist. Once Koop explains, again after the event, a mollified Ravdin confesses that "Your letter throws an entirely new light on the matter." Penn Box 23.

98 ACC Box 21.

99 Gauderer and Ziegler, "Charles Everett Koop MD."

100 Moritz Ziegler interview.

101 *Pennsylvania Medicine*, December 1985, 30. Whether by ironic accident or design, the facing page 31 includes a half-page ad for malpractice insurance! Koop's claim requires qualification. While the ultimate disposal of the case is unclear, Koop and another physician were sued for malpractice in the Superior Court of New Jersey by one Louise Brinson, on behalf of her infant son Donnell, on April 8, 1983. MSC 489 Box 74.

102 Transcript courtesy of Scott Adzick, MD, the Children's Hospital of Philadelphia. Transcript: "uncanningly."

103 The Evangelical Child and Family Service, founded in 1960 with Koop's friend and Children's Hospital nurse Erna Goulding as a trustee. The charity offered in addition to adoption services for "unwed mothers" foster homes and family counseling. ACC 2014–16 Box 22.

104 Ziegler/Koop, 38.

105 Ziegler/Koop, 36. He had never once had a former patient come back to him as an adult and say, "I wish I had never been born," 35.

106 *US News and World Report*, May 30, 1988, 57.

107 Paul Sweeney interview.

108 Easterbrook, *Surgeon Koop*, 27–29.

109 Shared by Carl Lingle.

110 "What I Tell the Parents of a Dying Child," *Reader's Digest*, February, 1968.

111 Nichols, *Roger's Textbook*, 90.

112 Ralston, "'Eyes and Ears . . . ,'" 276.

113 Ralston, "'Eyes and Ears . . . ,'" 276.

114 Zeller et al., "History of Pediatric Surgery."

115 Ralston, "'Eyes and Ears . . . ,'" 267–68.

116 This was the third grant that Koop had written for the purpose. The first two had not been funded. Ralston, "'Eyes and Ears . . . ,'" 268–69.

117 Gauderer and Ziegler, "Charles Everett Koop MD." Ralston notes that, reflecting usage at the time, "The documents in the archives themselves as well as the nursing personnel interviewed refer to the unit as the infant intensive care unit, or IICU." "'Eyes and Ears . . . ,'" 275.

118 Koop recollects the politics involved. "Eventually, we had Co-Chiefs [presumably, to manage the two units]. When we moved to the new building, I gave it up because I got tired of fighting." Koop to H. William Clatworthy, October 13, 1993. DA-698 Box 1965.

119 Society for Pediatric Anesthesia obituary: "In Memoriam, John J. 'Jack' Downes," https://pedsanesthesia.org/in-memoriam-john-j-jack-downes-md/.

120 Nichols, *Roger's Textbook*, 98.

121 ACC 2015–011 Papers 1942–2009 Box 1.

122 See https://www.guinnessworldrecords.com/news/2022/12/the-dark-history-of-the-original-siamese-twins-chang-and-eng-bunker-730957, where it is noted that they were also slaveholders.

123 See James O'Neill, Jr., and nine others, including Koop, "Surgical Experience with Thirteen Conjoined Twins," a review of thirty years of such surgeries at the Children's Hospital, *Annals of Surgery* 208 (1988). See Koop memoir, 110.

124 Ehrhart/Koop, 74.

125 Ehrhart/Koop, 80.

126 Koop to Earl L. Boyette, November 23, 1981. This generalization is of course not accurate. MSC 489 Box 68. In his memoir, Koop notes that he had been involved with "more than ten" conjoined twin separations in all, 110.

127 Gregg Easterbrook, "A Moral Precedent for the Siamese Twins Case," on Beliefnet, https://www.beliefnet.com/love-family/parenting/2000/09/a-moral-precedent-for-the-siamese-twins-case.aspx.

128 *New York Times*, September 20, 1974.

129 *New York Times*, September 19, 1974.

130 *Pennsylvania Gazette*, December 1974, 2.

131 Madeline Bell, *The Children's Hospital of Philadelphia* (Images of America) (Mount Pleasant, SC: Arcadia Publishing, 2015), 89.

132 Marlene Cimons, *Los Angeles Times Magazine*, September 14, 1986, 20.

133 Donald C. Drake, "Zealot for life," *Philadelphia Inquirer*, September 2, 1979.

134 Quinn to Koop, November 3, 1976. MSC 489 Box 79. Quinn was Canadian. Koop memoir, 112.

135 Quinn to Koop, February 11, 1977. MSC 498 Box 78.

136 The identity of the family was kept secret at the time. For reasons that are not clear, perhaps simply to enliven his narrative, Koop's colleague Jack Templeton—who would soon leave the practice of medicine to run his family's charitable foundation—decided to name them Brisk and identify them as boys in his memoir, *John M. Templeton Jr.* (Philadelphia: Templeton Press, 2008), 271–72. Koop confirms they were girls, memoir, 113.

137 Marlene Cimons, *Los Angeles Times Magazine*, September 14, 1986, 20.

138 Donald C. Drake, "Siamese Twins. The Surgery: An Agonizing Choice—Parents, Doctors, Rabbis In Dilemma," *Philadelphia Inquirer*, October 16, 1977.

139 On the play, see Chapter 18.

140 Marlene Cimons, *Los Angeles Times Magazine*, September 14, 1986, 20.

141 His memory has shifted slightly in a letter later that year to an inquiring naval chaplain; it took the rabbis fifteen days to decide, and took him fifteen minutes. Koop to Earl L. Boyette, October 14, 1981. MSC 489 Box 68.

142 Cited by Easterbrook, "A Moral Precedent for the Siamese Twins Case."

143 Marlene Cimons, *Los Angeles Times Magazine*, September 14, 1986, 20.

144 Drake, "Siamese Twins."

145 Josephine Templeton, oral history interview, https://collections.countway.harvard.edu/onview/files/original/a06d39447b975140218c7114407b09e0.pdf.

146 Moritz Ziegler interview.

147 Josephine Templeton, oral history interview, https://collections.countway.harvard.edu/onview/files/original/a06d39447b975140218c7114407b09e0.pdf.

148 Moritz Ziegler interview.

149 Koop notes for a book on Leadership. ACC Box 21.

150 *Shelby Sun Times*, 7 February, 1991, reporting the January 23 visit. https://profiles.nlm.nih.gov/spotlight/qq/catalog/nlm:nlmuid-101584930X381-img https://www.memphiszoo.org/primate-canyon.

151 Ehrhart/Koop, 85–86.

152 Biographical notes. ACC 2014–016 Koop papers Box 26/33. Also confidential communication. In another version of the story, the patient was the godfather's granddaughter.

153 Gauderer and Ziegler, "Charles Everett Koop MD."

154 Ziegler/Koop, 34–35.

155 C. Everett Koop, "Pediatric Surgery: The Long Road to Recognition," *Pediatrics* 92, no. 4 (1993), 619.

156 Koop, "Pediatric Surgery," 619.

157 Ziegler/Koop, 35–36.

158 Marlene Cimons, *Los Angeles Times Magazine*, September 14, 1986, 20.

159 Penn Box 15. The specialisms are: neurosurgery (two surgeons), cardiovascular (two), ophthalmology (four), orthopedic (nine), otorhinolaryngology (two), urology (three), plastic and reconstructive (three), with Koop and six others listed as general surgeons—his key colleagues: Harry C. Bishop, Louise Schnaufer, John M. Templeton, Jr., Moritz M. Ziegler, Gertrude J. Frishmuth, and Martin R. Eichelberger.

160 Gauderer and Ziegler, "Charles Everett Koop MD."

161 Koop to Schaeffer, August 22, 1980; Schaeffer to Koop, September 22, 1980. MSC 489 Box 78.

162 Koop to Rickham, November 7, 1979. ACC 2014–016 Box 26/33.

163 Koop to Rickham, January 7, 1981. ACC 2014–016 Box 26/33.

164 Koop to Chase N. Peterson, May 4, 1982, confirms the month of his formal retirement. MSC 489 Box 69. In a press report of the retirement dinner it is given as March 9, "to become deputy assistant secretary of health." *The Bulletin*, April 29, 1981. In a memo to the White House counsel, Koop gives it as February 28, 1981. August 6, 1981. MSC 489 Box 68.

165 Harry C. Bishop to Jonathan E. Rhoads, October 15, 1980. Penn Box 15.

166 Holcomb/O'Neill, 26. "So I was more or less resented, because they had a

fair-haired boy, who was not in Philadelphia at the time, that they wanted to have come back, who would have been an excellent choice, by the way. But be that as it may, they chose me. But the people there didn't like it."

167 The restaurant, which claims origins in the sixteenth century, continues to flourish. https://tourdargent.com/.

168 Michel Carcassonne to Koop, April 21, 1980; invitation from the Assemblée Nationale for June 4; menu. NLM Box 144. The *Légion d'honneur* is indeed a high award, though over the years it has been distributed with increasing liberality. There are currently between two and three thousand awardees each year, including several hundred foreigners. President Macron is reported to be seeking to cut the number to six hundred. See "Emmanuel Macron lance la réforme de la Légion d'honneur," *Figaro*, November 12, 2017. (By comparison, the Presidential Medal of Freedom, awarded to Koop by President Clinton in 1995, has around ten recipients a year.) *University of Pennsylvania Almanac*, August 14, 1980. Presentation by the president of the *Assemblée* is not typical and points up the importance of Carcassonne's friends (Barnhouse got his from a local official). Koop had not forgotten another of Carcassonne's parties, on a topless beach in Marseille, that had resulted in the arrest of "Iron Curtain" participants who got drunk in the old port later in the evening. Carcassonne had had to bail them out. Biographical notes. ACC 2014–016 Koop papers Box 26/33.

169 Peter-Paul Reichenheim was author of *Neonatal Surgery*, "for many years the standard text," per his London *Times* obituary, December 1, 2003.

170 Transcript of the dinner, courtesy of Scott Adzick, MD, and the Children's Hospital of Philadelphia.

171 ACC 2016–016 Koop Papers Box 26/33. Koop actually wrote (as he records) "but with a whimper."

Part III: CAMPAIGNER

1 An exception was a critical, unsigned editorial in *Christianity Today* for February 16, 1973, "Abortion and the Court." Its author was actually Harold O. J. Brown, then a young member of the editorial staff. Even the magazine itself has been confused by this outlier expression of opinion. "Most evangelical Christians at the time saw it as an appalling decision, disregarding the unalienable right of life," writes Daniel Silliman, citing that editorial, in a celebratory essay after Roe was overturned in 2022. This is completely misleading.

2 Walter O. Spitzer and Carlyle L. Saylor, ed., *Birth Control and the Christian. A Protestant Symposium on the Control of Human Reproduction* (Wheaton, IL: Tyndale House in association with the Christian Medical Society, 1969), 32.

3 Spitzer and Saylor, *Birth Control and the Christian.*

4 Spitzer and Saylor, *Birth Control and the Christian*, 33.

5 Quoted by Randall Balmer, "The Real Origins of the Religious Right," *Politico*, May 27, 2014. Criswell, like many more, would later revise his stance. See also Randall Balmer, *Bad Faith: Race and the Rise of the Religious Right* (Grand Rapids: Eerdmans, 2021).

6 See https://christiansforsocialaction.org/resource/the-importance-of-the-chicago-declaration/.

7   Randall Balmer interview. There was no strong voter political alignment on abortion until long after 1973. According to Linda Greenhouse and Reva B. Siegel in *Before Roe v. Wade*, "Only after 1988 does Gallup consistently show more Democrats than Republicans supporting access to abortion," (New York: Kaplan, 2010), 207. The striking exception among prominent evangelicals was Senator Mark Hatfield, who immediately introduced legislation to limit abortions. Interviews with Randall Balmer and Thomas Getman (former Hatfield staffer).

8   See Chapter 6.

CHAPTER 6: Advocate for Life

1   Wheaton College in Wheaton, Illinois, dates from 1860, when a struggling Wesleyan school was renamed by staunch abolitionist John Blanchard, though as a recent report has highlighted it soon abandoned its commitment to civil rights. "Wheaton College Releases Report on its History of Racism," *Christianity Today*, September 14, 2023.

2   So far as can be determined, this address, which represents the birth of the post-Roe evangelical pro-life movement, has never been published, except in an abbreviated version in the Tenth Presbyterian Church quarterly magazine, *Tenth*, for October 1973. It is archived in Box 1, Folder 10 of the papers Koop deposited in the Wheaton College Library Special Collections and footnoted as an unpublished address in his Ladd Speech that appeared in the *Human Life Review* 3(2), Spring 1977.

3   John P. Judis, "The Unlikely Celebrity of C. Everett Koop," *New Republic*, February 26, 2013. Brown played a key role in a wider process, in part enabled by growing practical collaboration between evangelicals and Catholics in the pro-life cause, an ecumenical dialog called Evangelicals and Catholics Together. Brown had been raised Catholic. See for example *First Things*, May 1994.

4   Elliot was the widow of one of the five missionaries to Ecuador whose killing by tribesmen in 1956 transfixed America and rapidly made her one of the best-known of evangelicals, especially after she followed her late husband to evangelize the tribespeople who had killed him. See *Time*, January 23, 1956. Robert Case interview and *National Right to Life News*, August 1975. See also, Jennifer Donnally, "The Politics of Abortion and the Rise of the New Right" (PhD diss., University of North Carolina, 2013).

5   Koop confirms that it was Catholic money that enabled this evangelical initiative. McFadden "put up the original money that made it possible." Koop to Joseph Stanton, June 17, 1980. ACC 2014–016 Box 26/33.

6   Koop to Robert Liken, October 21, 1977. ACC 2014–016 Box 18/33.

7   Robert Case, "Harold O. J. 'Joe' Brown, the Christian Action Council and Me," May 15, 2011. https://theaquilareport.com/harold-o-j-joe-brown-the-christian-action-council-and-me/.

8   The name of the Christian Action Council would later be changed to CareNet; there are now around eleven hundred "crisis pregnancy centers" in its network. See care-net.org.

9   Mike Mallowe, *Interview Magazine*, April 1982, 28. He continues: "That makes it easy to move on to the next classification of citizens who might not be seen as having a life worth living, and that's the elderly. There's three groups who have no

advocate—the unborn, the newborn and the aged. But believe me, as Surgeon General, I intend to give them an advocate." "A career switch to public affairs seemed an inviting prospect, and the antiabortion movement had what might be called job openings," noted Gregg Easterbrook in his essay *Surgeon Koop* (N.l., Whittle: 2001), 37.

10 Koop to Lindsell, November 19, 1976. Wheaton Koop Box 2.

11 Raymond S. Duff & A. G. M. Campbell, "Moral and Ethical Dilemmas in the Special-Care Nursery," *New England Journal of Medicine* 289 (1973), 890–94. The debate and its impact are helpfully reviewed in Mark R. Mercurio, "The Aftermath of Baby Doe and the Evolution of Newborn Intensive Care," *Georgia State University Law Review*, 2012.

12 Speaking with Koop many years later, Moritz Ziegler reminded him of the occasion—at which Ziegler, then a resident, had been present. He probes gently. "And there was a fair amount of controversy around it. Or, said a different way, there were those in the audience who were not aligned with you." Koop responds with a story about a British "Baby Doe" case in which he was informally involved. He does not address the furor his address provoked. Ziegler/Koop, 39.

13 *The Human Life Review*, May 1977.

14 Allan C. Carlson, *Godly Seed: Evangelicals Confront Birth Control, 1873–1973* (New Brunswick, Canada: Transaction, 2011), 154.

15 Confidential interview.

16 Matthew Miller, "'No Diga Mentiras': The Pivotal Role of Harold O.J. Brown in the Emergence of the Evangelical Pro-life Movement" (ThM diss., Erskine Theological Seminary, SC, 2015), 31, reporting an interview with Brown's widow, Grace.

17 Carl F. H. Henry, spoken to Robert Case. Case added: "Without Joe Brown, it never would have happened. Brown was the animating force. He was the guy that had all the passion. . . . The grey eminence was Chick Koop. But Schaeffer and Koop did their series, and of course that changed everything." Robert Case interview.

18 D. Michael Lindsay, *Faith in the Halls of Power* (New York: Oxford University Press, 2007), 20. Koop and Henry exchanged several letters arranging the dinner, finally scheduled for February 13, 1970. "I trust you won't mind this being a stag affair so we can get to [sic] the business at hand accomplished if possible." Koop to Henry, December 11; Henry to Koop, December 18, 1969. Trinity Henry archive.

19 Koop to Henry, October 4; reply, October 23, 1979. Trinity Henry archive.

20 Judis, "Unlikely Celebrity."

21 Robert Case interview.

22 "Religion: Mission to Intellectuals," *Time*, January 11, 1960.

23 Koop memoir, 266.

24 Linny Dey to Koop, May 31, 1977. MSC 489 Box 78 Cor.

25 E.g., Frank Schaeffer, *Crazy for God* (Boston: Da Capo Press, 2008).

26 Francis A. Schaeffer, *How Should We Then Live?* (Wheaton, IL: Crossway), 1976.

27 Frank Schaeffer interview.

28 Koop memoir, 267.

29 Frank Schaeffer interview. Koop would likely have regarded Schaeffer's characterization as exaggerated, but there's no question this was a major salient in his thinking.

30 Mike Stobbe, *Surgeon General's Warning* (San Francisco: University of California Press, 2014), 173–74.

31 Harold O. J. Brown, "Protestantism, America and Divine Law," *Chronicles* maga-zine, June 2007.

32 James Risen and Judy L. Thomas, *Wrath of Angels* (New York: Basic Books, 1998), 122. The authors, claimed on the book jacket as the leading journalist experts on the anti-abortion movement, spoil their sometimes insightful analysis by sloppy confusion of evangelicals and fundamentalists. The jacket also makes the interest-ing claim that they are chronicling the "rise and fall" of the movement.

33 Frank E. Ehrlich, MD, to Koop, November 16, 1979. Wheaton Koop Box 1 F 9.

34 Nadine Brozan, "Two Fundamentalists Crusade against Abortion," *New York Times*, September 29, 1979.

35 "Remembering the New Right," June 10, 2009, paper for Political Research Asso-ciates. See https://politicalresearch.org/.

36 CACE Forum, "Ethics of Activism, Protest, and Dissent," Dr. C. Everett Koop's Remarks. Undated, early 1990s, Wheaton CACE archive.

37 Marlene Cimons, *Los Angeles Times Magazine*, September 14, 1986, 16.

38 CACE Forum, "Ethics of Activism."

39 CACE Forum, "Ethics of Activism." This is a curious argument for him to make, since Koop had been a board member of Americans United for Life, the Chicago-based public interest law firm, since soon after it was established in 1971 precisely to aid legal and legislative action. He continued quietly supporting AUL when in office as Surgeon General and offered to rejoin the board thereafter.

40 Richard Doerflinger, email to the author, May 28, 2021.

41 Evangelical Child and Family Service, an adoption and counseling agency, was founded by Koop in 1960, with his friend Erna Goulding as one of the trustees. ACC 2014–16 Box 22.

42 Judis, "Unlikely celebrity."

43 Commencement address, Philadelphia College of Osteopathic Medicine, June 3, 1979. ACC 2014–16 Box 22.

Part IV: SURGEON GENERAL

1 Other key figures included Grover Norquist, Morton Blackwell, and Richard Viguerie.

2 Daniel K. Williams, *God's Own Party: The Making of the Religious Right* (New York: Oxford University Press, 2010), 159.

3 "Remembering the New Right," June 10, 2009, paper for Political Research Associates. See https://politicalresearch.org/. See also his "The 'Vast Right-Wing Conspiracy': Media and Conservative Networks," *New Political Science* 34, no. 4 (December 2012).

4 Williams, *God's Own Party*, 195. As we note later, Catholics scored rather better.

5 William Martin, *With God on Our Side: The Rise of the Religious Right in America* (New York: Broadway, 1996), 239.

6 Steven Hayward, *The Age of Reagan: The Conservative Counterrevolution* (New York: Random House, 2009), 42.

7 "Whether out of inspiration, writer's block or despair." Stephen R. Weisman, "The Hollow Man," *New York Times*, October 10, 1999, of Edmund Morris, *Dutch: A Memoir of Ronald Reagan* (New York: Random House, 1999).

8 Paul Kengor, *God and Reagan: A Spiritual Life* (New York: Regan Books, 2004). For

this section see also Kathleen M. Sands, *America's Religious Wars: The Embattled Heart of our Public Life* (New Haven, NJ: Yale University Press, 2019); Steven P. Miller, *The Age of Evangelicalism: America's Born-again Years* (New York: Oxford University Press, 2014); D. Michael Lindsay, *Faith in the Halls of Power: How Evangelicals joined the American Elite* (New York: Oxford University Press, 2007); Diane Winston, *Righting the American Dream: How the Media Mainstreamed Reagan's Evangelical Vision* (Chicago: Chicago University Press, 2023).

9 Randall Balmer, *Bad Faith: Race and the Rise of the Religious Right* (Grand Rapids: Eerdmans, 2021), 46–47.

10 Daniel K. Williams, *God's Own Party: The Making of the Christian Right* (Oxford: Oxford University Press, 2010), 7.

11 Many sources inaccurately give the date Koop took office as Thursday, January 21, 1982. This is the date of a repeat event—a common Washington device—in which Secretary Schweiker ceremonially re-administered the oath. Koop was actually "sworn in" as Surgeon General on November 17, 1981, "quietly and immediately," as he himself notes, the day following his confirmation. The NIH archive photo of the November 17 ceremony shows the oath being administered by an officer of the Commissioned Corps—both he and Koop are in uniform—though its identification of that officer as "James Mason, Assistant Secretary of Health" (properly, for Health) is likely in error. The officer does resemble Mason. Mason would become assistant secretary in 1989; in 1981 he was running Utah's Department of Health. Koop memoir, 146–47. https://www.upi.com/Archives/1982/01/21/Pediatric-surgeon-C-Everett-Koop-was-sworn-in-Thursday/4847380437200/, https://collections.nlm.nih.gov/catalog/nlm:nlmuid-101584932X875-img - photograph with "James Mason," https://geiselmed.dartmouth.edu/koop/c-everett-koop/.

12 The position was nominally combined with that of the assistant secretary for health, the Surgeon General's boss, as happened during most of 1981.

13 Mike Stobbe, *Surgeon General's Warning* (San Francisco: University of California Press, 2014), 282.

14 "U.S. Seamen's Hospitals still open in many cities," *New York Times*, October 27, 1981.

CHAPTER 7: Welcome to Washington

1 *Interview Magazine*, April 4, 1982, 28. In later interviews and his memoir Koop curiously omits this story and focuses on later calls he received from Reagan recruiters (though in an interview with Philip Yancey in 1989 he tells of a call in August of 1980. Yancey/Koop). "All I could think," Koop tells the interviewer, "was that . . . it would mean going to work for somebody else for the first time in my life"—a telling observation in light of his troubled relationship with his long-time boss at the Children's Hospital, I.S. Ravdin.

2 There would be a serious falling-out with Carl Anderson over AIDS policy. See Chapter 11.

3 Ziegler/Koop, 41–42.

4 Koop to Robert C. Grasberger, late November 1980. ACC 2014–016 Box 25/33.

5 Koop to Graham, January 6, 1981. ACC 2014–016 Box 25/33. The positions had been held together previously; taken together, they came close to re-stating the Surgeon General position before its mid-60s evisceration.

6 D. Michael Lindsay, *Faith in the Halls of Power* (New York: Oxford University Press, 2007), 28.

7 Confidential interview.

8 According to the March's own website, attendance that year was around 100,000. https://www.marchesforlife.com/Washington-2/1981.

9 Confidential interview.

10 For the announcement, see https://www.presidency.ucsb.edu/documents /nomination-c-everett-koop-be-surgeon-general-the-public-health-service-o.

11 The general failure of the evangelical "religious right" to get its people into top government positions during the Reagan years was a cause for heart-searching. Carl F. H. Henry (1913–2003), doyen of evangelical theologians who lived for many years near Washington, would later lament that "the evangelicals got their pictures taken with the President, while the Catholics got the cabinet positions." Commenting on Henry's statement, William Bennett (1943-), noted Roman Catholic and Reagan's Education Secretary from 1985 who clashed with Koop over AIDS, responded, "they were great days!" (Henry and Bennett comments both made to the author.)

12 See https://findingaids.nlm.nih.gov/repositories/ammp/resources/koop.

13 Confidential interview.

14 See for example his response to a Reagan recruiter in 1980, "This guy hasn't even been elected yet, nominated. How can he go around seeking his cabinet?" Ziegler/ Koop, 42. This illusion persists in quarters which should certainly know better, such as the influential Health Care Blog, which described Koop as "the most revered Surgeon General in history, perhaps even the most revered Cabinet member." https://thehealthcareblog.com/blog/2013/08/08/the-strange-case-of-the-c-everett -koop-national-health-award/. Even in his pre-mid-1960s hey-day, the Surgeon General was never in the cabinet. Hillary Clinton herself believed that Koop had been "in charge of overseeing the nation's Public Health Service," which of course he had not. *Living History*, 216.

15 For a history of the Surgeon General's role, see Mike Stobbe, *Surgeon General's Warning: How Politics Crippled the Nation's Doctor* (Oakland: University of California Press, 2014). The relevant US government website summarizes the office and its history: https://www.hhs.gov/surgeongeneral/about/history/index.html. On the NIH component: www.history.nih.gov.

16 Stobbe, *Surgeon General's Warning*, 17–18.

17 Stobbe, *Surgeon General's Warning*, 23.

18 Stobbe describes Woodworth and his two successors, John Hamilton and Walter Wyman, as "empire builders who built the core of what became the U.S. Department of Health and Human Services." *Surgeon General's Warning*, 16.

19 Periodic re-organizations took the Surgeon General's office in 1939 from the Treasury to the Federal Security Agency, and in 1953 to the Department of Health, Education and Welfare. In 1979 the Department of Education was spun off, leaving the Department of Health and Human Services. See Stobbe, *Surgeon General's Warning*.

20 A striking example of the diminution of the Surgeon General's role lies in the fact both Burney and Terry not only supervised but appointed the director of the National Institutes of Health, then required to be an officer of the Commissioned Corps. From 1971 it became a presidential appointment.

21 Appointed August 18, 1965.

22 Stobbe details the role of one Wilbur Cohen, the Department of Health, Education and Welfare's number three official, who had served as a "behind-the-scenes tactician" in the creation of Social Security in the 1930s and who wished to develop the department's various programs without reliance on Surgeons General of varied backgrounds and competencies. *Surgeon General's Warning*, 117.

23 Stobbe, *Surgeon General's Warning*, 5.

24 Arlen Specter, Senate Committee on Labour and HR, October 1, 1981, 3.

25 James Bowman, in Terry L. Cooper and N. Dale Wright, *Exemplary Public Administrators* (San Francisco: Jossey-Bass, 1992), 274. There is actually on file an extensive formal job description for the Surgeon General, characterized by its repeated focus on the advisory nature of his responsibilities, and need for direction from the assistant secretary for health. Exceptions are service on the boards of the National Library of Medicine and the Uniformed Services University of the Health Sciences. "The Surgeon General . . . Functions and Legal Responsibilities." ACC 2014–016 Box 22.

26 The complex modern history of the office is briefly captured in this extract from the relevant statute, qualified by subsequent changes as noted. https://www.govinfo.gov/content/pkg/USCODE-2019-title42/html/USCODE-2019-title42-chap6A-subchapI-partA-sec206.htm.

27 Edward Brandt interview with James Bowman, August 7, 1990, in Cooper and Wright, *Exemplary Public Administrators*, 274.

28 James Bowman interview with Schweiker, August 23, 1990, in Cooper and Wright, *Exemplary Public Administrators*, 274.

29 Stobbe, *Surgeon General's Warning*, 175.

30 Mullan/Koop, 30–31, cited by Stobbe, *Surgeon General's Warning*, 176.

31 James Bowman, citing an anonymous source, interview, June 22, 1990, in Cooper and Wright, *Exemplary Public Administrators*, 274.

32 Koop to Brandt, May 4, 1982. MSC 487 Box 69. Koop to HHS Secretary, August 26, 1981. MSC 409 Box 68.

33 For the delegation, see: https://www.reaganlibrary.gov/public/2022-03/40-654-IT102-036-003-2022.pdf.

34 Koop to Gordon Jacobs, July 23, 1981. MSC 489 Box 68.

35 Koop to David Newhall III, October 9, 1981. MSC 489 Box 68.

36 Senate nomination hearing, Committee on Labour and HR, Senate, Oct 1, 1981, 42.

37 Memorandum (undated) re October 26–30, 1981, trip. Oddly, in his memoir and other subsequent comments, Koop recalls this visit as relating to the Spanish cooking oil scandal (Toxic Oil Syndrome), to which his six-page memo makes no reference. See NLM Unique ID 101584930X506.

38 Koop had never been seriously politically engaged before, though he does appear in the *Congressional Record* for July 17, 1979. Representative Robert K. Dornan had heard him speak, likely at a *Whatever Happened to the Human Race?* event, and placed his speech on "The Silent Domino: Infanticide" in the *Record*.

39 See Chapter 18 for more on their friendship. For more on Kessel's bio, see: http://www.global-partners-united.com/member/woodie-kessel-md-mph.

40 Woodie Kessel interview.

41 Woodie Kessel interview.

42 For more details of his bio, see http://www.martin-blanck.com/bio_edward-martin .php. See Chapter 8 for more on Martin's role.

43 Anthony Fauci interview.

44 Anthony Fauci interview.

45 *Atlantic*, March 4, 2013. Easterbrook notes the sloppy journalism around Koop's religion: "most journalists failed to grasp the difference between an evangelical Christian (Koop) and a fundamentalist." Gregg Easterbrook, *Surgeon Koop* (N.l.: Whittle, 2001), 41. We discuss this issue in the Introduction.

46 A Google search establishes that there actually are American physicians and dentists with this unfortunate name.

47 Ziegler/Koop, 42–43.

48 James Bowman, in Cooper and Wright, *Exemplary Public Administrators*, 274.

49 Confidential interview.

50 IFACS was the Institute for Advanced Christian Studies, a network of evangelical academics, now defunct. Henry to Koop, February 14, 1981. ACC 2014–016 Box 22/33.

51 Pollack to Koop, April 13, 1981; Koop to Pollack, April 16, 1981. MSC 487 Box 68.

52 Koop memoir, 123.

53 The testimony is available here: https://collections.nlm.nih.gov/catalog/nlm:nlmuid -101584930X512-doc.

54 See *Washington Post*, October 22, 1981.

55 Koop to McBeath, December 16, 1981. Interestingly, Koop adds that he knows McBeath has read *Sometimes Mountains Move*. MSC 487 Box 70. Also, Woodie Kessel interview.

56 Easterbrook, *Surgeon Koop*, 41. Paul Kengor challenges this widespread take on Reagan's religious life in *God and Reagan: a Spiritual Biography* (New York: Perfect bound/HarperCollins, 2004).

57 Easterbrook, *Surgeon Koop*, 42.

58 Pub. L. 32 86–415-APR. 8 1960, available at https://www.govinfo.gov/content/pkg /STATUTE-74/pdf/STATUTE-74-Pg32.pdf#page=1.

59 Pub. L. 97–25 available at https://www.govinfo.gov/content/pkg/USCODE-2019-title 42/html/USCODE-2019-title42-chap6A-subchapI-partA-sec205.htm.

60 Cited in the *Boston Globe* obituary, February 25, 2013.

61 Details are given in *CQ Almanac* 1981, available at https://library.cqpress.com /cqalmanac/document.php?id=cqal81-1173347.

62 See, https://www.presidency.ucsb.edu/documents/nomination-c-everett-koop-be -surgeon-general-the-public-health-service-0. The process through House and Senate is helpfully characterized here in the *Congressional Quarterly*: https:// library.cqpress.com/cqalmanac/document.php?id=cqal81-1173347.

63 *New York Times* obituary, February 26, 2013.

64 See https://www.upi.com/Archives/1981/11/16/Senate-confirms-Koop-as-surgeon -general/4106374734800/.

65 Confidential interview.

66 Heininger/Koop, 4.

67 Woodie Kessel interview. Full voting details: https://www.govtrack.us/congress /votes/97-1981/s379.

68 Mona Khanna interview. In his memoir, Koop plays down the unpleasantness of their

first connections—there's no reference to the cigar or the handshake refusal. Koop memoir, 143. He too recalls the daily meetings with Kennedy in the White House grounds but places them in 1997 when the topic was tobacco. Heininger/Koop, 6.

69 Easterbrook, *Surgeon Koop*, 45, and see above.

70 Easterbrook, *Surgeon Koop*, 45, and see above.

71 Rhoads Senate testimony October 1, 1981. Penn R474 Box 28 F 12 Rhoads papers.

72 Rhoads testimony.

73 Rhoads testimony.

74 Rhoads testimony.

75 Donya Currie Arias, "C. Everett Koop, the Nation's Health Conscience," *American Journal of Public Health* 98, no. 3 (March 2008), 396. The population of the United States in 1981 was of course not 347 million, but around two-thirds that number. By 2022 it had risen to more than 330 million. Koop was usually very precise in his use of numbers. See Office of the Census: https://www2.census.gov/library /publications/1981/demographics/P25-898.pdf.

76 *US News and World Report*, May 30, 1988, 60.

77 James S. Bowman and Brent Wall, "Koop as an Exemplar of Moral and Democratic Decision Making," in *Administration and Society* 29, no. 3 (July 1997), 256.

78 Philip Yancey, *Christianity Today*, February 25, 2013.

79 Koop to Joseph Stanton, April 14, 1981. ACC 2014–016 Box 26/33.

80 Martin Eichelberger interview.

81 Koop was originally thinking in terms of a single four-year appointment. He tells the realtor who sold their home in Philadelphia that by 1985 they will perhaps be "living on Cape Cod." Koop to Ethel Sanders, July 16, 1982. MSC 487 Box 70.

82 Ziegler/Koop, 42.

83 John P. Judis, "The Unlikely Celebrity of C. Everett Koop," *New Republic*, February 26, 2013.

84 Confidential interview. It was "pretty much our impression that Dr. Koop had, you know, settled for some sort of agreement . . . an acknowledgement from Dr. Koop that he was not going to be speaking . . . about abortion." This represents an understandable effort to make sense of Koop's decision, but plainly it is not what happened.

85 He would continue to be oddly troubled by the idea of associating the office of the Surgeon General with the pro-life agenda, even in the case of Americans United for Life. One time he scolds AUL for using his Surgeon General title under statements he made when he was a private citizen. "My concern is for historical accuracy and the avoidance of any criticism of AUL . . . for misrepresentation." Koop to Paige Comstock Cunningham, January 5, 1984. MSC 489 Box 72.

86 Koop to Elizabeth Chepules, June 5, 1981. MSC 487 Box 68.

87 Elaine Bratic to Frank H. King, July 7, 1982. MSC 489 Box 70.

88 Details here: https://profiles.nlm.nih.gov/spotlight/qq/catalog/nlm:nlmuid-10158 4930X482-doc.

89 Details here: https://profiles.nlm.nih.gov/spotlight/qq/catalog/nlm:nlmuid-10158 4930X75-doc.

90 Grant had written the speech. Edward Grant interview. *Journal of Law, Ethics, and Public Policy* 2 (1986).

91 Koop to Joe and Holly Coors, July 21, 1986; Koop to Guy Condon, July 23, 1986.

ACC Box 82. Letter from Guy Condon to Koop, October 5, 1988. ACC Box 22 Pro-Life Letters.

92 Koop to Condon, undated, likely 1987 or 88. NLM Box 86 Cor. For some reason this did not happen. Edward Grant interview.

93 Arias, "C. Everett Koop, the Nation's Health Conscience," 396.

94 Sandy Roberts email, November 12, 2022.

95 Richard Kluger, *Ashes to Ashes* (New York: Knopf, 1996), 537–38.

96 Koop to Admiral Walter Welham, February 25, 1982. MSC 489 Box 69.

CHAPTER 8: Bully Pulpit

1 "He was a dramatist. I mean, he was an actor. And I don't mean that as a criticism, but he had a role to play," observed one activist who had worked closely with him. Confidential interview. Koop later described this press conference as "one of the best things that happened to me in Washington." Heininger/Koop, 8.

2 At least until the end of 1984, relations between Koop and Helms were warm. Helms to Koop, December 21, 1984. ACC 2014–016 Box 22/33.

3 "New Report Links Cigarette Smoking to Additional Cancers," *Washington Post*, February 23, 1982. Edward Martin, who knew them both well, comments: "Ed Brandt was the assistant secretary, and was his boss. The fact of the matter was, that Chick, got all the publicity, he got all the notoriety. So he sort of out-shadowed Ed Brandt. Well, Ed was such a good person that he didn't allow it to get to him. But there were people that worked for Ed that didn't like it." Edward Martin interview.

4 Edward Martin, a top HHS official and later Koop's chief of staff, noted that the relationship between Koop and Brandt was "formal." Edward Martin interview.

5 Remarks, available at www.collections.nlm.nih.gov.

6 Mike Stobbe, *Surgeon General's Warning* (Oakland: University of California Press, 2014), 177.

7 As Richard Kluger reports in his history of tobacco policy, "When Shopland returned to Koop's office a few days after presenting him with the final manuscript, he was astonished to see that the pages were dog-eared and speckled with inquiries that the Surgeon General wanted answered before signing off on the hefty document and publicly endorsing its findings in strong language." Kluger, *Ashes to Ashes* (New York: Knopf, 1996), 539. On August 11, 2000, Koop presented Shopland with the first Unsung Hero's Award. ACC 2015–011 Box 3.

8 According to one historian of the office, Stobbe, *Surgeon General's Warning*, 176.

9 Remarks, available at https://profiles.nlm.nih.gov/spotlight/qq/catalog/nlm:nlmuid -101584930X6-doc.

10 Koop would later refuse to debate the industry, as he did not believe they were serious about science and held that to do so would diminish the stature of his office. James Bowman, in Terry L. Cooper and N. Dale Wright, *Exemplary Public Administrators* (San Francisco: Jossey-Bass, 1992), 276.

11 Jim Shahin, "Koop Uncooped," in *American Way*, June 15, 1989, cited by James Bowman, in Cooper and Wright, *Exemplary Public Administrators*, 276. And this despite the fact that the Reagan administration had just chopped the budget of the Office on Smoking and Health by 27 percent.

12 Interview in Mike Stobbe, "The Surgeon General and the Bully Pulpit" (DPH diss.,

University of North Carolina, 2008), 87. Available at: https://core.ac.uk/download/pdf/210600474.pdf.

13 Cited by James Bowman, in Cooper and Wright, *Exemplary Public Administrators*, 276, from the 1989 PBS *Nova* presentation, "The Controversial Doctor Koop."

14 Interview in Stobbe, "Bully Pulpit," 86.

15 James S. Bowman and Brent Wall, "Koop as an Exemplar of Moral and Democratic Decision Making," in *Administration and Society* 29, no. 3, July 1997, 263, citing Koop, personal communication, September 5, 1990.

16 See his reminiscence at https://profiles.nlm.nih.gov/spotlight/qq/catalog/nlm:nlmuid-101584930X205-doc.

17 See https://budgetcounsel.files.wordpress.com/2017/11/the-budget-of-the-united-states-government-fiscal-year-1981.pdf 454. The comparable figure for 2022 is $131.8 billion in discretionary funding, plus $1.5 trillion in mandatory funding. See https://www.hhs.gov/about/budget/fy2022/index.html#:~:text=The%20FY%202022%20budget%20proposes,%241.5%20trillion%20in%20mandatory%20funding.

18 Ziegler/Koop, 30–31.

19 During more than eight years in office Koop served three assistant secretaries for health, Edward Brandt, Jr. (1981–84), Robert E. Windom (1986–89), and James O. Mason (1989–93; Mason also served as acting assistant secretary between Brandt and Windom); and four secretaries—Robert S. Schweiker (January 22, 1981–February 3, 1983), Margaret Heckler (March 10, 1983-December 13, 1985), Otis Bowen (December 13, 1985–March 1, 1989), and finally Louis W. Sullivan (March 1, 1989-January 20, 1993).

20 Mason's background was unusual, in that he was a leader of the Mormon Church and earlier in his career had administered the church's hospital system. During the Reagan administration he served as director of the Centers for Disease Control. He was a commissioned officer of the PHS, which meant that on being confirmed as assistant secretary he also moved up to the rank of four-start admiral. It must have rankled Koop that his fellow Reagan appointee was not only retained in the incoming Bush administration, but promoted over his head, though during the interregnum he had established a good working relationship with Mason.

21 B. A. Williams, "Surgeon General Nominee Faces New Congressional Obstacles," Associated Press wire, June 18, 1981, cited by Stobbe, "Bully Pulpit," 162.

22 Stobbe, "Bully Pulpit," 82.

23 There would be two further acting assistant secretaries during that time, for brief periods: James F. Dickson and Donald I. McDonald.

24 Koop memoir, 202.

25 Edward Martin interview. "Bob Windom was a commissioned officer, he was a two star officer. And Chick was a three star. And Bob Windom was a physician. He had enormous respect for Chick. So they got along famously. . . . Dr. Koop loomed way above any of those people. I mean, he was just a very, very big figure." There could however be friction, or at least its appearance, likely staff-generated. The *New York Times* reports "strong rivalry between Dr. Koop and Dr. Robert E. Windom" at the height of the AIDS controversies, June 12, 1987.

26 Heckler departed in December of that year. Art Buchwald summed it up in his *Washington Post* column for October 8, 1985. His White House source had told him, with a straight face: "We didn't knock her out of a job. All we did was give her

a better one. This administration has never stopped anyone from getting ahead." Haddow recalls her sending him to Ireland ahead of her move—to check out the living quarters at the embassy. He reported back that they were in poor repair. Mac Haddow interview.

27 Stobbe, "Bully Pulpit," 90.

28 Koop memoir, 132.

29 Our final chapter paints a portrait of Koop the man and will pick up some of the threads of this discussion.

30 Available at https://profiles.nlm.nih.gov/spotlight/qq/catalog/nlm:nlmuid-10158 4930X779-doc.

31 Mullan/Koop. He is being unduly modest. The file is actually called "A really terrific sermon." See https://profiles.nlm.nih.gov/spotlight/qq/catalog/nlm:nlmuid-10158 4930X294-doc.

32 See https://profiles.nlm.nih.gov/spotlight/qq/catalog/nlm:nlmuid-101584930 X779-doc.

33 Koop memoir, 259. The case is helpfully summarized in her mother Julie's obituary in the *New York Times* for May 25, 2022. Koop discusses it in his Glasgow speech: https://profiles.nlm.nih.gov/spotlight/qq/catalog/nlm:nlmuid-101584930X779 -doc. The Becketts, mother and daughter, became vocal advocates for the disabled. Katie died at 34. https://www.npr.org/templates/story/story.php?storyId= 131145687. See also: https://www.readkong.com/page/katie-beckett-waiver-proposal -allison-lesmann-meaghan-9710963.

34 *LaSalle Magazine*, Summer 1984, 6.

35 Koop to Brown, January 8, 1982, and March 1, 1982. MSC 489 Box 69.

36 Koop to friend (name withheld for privacy), late 1991. MSC 489 Box 68.

37 The Office of Presidential Personnel routinely staffs scores of advisory boards and commissions with hundreds of supporters of the administration of the day.

38 Koop to Ray Lett, USDA, July 22, 1982. MSC 489 Box 70.

39 Koop to Schweiker, July 1, 1882. MSC 489 Box 70. The Schweikers were members of this very small, originally German, sect.

40 For example, Koop to Krol, November 27, 1986. MSC 489 Box 79.

41 Koop to Dean Daniel Tosteson, July 22, 1981. MSC 489 Box 68.

42 Koop to Didier Schott, July 10, 1984. MSC 489 Box 74.

43 See https://profiles.nlm.nih.gov/spotlight/qq/catalog/nlm:nlmuid-101584930 X206-doc.

44 Alfred M. Bongiovanni to Koop, March 18, 1981; Koop to Bongiovanni, March 23, 1981. ACC 2014–016 Box 24/33.

45 Koop shared this at a 1988 meeting with Forrest Peebles, Capt. USPHS retired; Peebles email November 16, 2022.

46 Koop to Kabelka, July 21, 1981. MSC 487 Box 68.

47 Koop to Wood, April 30, 1982. MSC 489 Box 69.

48 Confidential interview.

49 By email, from USPHS Captain William Hess, May 14, 2021. Hess was MC at the dinner.

50 Mac Haddow interview.

51 Young/Bowen, 16.

52 Mac Haddow interview.

53 Mullan/Koop, 32, 33.

54 After being trimmed down under budget-cutting pressure, this office has more recently grown in significance and size, renamed first the Office of Global Health Affairs and then Office of Global Affairs; from 2012 it has had its own assistant secretary (again), and around fifty staff. https://www.hhs.gov/about/agencies/oga/index.html.

55 "Resolutions and Decisions," https://apps.who.int/iris/bitstream/handle/10665/155679/WHA34_1981-REC-1_eng.pdf?sequence=1&isAllowed=y. A year earlier, in his capacity as deputy assistant secretary, he had joined the US delegation to the World Health Assembly meeting May 4–22, the first of eight or nine occasions when he would represent the United States at the Assembly. (It's unclear whether Koop was part of the 1988 delegation; an undated memo to the secretary suggests otherwise.) MSC Box 87 Cor.

56 Memorandum to Agency Heads et al., April 8, 1982. MSC 489 Box 143 F12 Cor.

57 This highly prestigious award, for outstanding achievements in "social medicine," had been presented to one previous Surgeon General, Dr. Thomas Parran, in 1958. https://apps.who.int/gb/awards/e/Bernard.html.

58 Given the hostility toward Koop displayed by the incoming Bush administration, it's surprising that he continued to serve as director of the Office of International Health, a position from which he could have been easily removed, and to represent the United States at the 1989 Assembly.

59 The text actually says "enervative," doubtless a dictation error. Available here: https://collections.nlm.nih.gov/ocr/nlm:nlmuid-101584930X786-doc.

60 Bowman, in Cooper and Wright, *Exemplary Public Administrators*, 287.

61 As Koop later put it, "nearly a dozen." https://www.ojp.gov/pdffiles1/Digitization/118732NCJRS.pdf.

62 From one of the reminiscences Koop wrote to introduce files he passed to the National Library of Medicine, in this case the workshop on drunk driving. https://collections.nlm.nih.gov/ocr/nlm:nlmuid-101584930X786-doc.

63 He sent a copy of the outcomes report to the President, who replied with a letter of thanks on May 20, 1983, at https://profiles.nlm.nih.gov/spotlight/qq/catalog/nlm:nlmuid-101584930X744-doc.

64 December 13–14, 1982. NLM Box 146 F 30.

65 Winchester, Virginia, June 7–9, 1983.

66 Rochester, New York, June 11–12, 1984.

67 Leesburg, Virginia, October 27–29, 1985.

68 June 22–24, 1986.

69 Los Angeles, September 20–22, 1987.

70 The Children's Hospital of Philadelphia, April 6–8, 1987.

71 Mayflower Hotel, Washington, DC, March 20–23, 1988.

72 Jennifer M. Hazen, "Reducing armed violence: the public health approach," at https://www.smallarmssurvey.org/sites/default/files/resources/Small-Arms-Survey-2008-Chapter-07-EN.pdf.

73 Shared by Joshua Nelson, interview.

74 *New York Times*, April 7, 1987.

75 *Los Angeles Times*, May 10, 1988. Barron Lerner, *One for the Road: Drunk Driving since 1900* (Baltimore, MD: Johns Hopkins University Press, 2011), 115.

76 Howard Filston interview. Koop relented, and invited the Filstons to join. Workshop details: Available at https://files.eric.ed.gov/fulltext/ED332595.pdf. Lerner, in his history of drunk driving, is critical of the Workshop for its exclusion of representatives of the alcohol industry (Koop said that was to aid consensus), and what he sees as moves to jump to conclusions. Koop was warned shortly before the event that the evidence then current did not support the idea that alcohol advertising has an effect on the level of drunken driving, though this was ignored. This workshop was held at the Mayflower Hotel in Washington, DC, December 14–16 of 1988. An industry group unsuccessfully filed suit to seek to have the event delayed. See Lerner, *One for the Road*, 118 and 93.

CHAPTER 9: Saving Baby Doe

1 See Chapter 6; his lecture is available at https://humanlifereview.com/the-slide-to-auschwitz/.

2 Fred Barbash and Cristine Russell, "The Demise of 'Infant Doe': Permitted Death Gives New Life to an Old Debate," *Washington Post*, April 17, 1982.

3 Raymond S. Duff and A.G.M. Campbell, "Moral and Ethical Dilemmas in the Special-Care Nursery," *New England Journal of Medicine* 289 (1973), 890.

4 Nat Hentoff, "The Awful Privacy of Baby Doe," *Atlantic*, January 1985.

5 Norman L. Geisler and Frank Turek, *Legislating Morality: Is It Wise? Is It Legal? Is It Possible?* (Eugene, OR: Wipf and Stock, 2003), 180.

6 *Indianapolis Star*, April 17, 1982.

7 The U.S. Civil Rights Commission would conduct an extensive inquiry into this case and the wider issues it raises for medical discrimination against the handicapped. *Report of the U.S. Commission on Civil Rights on Medical Discrimination against Children with Disabilities*, September 1989. It handily includes a number of additional pertinent documents, including the "Circuit Court Declaratory Judgment in the Infant Doe Case," of April 10, 1982. The report and the judgment are the source for many details noted here. Available at https://files.eric.ed.gov/fulltext/ED326018.pdf 389–92.

8 *Report of the U.S. Commission on Civil Rights on Medical Discrimination against Children with Disabilities*, September 1989, 323–24.

9 "Charges Weighed for Parents Who Let Baby Die Untreated," *New York Times*, April 17, 1982.

10 Koop memoir, 243. This is not noted in other sources.

11 *Indianapolis Star*, April 20, 1982.

12 "Down's Syndrome Baby Barred from Food Dies," *Washington Post*, April 16, 1982.

13 Barbash and Russell, "Demise." "Charges Weighed for Parents Who Let Baby Die Untreated," *New York Times*, April 17, 1982.

14 *Indianapolis Star*, April 20, 1982. Koop points out that there remained uncertainties as to the exact medical condition of the baby: "we did not have the complete medical record. . . . Baby Doe does not fit neatly into any of the legal or medical or ethical pigeonholes we have all so carefully constructed for ourselves over time." Glasgow speech, 24. https://profiles.nlm.nih.gov/spotlight/qq/catalog/nlm:nlmuid-101584930X779-doc.

15 "'Private' Death," *New York Times*, April 27, 1982.

16 Koop Glasgow speech, 30. https://profiles.nlm.nih.gov/spotlight/qq/catalog/nlm: nlmuid-101584930X779-doc.

17 "Reagan Says Allowing Retarded Child to Die Breaks Federal Law," *Washington Post*, May 1, 1982. Koop later commented acidly: "I was a pediatric surgeon, and I had probably operated on more Baby Does than anybody in the world, and yet nobody in the government ever asked me what I thought about it at all. Things all took place around me. And suddenly we had a crisis on our hands, with a doctor who didn't know what he was doing, a judge who didn't know what he was doing, making the decision that the family could do what they wanted to do, and of course having a 'blob' with an operative mortality of fifty per cent, said, We don't want our child to be operated upon." Koop added: "I should just tell you that my operative mortality for the previous eight years, in a full-term baby like that, was zero." Center for Applied Christian Ethics (CACE), Wheaton College, 2002. https://www .youtube.com/watch?v=Pm0NqPXAqaY.

18 See Chapter 3.

19 See https://www.upi.com/Archives/1984/10/10/Baby-Jane-a-year-old/4587466 228800/.

20 See https://profiles.nlm.nih.gov/spotlight/qq/feature/babydoe.

21 Available at https://www.newsday.com/news/health/baby-jane-doe-at-30-happy-jok ing-learning-u93680. This report would seem to contradict the National Library of Medicine description of her as "severely retarded." https://profiles.nlm.nih.gov /spotlight/qq/feature/babydoe.

22 PBS *Nova*, "The Controversial Dr. Koop."

23 Center for Applied Christian Ethics (CACE), Wheaton College, 2002. https://www .youtube.com/watch?v=Pm0NqPXAqaY.

24 Mac Haddow interview.

25 James Bowman, in Terry L. Cooper and N. Dale Wright, *Exemplary Public Administrators* (San Francisco: Jossey-Bass, 1992), 278–79.

26 See https://embryo.asu.edu/pages/baby-doe-rules-1984.

27 CACE, Wheaton College, 2002. https://www.youtube.com/watch?v=Pm0NqPX AqaY.

28 CACE Forum, "Ethics of Activism, Protest, and Dissent," Dr. C. Everett Koop's Remarks. Undated, likely early 1990s, Wheaton CACE archive.

29 Bowman, in Cooper and Wright, *Exemplary Public Administrators*, 278–79.

30 Bowman, in Cooper and Wright, *Exemplary Public Administrators*, 278–79.

31 Quoted by Nat Hentoff, *Atlantic*, January 1985.

32 Alyssa Burgart interview.

33 Glasgow speech, 27. https://profiles.nlm.nih.gov/spotlight/qq/catalog/nlm: nlmuid-101584930X779-doc.

34 Glasgow speech, 34, 35. https://profiles.nlm.nih.gov/spotlight/qq/catalog/nlm: nlmuid-101584930X779-doc.

CHAPTER 10: Smoke-free Society?

1 Koop memoir, 180.

2 See NLM Box 105 F 8.

3 Julia M. Jones was a physician who spent most of her professional life working with tuberculosis patients at Bellevue and Harlem hospitals in New York. She died at the age of 64 in 1973. See *New York Times* obituary, April 24, 1973.

380 NOTES TO PAGES 183–190

4 See Charles A. LeMaistre and Donald R Shopland, *Clearing the Air: The Untold Story of the 1964 Report on Smoking and Health* (Berkeley: UC Medical Humanities Press, 2024).

5 Surgeon General's report, 1982, 2.

6 Julia M. Jones Memorial Lecture: Presented to a Joint Annual Meeting of the American Lung Association and the American Thoracic Society, Miami Beach, Florida, 5. NLM https://collections.nlm.nih.gov/catalog/nlm:nlmuid-101584930X61-doc.

7 Jones Lecture, 9.

8 Jones Lecture, 12–13.

9 Jones Lecture, 13–16.

10 Jones Lecture, 17.

11 James S. Bowman and Brent Wall, "Koop as an Exemplar of Moral and Democratic Decision Making," in *Administration and Society*, 29, no. 3 (July 1997), 263, citing Matthew Meyers (personal communication, July 12, 1990), of the Coalition on Smoking and Health. (It is referred to elsewhere as the Coalition on Smoking OR Health.)

12 PBS *Nova*, "The Controversial Dr. Koop."

13 Dean E. Schraufnagel, *Annals of the American Thoracic Society* 10, no. 3 (June, 2013), 276.

14 Sarah Milov, *The Cigarette: A Political History* (Cambridge, MA: Harvard University Press), 6.

15 Milov, *The Cigarette*, 6.

16 Surgeon General's report for 2000, chapter 2, "A Historical Review of Efforts to Reduce Smoking in the United States," 43, available at https://www.cdc.gov/tobacco /sgr/2000/complete_report/pdfs/chapter2.pdf CDC, 2000.

17 CDC, Surgeon General's report for 2000, 45.

18 CDC, Surgeon General's report for 2000, 45.

19 See the Koop will, available from Haverhill Probate Division, NH, case 315–2013-ET -00182.

20 "Where there's smoke: Problems and policies concerning smoking in the workplace, a BNA special report," 2nd edition, 1987, 6. I am grateful to Sarah Milov, *The Cigarette*, 303, for this reference. The report is available here in the archives of the University of California San Francisco: https://www.industrydocuments.ucsf. edu/docs/#id=yzhv0060. The report notes that 54 percent of firms surveyed had smoking policies, up from 36 percent the year before. At that time Bloomberg was known by the curious name the Bureau of National Affairs (BNA).

21 "Where there's smoke," 5.

22 "Where there's smoke," 6.

23 "Where there's smoke," 7.

24 "Where there's smoke," 7.

25 "Where there's smoke," 1.

26 "Where there's smoke," 2.

27 "Where there's smoke," 5.

28 "Where there's smoke," Appendix G-4.

29 "Where there's smoke," 6.

30 "Where there's smoke," 6.

31 CDC, Surgeon General's report for 2000, chapter 2, "A Historical Review of Efforts to Reduce Smoking in the United States," 38, available at https://www.cdc.gov/tobacco/sgr/2000/complete_report/pdfs/chapter2.pdf.

32 Leon Festinger, *A Theory of Cognitive Dissonance* (Stanford: Stanford University Press, 1957).

33 HHS bio archived here: https://web.archive.org/web/20080916014425/http://surgeongeneral.gov/about/previous/bioburney.htm.

34 Burney went significantly further in a follow-up article in the *Journal of the American Medical Association*, titled "A statement of the Public Health Service." "The weight of evidence at present implicates smoking as the principal etiological factor in the increased incidence of lung cancer." See https://famri.org/surgeon-general-reports-on-smoking-and-health/. See also: CDC, Surgeon General's report for 2000, 39.

35 See Charles LeMaistre and Donald R. Shopland, *Clearing the Air: The Untold Story of the 1964 Report on Smoking and Health* (San Francisco: UC Health Humanities Press, 2024).

36 Allan M. Brandt, *The Cigarette Century* (New York: Basic Books, 2007), 219.

37 Brandt, *The Cigarette Century*, 220. Terry himself quit cigarette smoking shortly before the report was published (he moved to a pipe). Some other members made similar personal choices; one only after losing a lung. Brandt, *The Cigarette Century*, 229.

38 Luther Terry, *New York Times* obituary, March 31, 1985.

39 See *New York Times*, January 12, 1964.

40 CDC, Surgeon General's report for 2000, 39.

41 CDC, Surgeon General's report for 2000, 41. The others were: Dr. Paul Kotin, director of the Division of Environmental Health Sciences of the NIH, Dr. Kenneth Milo Endicott, director of the National Cancer Institute, and Dr. Daniel Horn, director of the National Clearinghouse on Smoking and Health. Stewart was puffing his pipe as he told an interviewer that "there is very little evidence of anything with pipe smoking or cigar smoking." McComb/Stewart, 17. It would take the 1973 report formally to explode this comforting myth. Koop at this stage was still a pipe smoker.

42 All the reports plus commentary are conveniently available from the Flight Attendant Medical Research Institute, formed after a class action suit by flight attendants against the tobacco industry in October 1991. "The suit sought damages for diseases caused to Flight Attendants from their exposure to secondhand tobacco smoke in airline cabins." https://famri.org/surgeon-general-reports-on-smoking-and-health/. And here: https://www.ncbi.nlm.nih.gov/books/NBK294311/table/ch3.t1/?report=objectonly. This article explains how the reports were compiled: https://www.ncbi.nlm.nih.gov/books/NBK294311/.

43 See "FBI investigated threat to kill Surgeon General C. Everett Koop over cigarette labels," https://www.muckrock.com/news/archives/2013/nov/12/koop-files-look-vetting-presidential-nominees/.

44 There was no report published for 1987. The Office on Smoking and Health was transferred from HHS to CDC, and this occasioned some disruption. Donald Shopland interview.

45 Brandt, *The Cigarette Century*, 297.

46 Koop to Berenstains, February 20, 1985. MSC 489 Box 76.

47 Koop to Schweiker, November 29, 1985. MSC 489 Box 78. He handwrites a post-script: "My second confirmation was very easy!"

48 Names withheld for privacy. Koop letters June 21, 1984, August 7, 1984. MSC 489 Box 74. We do not know if this high-level intervention was successful.

49 Ziegler/Koop, 52–53. He had begun the process with an informal experiment using scientists flying to a conference as volunteers. On January 23, 1987, he reports on a feasibility study. ACC Papers 42–44 Box 22.

50 See Douglas Jehl, "Senate Acts to Ban Smoking on 70% of American Flights," *Los Angeles Times*, October 30, 1987.

51 Brandt, *The Cigarette Century*, 306.

52 Robin Toner, "Senate Approves a Ban on Smoking on all U.S. flights," *New York Times*, September 1, 1989.

53 Kluger, *Ashes to Ashes*, 540.

54 *New York Times* obituary, February 26, 2013.

55 See https://www.lung.org/research/trends-in-lung-disease/tobacco-trends-brief/overall-tobacco-trends.

56 See https://news.gallup.com/poll/1717/tobacco-smoking.aspx.

57 James S. Bowman and Brent Wall, "Koop as an Exemplar of Moral and Democratic Decision Making," 264.

58 Michael Fiore interview.

59 Joseph O'Donnell interview.

CHAPTER 11: Confronting AIDS

1 *Los Angeles Times*, June 5, 1989. *Washington Post*, February 27, 2013. Younger readers may find it hard to grasp how recently the gay community has been habil-itated within mainstream American society. As recently as 2008 Barack Obama campaigned for the presidency as an opponent of federal endorsement of gay/equal marriage. See Juliet Eilperin, "How Attitudes Towards AIDS have Changed," *Washington Post*, December 4, 2013.

2 Koop, Introduction to AIDS Archive, NLM, https://collections.nlm.nih.gov/catalog/nlm:nlmuid-101584930X516-doc.

3 Williams/Fauci, 5.

4 Koop, Introduction to AIDS Archive, NLM, https://collections.nlm.nih.gov/catalog/nlm:nlmuid-101584930X516-doc.

5 When Mason took over as acting assistant secretary for health, he confirmed to Koop that Brandt had "very deliberately" prevented his being involved in AIDS matters. Koop notes for a book on AIDS. ACC Box 21.

6 As late as April, 1987, HHS was still referring to the virus as HTLV-III or indeed HTLV-III/LAV. Windom switched to HIV in an April 17 memo. Windom to Agency Heads et al. MSC 607 Box 3/10.

7 Anthony Fauci interview.

8 See https://www.pbs.org/wgbh/pages/frontline/aids/interviews/heckler.html.

9 Mac Haddow interview.

10 Mac Haddow interview.

11 Koop, notes for book on Leadership. ACC Box 21.

12 Koop, Introduction to AIDS Archive, NLM, https://collections.nlm.nih.gov/catalog
/nlm:nlmuid-101584930X516-doc. In this essay he mistakenly cites the date of 1987.
Report on Acquired Immune Deficiency Syndrome, available at https://www.ojp
.gov/ncjrs/virtual-library/abstracts/surgeon-generals-report-acquired-immune
-deficiency-syndrome#:~:text=This%20report%20discusses%20how%20acquired,
attacks%20certain%20white%20blood%20cells.

13 *British Medical Journal*, obituary March 15, 2013.

14 William F. Buckley, Jr., "Crucial Steps in Combating the AIDS Epidemic," *New York
Times*, March 18, 1986.

15 John-Manuel Andriote, Koop obituary, *Atlantic*, March, 2013.

16 Smith/Brandt, 63.

17 Confidential interview.

18 Smith/Brandt, 63. The writer who did interview him ("that gal," he calls her on
the tape as they try and recall her name) was Sandra Panem, author of *The AIDS
Bureaucracy* (Cambridge, MA: Harvard University Press, 1988). She quotes him
extensively, though, frustratingly, never on this matter.

19 Edmund Morris's view is that Reagan's moral framework was rather simple. "To be
fair to him, he made no moral distinction between homosexuality, heterosexuality
out of wedlock, or abortion on demand. All three were abhorred by God, in his
opinion. The best that could be said about the first 'sin' was that its consequence
was, perhaps, a caution against the other two: I think people were happier and
better off when there wasn't the tremendous plague of single motherhood cases or
abortions—the thousands and thousands and thousands that take place regularly
now and, uh, whether it's going to take such a tragic thing as that disease . . . that
horrible disease to return us to a sense of values that were very much a part of our
generation." Edmund Morris, *Dutch: A Memoir of Ronald Reagan* (New York:
Random House, 1999). Kindle Edition, at 8982.

20 Reported in *The Dartmouth*, July 1, 2004.

21 See *Los Angeles Times*, December 24, 1985. This was in the 1987 budget proposal,
to take effect from October 1987.

22 Panem, *The AIDS Bureaucracy*, 71. A year later there would be continuing discussion of the need for a "National Center for AIDS" within the office of the assistant
secretary for health, in part since this would send a good message to the public;
though with "continuation of its component activities remaining in the appropriate
agencies." Note to Robert Helms from Robert E. Windom, January 12, 1987. MSC
607 Box 5/10 AIDS Cor. 1982–90.

23 Albert R. Brashear to Stephanie Lee-Miller, December 17, 1985. MSC 607 Box 4.

24 Donald Ian Macdonald to Thomas Burke, January 9, 1986. MSC 607 Box 4.

25 At 11.39 EST on the morning of January 28, 1986, the Space Shuttle Challenger took
off from Cape Canaveral in Florida; 73 seconds later it broke apart in flight, killing
all seven crew members. The State of the Union scheduled for that evening was
postponed, and instead the President gave a brief 5:00 p.m. address to the nation.
"Today is a day for mourning and remembering. . . . The crew of the space shuttle
Challenger honored us by the manner in which they lived their lives. We will never
forget them, nor the last time we saw them, this morning, as they prepared for their
journey and waved goodbye and 'slipped the surly bonds of earth' to 'touch the face
of God.'" Available at https://history.nasa.gov/reagan12886.html#:~:text=The%20

384   NOTES TO PAGES 204–207

future%20doesn't%20belong,t%20hide%20our%20space%20program. The quotation is from a 1941 sonnet by Canadian war poet and air force pilot John Gillespie McGee. The sonnet is given in full on the Challenger memorial at Arlington, VA. McGee was killed three months after he wrote it. He was nineteen.

26 Available at presidency.ucsb.edu/people/president/ronald-reagan.

27 Confidential interview.

28 James S. Bowman and Brent Wall, "Koop as an Exemplar of Moral and Democratic Decision Making," in *Administration and Society* 29, no. 3 (July 1997), 258.

29 *Los Angeles Times Magazine*, September 14, 1986, 23.

30 Jeffrey Levi interview.

31 What remains curious is that the DPC in passing this hugely significant task to Koop seems never to have met with him to discuss the matter beforehand, just as those who recruited him to his position in the first place failed to discuss abortion, as noted in chapter 2.

32 Jennifer Brier, *Infectious Ideas: U.S. Political Responses to the AIDS Crisis* (Chapel Hill: University of North Carolina Press, 2009), 80.

33 Brier, *Infectious Ideas*, 80–81. Watkins' Commission was off the reservation for quite another reason also. "The presidential commission . . . presented sharp criticisms of the eviscerated welfare state, a position that put the commission in direct opposition to those who called for economic conservatism in the form of less governmental spending."

34 January 27, 1987. https://www.presidency.ucsb.edu/documents/message-the-congress -quest-for-excellence.

35 Highly influential were three officials who would be critical of Koop's approach. Gary Bauer was undersecretary at the Department of Education until the end of January 1987, when he became domestic policy advisor to the President. Anderson had earlier worked with Senator Helms when he was instrumental in Koop's nomination as Surgeon General and then as acting director of the White House Office of Public Liaison; he was close to Koop over several years. He went on to become the thirteenth Supreme Knight of the Knights of Columbus, a Roman Catholic fraternal and charitable organization, before his retirement in 2021. Anderson has not responded to several invitations to be interviewed for this book; Baur declined, through a third party. William J. Bennett was secretary of education 1985–88.

36 It's not uncommon for White House meetings with outsiders on sensitive issues to be held off-site, either to avoid attention from colleagues or press, or to avoid record-keeping; these latter tend to be in coffee houses.

37 Brier, *Infectious Ideas*, 83.

38 Brier, *Infectious Ideas*, 78.

39 Brier, *Infectious Ideas*, 78. She notes that of twenty-five meetings of the DPC during the Reagan administration's first term, five had been attended by the President in person.

40 Brier, *Infectious Ideas*, 79.

41 Brier, *Infectious Ideas*, 88.

42 Memorandum from the director, CDC, to the assistant secretary for health, February 3, 1987. MSC 607 AIDS Cor. 1982–90 Box 5/10. It's interesting to note that Mason signs the memo using his title as Assistant Surgeon General.

43 Brier, *Infectious Ideas*, 93.

44 Brier, *Infectious Ideas*, 93; the Executive Order is dated June 24. https://archive.org /details/4732393.1987.001.umich.edu/page/717/mode/2up. Koop had weighed in against the Presidential Commission plan as too slow a vehicle and favored a commission under the HHS secretary. See Note to Bill Roper with the caveat Eyes Only, February 5, 1987. NLM Box 84 Cor.

45 "Bennett's Far-flung Opinions Make Him Subject of Debate," *Washington Post*, August 3, 1987.

46 The statement is found here: Departments of Labor, Health and Human Services, Education, and Related Agencies Appropriations for 1988: Hearings Before a Sub-committee of the Committee on Appropriations, House of Representatives, One Hundredth Congress, First Session, Part 7, 427. NLM Box 84 Cor.

47 Koop memoir, 42.

48 D. Michael Lindsay, *Faith in the Halls of Power* (New York: Oxford University Press, 2007). Lindsay wrongly claims that evangelical leaders, including evangelical White House staff, were against Koop's writing the report in the first place. He is also mistaken in suggesting that opposition to the Salute to the Surgeon General was led by evangelicals. Neither Phyllis Schlafly not Paul Weyrich was one. 63–64.

49 *New York Times* January 20, 1987. Koop's AIDS role is helpfully reviewed in William Martin, *With God on Our Side: The Rise of the Religious Right in America* (New York: Broadway, 1996), 238–257.

50 Philip Yancey, *Christianity Today*, February 25, 2013.

51 Dugan to Koop, March 19, 1987. NLM Box 86 Cor.

52 Falwell to Koop, October 1, 1987; Koop to Falwell, November 3, 1987. NLM Box 86 Cor.

53 Michael Horton interview.

54 Koop writes of Anderson as "my early Washington friend and mentor." Koop memoir, 222.

55 Koop memoir, 223.

56 Note to Don Newman, July 31, 1987. NLM Box 86 Cor. See also Stobbe, *Surgeon General's Warning*, 184.

57 Stobbe, *Surgeon General's Warning*, 185.

58 Brier, *Infectious Ideas*, 90.

59 "Koop Defends Views on AIDS Education," *New York Times*, February 3, 1987.

60 *New York Times*, March 25, 1987.

61 *New York Times*, February 11, 1987.

62 *New York Times*, October 1, 1987. Inimitable wordsmith William Safire took the opportunity to discourse on the etymology of the word, which is obscure but seems not to depend on an historical Colonel Cundum in seventeenth century England. *New York Times*, December 14, 1986.

63 Edwin Meese interview.

64 Michael DellaVecchia interview.

65 Brier, *Infectious Ideas*, 94.

66 Brier, *Infectious Ideas*, 95.

67 Brier, *Infectious Ideas*, 98.

68 Bruce Lambert, "AIDS Panel to Organize after Delay of Seven Months," *New York Times*, July 31, 1989.

69 Brier, *Infectious Ideas*, 98.

70 Edward Martin interview.

71 Edward Martin interview.

72 "Belated as it was, the speech did mark a turning point for both of the Reagans. They finally began drawing the spotlight that followed them to the plight of AIDS victims and the stigma they faced. In July, not quite two months after his amfAR address, Ronnie visited the National Cancer Institute's pediatric ward and cuddled a fourteen-month-old baby infected with HIV. The photo made the front page of the next day's New York Times. In May 1988 Nancy became honorary chairman of the first international event at the United Nations for children affected by AIDS." Karen Tumulty, *The Triumph of Nancy Reagan* (New York: Simon and Schuster, 2021), 425–26.

73 amfAR, the American Foundation for AIDS Research, cofounded by actress Elizabeth Taylor in 1985. https://www.amfar.org/.

74 Landon Parvin interview.

75 Landon Parvin interview. See also Tumulty, *Triumph of Nancy Reagan*, 422.

76 Koop memoir, 229.

77 Koop memoir, 230.

78 Koop wrote the following day to thank the President and share his regret at the boos. Letter to the President, June 1, 1987. NLM Box 86 Cor.

79 See: https://www.presidency.ucsb.edu/documents/remarks-the-american-founda tion-for-aids-research-awards-dinner.

80 Randy Shilts, *And the Band Played On* (New York: St. Martin's Press, 1987), 592.

81 Heininger/Koop, 24.

82 *Understanding AIDS* is available at: https://stacks.cdc.gov/view/cdc/6927. See: https:// www.upi.com/Archives/1988/01/28/A-brochure-on-AIDS-will-be-mailed-to -every/6911570344400/

83 Brier, *Infectious Ideas*, 100–101.

84 The funding had of course been specially appropriated by Congress.

85 Available at https://digitalcommons.usf.edu/fl_public_health_ohp/10/.

86 Sandra G. Boodman, *Washington Post*, May 5, 1988.

87 Anthony Fauci interview.

88 Koop memoir, 235.

89 Mailer available at: https://stacks.cdc.gov/view/cdc/6927.

90 Elizabeth Fee and Theodore M. Brown, "Michael S. Gottlieb and the Identification of AIDS," *American Journal of Public Health* 96, no. 6 (June 2006), 982–83.

91 Michael Gottlieb interview.

92 *New York Times*, April 6, 1987.

93 Joshua Green, "Former Surgeon General Koop: An Unsung Hero in the Fight against AIDS," *Washington Post*, February 27, 2013.

94 Quoted by John-Manuel Andriote, *Atlantic*, March 4, 2013.

95 *New York Times*, February 26, 2013.

96 PR Newswire March 31, 2011, available at https://www.prnewswire.com/news -releases/journal-publishes-dr-koops-personal-account-of-the-aids-controversy -118977359.html.

97 Michael Getman interview. PEPFAR, the President's Emergency Plan for AIDS Relief, was initiated in 2003 by President George W. Bush to address AIDS in Africa. "[Koop] was undoubtedly influential in George W. Bush's initiative to provide AIDS care and detection in Africa, considered one of the most important achievements

of the 43rd President." Plarr's Lives of the Fellows, Royal College of Surgeons (of England), of which Koop was a Fellow. https://livesonline.rcseng.ac.uk/client/en _GB/lives/search/results?qu=Koop&te=ASSET.

98 Shilts, *And the Band Played On*, 585.

99 Shilts, *And the Band Played On*, 588.

100 David France, *How to Survive a Plague* (New York: Vintage Books, 2016).

101 France, *How to Survive a Plague*, 458.

CHAPTER 12: Revitalizing the Corps

1 Mike Stobbe, *Surgeon General's Warning* (Cambridge, MA: Harvard University Press, 2014), 181.

2 Mike and Sandy Roberts interview.

3 Mullan/Martin, 39–40.

4 Ad Hoc Committee on the Public Health Service Mission for the Future, Report to the Surgeon General, April 5, 1984. The committee consisted of Deputy Surgeon General Faye Abdellah together with five Assistant Surgeons General, including Edward Martin. ACC 2014–016 B3.

5 The memo is undated but likely contemporary with the report, since they are filed together. ACC 2014–016 Box 3.

6 Memorandum from Surgeon General to PHS Assistants Surgeon General, PHS Chief Professional Officers, September 12, 1984. "Assistants Surgeon General" is, amusingly, the plural selected in the original, here and elsewhere in the document. ACC Box 3. The title "Assistant Surgeon General" (ASG), a hangover from the time before the mid-1960s when the Surgeon General was in actual command of the Public Health Service, including CDC and the NIH. This title was still in use, in many cases for personnel who were actually more senior in the government hierarchy than the Surgeon General himself. Koop's first boss, assistant secretary for health Edward Brandt, who had early on declared the Surgeon General's role an anachronism, nonetheless found time in May of 1983 to issue a memo clarifying the criteria for the use of the Assistant Surgeon General honorific. It did not usually have anything to do with assisting the Surgeon General. First on the list was Brandt himself, the Surgeon General's boss! Then, the heads of NIH and CDC and the other PHS agencies. Then, bizarrely, the Deputy Surgeon General, who is also an Assistant Surgeon General, and in fact the only one whose job is actually to assist the Surgeon General. Then deputy assistant secretaries, then deputies to agency heads, then directors of bureaus, NIH institutes, and CDC centers. After that, it all depended on how many ASG titles there were left to be handed out. Edward Brandt memorandum, May 1983. ACC 2014–016 Box 3/33. The Public Health Service Act, Section 205(c), states that up to one per cent of the active duty strength may carry this title. On July 18, 1986, for example, the strength of the Corps was 5228 officers; therefore the maximum number of Assistant SGs was fifty-two. On that date, there were forty-nine positions filled.

7 Richard Kluger, *Ashes to Ashes* (New York: Knopf, 1996), 95–96.

8 The annual cost to the budget of an officer in the Corps was estimated to be 10–30 percent higher than that of a comparable civil service position. In addition to various housing and related benefits that echoed those of the military, Corps

officers were eligible for retirement after thirty years' service, at 75 percent of their regular pay. See Ronald Hamowy, *Government and Public Health in America* (Northampton, MA: Elgar, 2007), 76–77. It happened to be Martin's bureau that was tasked with managing the hospital disposals and associated retirements of large numbers of officers. Edward Martin interview.

9   The HHS *Green Sheet* for February 18, 1987, includes a fine profile of "bluff, blunt-spoken" Burke.

10 Koop continued to collaborate with Burke after he stepped down; see Chapter 15. An economist, Burke had trained green berets in counterinsurgency. Chief of staff under Bowen from 1986–1989, he died at 57 in 1996. https://www.nytimes.com/1987/02/18/us/washington-talk-working-profile-man-behind-medicare-expansion-plan-thomas-r.html. See *Washington Post* obituary, July 3, 1996.

11 Edward Martin interview.

12 Mullan/Martin, 43. The typescript of the interview has "the plan," corrected by hand by Martin to "Dr. Koop's." Of course Martin (and Burke) had much to do with it. Mullan/Martin. NLM Box 144 F33 39–40. Koop and PHS colleague Harold M. Ginzburg wrote a review of the revitalization effort for *Public Health Reports*, March–April 1989.

13 Mullan/Martin, 44.

14 Edward Martin interview.

15 Proposed Reorganization within the Office of the Surgeon General, April 21, 1988. NLM Koop Papers Box 143 F17.

16 Mullan/Martin, 46.

17 Mullan/Martin, 45.

18 Wyngaarden to Windom, June 9, 1987. MSC 489 Box 86.

19 Wyngaarden to Windom, June 7, 1987. MSC 489 Box 86.

20 "Koop seeks health corps 'uniformity,'" *The Scientist*, June, 1987.

21 "Health corps 'uniformity.'"

22 "Health corps 'uniformity.'" The writer notes that the cost of a full dress uniform is about $250. Corps members required summer whites and dress blues.

23 Mullan/Martin, 45.

24 Robert Mecklenburg interview.

CHAPTER 13: Abortion Again

1   Editorial, "Dr. Koop's Legacy of Principle," *New York Times*, May 6, 1989.

2   John B. Judis, "The Unlikely Celebrity of C. Everett Koop," *New Republic*, February 26, 2013. It is of course doubtful that anyone actually thought this. But evidence for negative sequelae would be grist to the mill.

3   *Los Angeles Times*, November 19, 1989. MSC 489 Box 70.

4   Koop to Mary Alice Duffy, July 23, 1981. MSC 487 Box 68.

5   Koop to Matthew J. Bulfin, September 23, 1982.

6   Koop to the assistant secretary for health, undated. MSC Box 86 Cor.

7   Koop to Thomas R. Burke, HHS chief of staff. MSC Box 86 Cor.

8   Untitled and undated memo to file, October 15, 1987. ACC 2014–016 Box 26/33. Emphases ours.

9 Michael E. Samuels to Koop, "Through Dr. Edward Martin," August 19, 1987. MSC Box 86 Cor.

10 Meanwhile, he felt he should end his occasional efforts to raise money for the pro-life law firm, American United for Life. Koop to Guy Condon, December 4, 1987. NLM Box 86 Cor.

11 *Science*, Vol. 243, 730.

12 Intergovernmental Relations and Human Resources Subcommittee of the House Government Operations Committee. The hearing is available on C-SPAN: https://www.c-span.org/video/?6668-1/surgeon-generals-report-abortion.

13 *New York Times*, January 11, 1989.

14 Edwin Meese interview.

15 See Reaganfoundation.org.

16 Philip Yancey, *Christianity Today*, October 20, 1989. An immediate follow-up was a call from Edith Schaeffer, asking if he had changed his opposition to abortion. Yancey/Koop.

17 *New York Times*, March 17, 1989. "The draft report, which Dr. Koop said he never approved, was made public today as part of the hearing record after the Intergovernmental Relations and Human Resources Subcommittee of the Government Operations Committee subpoenaed it and supporting documents. The subcommittee, which oversees some federal health budgets, has had periodic hearings on abortion policy." U.S. Government Printing Office, Washington, 1989. The March 16 hearing is available on C-SPAN: https://www.c-span.org/video/?6668-1/surgeon-generals-report-abortion.

18 James Bowman, in Terry L. Cooper and N. Dale Wright, ed. *Exemplary Public Administrators* (San Francisco: Jossey-Bass, 1992), 286.

19 Bowman, in Cooper and Wright, ed., *Exemplary Public Administrators*, 285.

20 Bowman, in Cooper and Wright, ed., *Exemplary Public Administrators*, 261, citing a personal communication from speechwriter Ted Cron, July 12, 1990.

21 Bowman, in Cooper and Wright, ed., *Exemplary Public Administrators*, 261.

22 Koop to President-elect George H. W. Bush, January 5, 1989. NLM Box 89 Cor.

23 Bowman, in Cooper and Wright, ed., *Exemplary Public Administrators*, 286.

24 Interview with Koop, *Rutherford Institute Magazine*, Spring 1989, 32.

25 Bowman, in Cooper and Wright, ed., *Exemplary Public Administrators*, 285–86.

26 Bowman, in Cooper and Wright, ed., *Exemplary Public Administrators*, 262.

27 See Reaganfoundation.org. The draft report is available in various places, e.g. https://www.priestsforlife.org/library/9550-the-koop-non-report.

28 *New York Times*, January 10, 1989.

29 Philip Yancey, *Christianity Today*, October 20, 1989.

30 By email, September 29, 2023.

31 Confidential interview.

32 *New York Times*, March 21, 1989.

33 Diana Greene Foster, *The Turnaway Study* (New York: Scribner's, 2020).

34 Foster, *Turnaway Study*, 14–15.

35 This is the precise issue addressed in *The Turnaway Study*, a book-length report on research conducted from 2007 on. Foster, *Turnaway Study*.

36 Foster, *Turnaway Study*, 16.

37 Foster, *Turnaway Study*, 108. One is reminded of Koop's focus on the extraordinary love of (most) parents for their children, handicapped or not.

38 This is what they had been watching the previous evening: the Intergovernmental Relations and Human Resources Subcommittee of the House Government Operations Committee. The March 16 hearing is available on C-SPAN: https://www.c-span.org/video/?6668-1/surgeon-generals-report-abortion.

39 Udo Middelmann to Koop, March 17, 1989; reply from Koop, date unclear. MSC 489 Box 89 Cor. He received other boosts from thoughtful leaders in the religious/pro-life community, such as Ronald Sider, head of Evangelicals for Social Action (a significant religious network, but not "religious right"). "I want to let you know that you make me proud to be an evangelical."

CHAPTER 14: Stepping Down

1 *New York Times*, May 1, 1987.

2 UPI, December 27, 1987, and D. Michael Lindsay, *Faith in the Halls of Power* (New York: Oxford University Press, 2008), 110.

3 Mullan/Martin. NLM Box 144 F33, 37. Interestingly, one major political figure who was there recalled it as a farewell dinner. Confidential interview.

4 *New York Times Good Health Magazine*, October 9, 1998, 30. McFadden and his committee had earlier played a key role in funding the early days of the Christian Action Council. Robert Case interview.

5 John P. Judis, "An Officer and a Gentleman," *The New Republic*, January 23, 1989.

6 Harold O. J. Brown, *Religion and Society Report*, 1989.

7 Judis, "An Officer and a Gentleman."

8 Anthony Fauci interview.

9 Koop memoir, 309–10.

10 When approached about this exchange, Baker confessed that he did not remember the circumstances well enough to comment. Email from aide John Williams, March 14, 2023.

11 Edward Martin interview.

12 Edward Martin interview.

13 Koop memoir, 310.

14 Jack Henningfield interview. There were of course other factors. For example, columnist Jack Anderson quotes a Koop colleague concerned that Koop's saying "Bush was a wimp" for failing to discuss AIDS on the campaign trail had got back to the President-elect. *Washington Post* column, May 23, 1989.

15 Ziegler/Koop, 49–50. These comments show that, despite the efforts of his friends to explain. he never understood the way senior political appointments are made in Washington.

16 Koop memoir, 311.

17 Koop memoir, 312.

18 Heininger/Koop, 23.

19 PBS *Nova*, "The Controversial Dr. Koop."

20 Koop memoir, 313.

21 Otis R. Bowen and William Du Bois, *Doc: Memories from a Life in Public Service* (Bloomington: Indiana University Press, 2000), 194. He ruefully reflects that he

had actually helped get the unknown Sununu elected governor in the first place! The incident sealed his view of life in Washington. "Rose and I were eager for a slower, less complicated life in Bremen. . . . Through no fault of my good friend President Reagan, serving as HHS secretary ranks only slightly ahead of being Marshall County coroner and far below being a family doctor, governor, IU Medical School professor, House speaker, or legislator. Perhaps all that this proves is that Washington is no place for a Fulton County boy to hang his hat."

22 Koop memoir, 313–14.

23 This led to a rather complex arrangement to manage incoming mail. Another staffer would log letters, then deliver to his office in the Humphrey Building. Then "I will read them, sort them, and assign one of the several form letters for the answer." The resulting replies will then go to his Parklawn office "for personalizing the salutation and the envelope." Then back to the Humphrey Building for signature and filing. Koop to staff, April 24, 1989. NLM Box 90 Cor.

24 Jack Anderson and Dale Van Atta's *Washington Post* column, May 23, 1989.

25 *Newsweek*, May 15, 1989.

26 As their "token Republican." Yancey interview with Brown, copy with the author.

27 Koop memoir, 312.

28 Knott/Sullivan, 45.

29 Koop to President Bush, May 4, 1989. See https://www.upi.com/Archives/1989/05/04 /Koop-resigns-as-surgeon-general/4486610257600/.

30 Koop to the President, May 4, 1989. ACC 2014–016 Box 26/33.

31 James Bowman, in Terry L. Cooper and N. Dale Wright, *Exemplary Public Administrators* (San Francisco: Jossey-Bass, 1992), 290–91; President Bush to Koop, May 4, 1989. The "seven and a half years" is curious. It would be eight minus six weeks as Surgeon General; including his time as deputy assistant secretary he was in government from February of 1981 until the end of September 1989, eight years and eight months.

32 *New York Times*, May 5, 1989. Koop took the view that the only reason Sullivan got the job was his skin color. Sullivan actually agreed with him. "I wasn't naïve . . . . I felt he wanted to have an African American in his Cabinet." Knott/Sullivan, 19.

33 Anderson and Van Atta, in the *Washington Post*.

34 PBS *Nova*.

35 Howard Filston interview.

36 PBS *Nova*.

37 Koop to Mrs. James E. Johnson, date uncertain (May/June 1989). Betty was in the hospital for ten days on return stateside. "She has recovered," Koop writes, "but still is extraordinarily weak." MSC Box 90 Cor.

38 Surgeon General's Medal/Medallion. For details see https://www.kennedy-center. org/news-room/press-release-landing-page/OSG2023/.

39 Paula Aspel to Koop, June 30, 1989; reply from Koop, July 5, 1989. MSC Box 94 Cor.

40 MSC Box 90 Cor.

41 Koop to Thomas C. Everding, April 14, 1989. MSC Box 90 Cor. Federal employees are generally forbidden to receive other earned income.

42 Statement of Senator Edward M. Kennedy, May 4, 1989. MSC Box 143 F 22.

43 Presentation speech, June 11, 1989. ACC 2015–011 Box 2. Koop was surely reminded

of his finally fruitless efforts, a third of a century before, to secure an honorary degree for his mentor and boss in Philadelphia, I.S. Ravdin. See Chapter 5.

44 Remarks by Louis B. Sullivan, American Health Foundation, May 24, 1989. MSC Box 143 F 23. "Baby Ruth" is an amusing confusion for the name of the famous ball player Babe Ruth. Baby Ruth was a controversial chocolate bar, whose branding led to litigation. The company claimed implausibly it was named after the dead baby daughter of President Cleveland. See https://www.tastingtable.com/1197586 /the-1920s-dispute-between-mlb-legend-babe-ruth-and-baby-ruth-candy/.

45 Remarks by Louis B. Sullivan, American Health Foundation, May 24, 1989. Emphases, and somewhat bizarre punctuation, original. MSC Box 143 F 23.

46 Koop memo to file, undated. DA Box 1270.

47 William Morris Agency Press Release, May 8, 1989, "Dr. C. Everett Koop selects the William Morris Agency for representation. Surgeon General to write book." DA Box 1270.

48 Brokaw would be named company president in the spring of 1989.

49 Koop notes, April 3, 1989. DA Box 1270.

50 Koop memo to file, undated. DA Box 1270.

51 Norman R. Brokaw to Koop, June 26, 1989. DA Box 1270.

52 Less than two months later, he died of AIDS. https://www.nga.gov/collection /artist-info.6517.html.

53 Invitation. MSC Box 90 Cor.

54 Yancey/Koop.

55 Edward N. Brandt to Koop, June 26, 1989. ACC Papers 42–44 Box 22.

56 Koop to Otis N. Bowen, undated (late January 1989), mailed to his Indiana home address. MSC Box 89 Cor. Bowen's wall: Young/Bowen, 24.

Part V: CITIZEN KOOP

1 "Just Who Brought Those Duds To Market?" asked Andrew Ross Sorkin in the *New York Times*, April 15, 2001, noting that Bear Stearns had the worst record among merchant banks, with at that date one-quarter of its companies in difficulties. It enjoyed a reputation as the most gung-ho of the banks. Bear Stearns itself, founded in 1923, finally collapsed under the weight of the 2007 subprime mortgage crisis, the same crisis that we note sank Dartmouth's Koop Building; two of its executives were the first Wall Street arrests of the crisis. Landon Thomas, Jr., "Prosecutors Build Bear Stearns Case on E-Mails," *New York Times*, June 20, 2008. (They were later acquitted.)

2 Technically, the new millennium did not begin until 2001, since in the western calendar there is no year zero.

3 See macrotrends.net/1320/Nasdaq-historical-chart.

4 *New York Times Book Review*, September 8, 1991.

5 *Los Angeles Times* profile, November 19, 1989.

6 Fiscal 1989 salary quoted by Bloomberg. https://www.bloomberg.com/news/articles/1994-12-18/now-its-c-dot-everett-koop-inc-dot. In 1986, for example, he had been forced to halve his 1980 pledge to the Children's Hospital. Koop to Richard D. Wood, December 11, 1986. NLM Box 83 Cor.

7 "He has received hundreds of promotional offers, among them a $2 million opportunity to appear in an advertisement for a Japanese condom maker and a $1 million

offer to endorse a well-known breakfast cereal. Never one to seek personal gain while in government, nothing has changed for Koop: to protect the integrity of the office, all of these overtures were turned down flat." James Bowman, in Terry L. Cooper and N. Dale Wright, ed. *Exemplary Public Administrators* (San Francisco: Jossey-Bass, 1992), 300.

8 "CITIZEN KOOP: Former Surgeon General's New Shingle Could Read: 'America's Family Doctor,'" *Los Angeles Times*, November 19, 1989.

9 Walter Goodman, reviewing for the *New York Times*, liked it, but ended on a reflective note. "I found myself wondering whether the public broadcasting producers, who are not known for delivering eulogies to conservatives, would have paid this deserved tribute to Dr. Koop if, though honest and committed to his beliefs, he had not proved so congenial to liberal positions." *New York Times*, October 10, 1989.

CHAPTER 15: In Washington

1 Government officials are often stunned to discover how insignificant they become once they no longer hold office, even if some are able to morph their government career into one in lobbying; but Koop found himself in a different category, since his activities during his government career had transformed him into a household name.

2 Brokaw also served as Cosby's agent, see *New York Times* Brokaw obituary, October 29, 2016. It's unclear if there was follow-up. Koop was frustrated that, despite his access, he was ineffective at raising money. Someone who worked with Koop commented to me that wealthy people like to be approached as the most important person around; Koop's ego could get in the way. Confidential interview. And a lesson Koop may never have learned is how much wealthy and famous people dislike being pitched to by people who take advantage of random meetings like this one.

3 Gospel Films had developed *Whatever Happened to the Human Race?*

4 Koop letter to Richard DeVos, May 9, 1990. DA-698 Box 1270.

5 Koop to Timothy Johnson, May 9, 1990. DA-698 Box 1270.

6 Johnson and Koop, *Let's Talk* (Grand Rapids: Zondervan, 1992). An effort a couple years soon after to persuade the publisher to issue a revised edition including healthcare reform was unsuccessful. Zondervan's Lyn Cryderman writes to Johnson, "health care reform is not a topic that drives book sales," and offers to return the rights. The original edition has anyway had disappointing sales of only twenty-five thousand copies. "The topics . . . just do not sell . . . . They are inevitably viewed as 'political,' and unless your name is Newt, books about politics don't sell." Even their Newt (Gingrich) book is selling below projections. December 8, 1995? (Year unclear) DA-698 Box 1270.

7 Koop to publicist, November 17, 1991. DA-698 Box 1270.

8 *New York Times*, December 6, 1991. A fair amount of money was involved in this contract. The *New York Times* dryly observed, "Publishers at several other houses said they had tried to sign Mr. Johnson to write a book but backed out when they were told that $5 million was not enough."

9 See the NLM profile: https://profiles.nlm.nih.gov/spotlight/qq/catalog/nlm:nlmuid -101584930X973-doc.

10 The Nantucket Cove recalled: https://www.stlmag.com/dining/memory-lane%3A -nantucket-cove/.

11 *St Louis Post-Dispatch*, October 13, 1991.

12 Koop stepped away from involvement in public debate about euthanasia and assisted suicide. It's plain he has re-ordered his priorities. He declined an invitation to record pro-life messages: "I feel absolutely no guilt about this in reference to the issue you raise. I have written two books, done five movies, and talk [*sic*] all over the world on this subject, I do believe I have stated my position." He adds, on the matter of his current priorities: "Therefore, I am leaving behind other things that I still have an interest in, but do not feel I can take an active part in." Koop to Robert J. Raubach, undated, DA-698 KI Cor. Jan–July 1993. Declining an invitation to participate in a legal case in April of 1996: "I am involved with several commercial enterprises where I feel morally bound to discuss this before moving into the limelight, as I certainly would." Koop to Ken Carozza, April 8, 1996. DA-698, Box 1273. He had earlier declined a collaborative book proposal on the same subject. Letter to the author, December 22, 1993. DA-698 Box 1965.

13 See Chapter 10.

14 Yancey/Koop.

15 Editor of *Good Housekeeping* to Koop, May, 1980, forwarded to Brokaw.

16 Yancey/Koop. Yancey's Koop profile appeared in *Christianity Today*, October 20 and November 3, 1989.

17 *Los Angeles Times* profile, November 19, 1989.

18 *Los Angeles Times*, November 19, 1989.

19 *Los Angeles Times*, November 19, 1989.

20 See NLM profile: https://profiles.nlm.nih.gov/spotlight/qq/catalog/nlm:nlmuid -101584930X917-doc.

21 *Los Angeles Times*, November 19, 1989.

22 Daniel Cerone, "Dr. Koop Finds His Bulliest Pulpit Yet: Television," *Los Angeles Times*, June 3, 1991.

23 Title and original airdates: 1 "Children at Risk," June 4, 1991; 2 "Listening to Teenagers," June 9, 1991; 3 "Forever Young," June 16, 1991; 4 "Hard Choices," June 23, 1991; 5 "A Time for Change," June 30, 1991.

24 *Deseret News*, June 3, 1991.

25 Letter from Koop to Norman Brokaw, October 28, 1992. DA-698 Box 1964.

26 See Chapter 17.

27 Daniel Cerone, *Los Angeles Times*, June 3, 1991. Of course, it is not the case that he got out of the administration because of its lack of focus on healthcare. He got out because his contract ran out.

28 Koop to Waxman, October 5, 1988. MSC 489 Box 87 Cor.

29 Koop to Constance Clark, July 28, 1988. MSC Box 94 Cor.

30 Koop to John Van Dienst, August 14, 1989. MSC Box 94 Cor.

31 Koop to Jacqueline Kennedy Onassis, July 6, 1989. DA-698 Box 1270.

32 Koop to Owen Laster, February 24, 1993. DA-698 Jan-July 93 KI Cor.

33 Later, Koop tried unsuccessfully to get the publishers of his medical text, *Visible and Palpable Lesions in Children* (New York: Grune and Stratton, 1976) to reissue it under the title, *Lumps, Bumps, and Kids*. See Ehrhart/Koop, 79.

34 *Los Angeles Times*, November 19, 1989. In 1992–93 he reports having given fifty-two

lectures, "to audiences of between two hundred and five thousand all over the country." Koop to Dartmouth dean Andrew. G. Wallace, May 3, 1993. DA-698 KI Cor. Box 93. It is not clear how many of these were paid; Koop would adjust his fee, and sometimes speak pro bono. Fees noted in Koop's files for 1990–91 range from $10,000 to $25,000, with $20,000 the norm, plus first class travel for him and an aide. ACC 2015–011 Koop Papers 1942–2009 Box 2.

35 Confidential interview.

36 *Los Angeles Times*, November 19, 1989.

37 *Los Angeles Times*, November 19, 1989.

38 The National Safe Kids Campaign is now a global non-profit, Safe Kids Worldwide. https://www.safekids.org/our-history.

39 Koop to Martin H. Eichelberger, May 5, 1988. MSC 498 Box 87 Cor.

40 As we noted, in 1955 Koop was the "surgical member" of the American Academy of Pediatrics Committee on Accident Prevention. AAP Board minutes, March 31, 1955.

41 Martin Eichenberger interview. In fall of 1992 the Children's National Medical Center, which hosted Safe Kids, agreed to fund 50 percent of a secretary for Koop. Koop to Don Brown, October 7, 1992. DA-698 Box 1964.

42 See *New York Times*, September 9, 1992. For reasons that are unclear, the Carnegie effort was short-lived.

43 Susan Okie, "Koop's Campaign to Rescue a Museum," *Washington Post*, September 7, 1989.

44 Quoted in Susan Okie, "Koops Campaign to Rescue a Museum," *Washington Post*, September 8, 1989 See also Nathan Abse, "Push is on for New Medical Museum as Old Collection is Modernized," *Washington Post*, December 16, 1997.

45 Mullan/Koop, 99. Sadly, Koop efforts at private fund-raising and an effort by Senator Kennedy to secure federal funding all came to nothing. The existing museum remains in the Washington suburbs (now in Silver Spring, Maryland). https://medicalmuseum.health.mil/. An announced new site in Atlanta, ironically under the chairmanship of Louis Sullivan, who was made HHS secretary when Koop wanted the job, has yet to come to fruition. See https://www.health leadersmedia.com/strategy/health-museum-be-built-atlanta and https://www .national-health-museum.org/.

46 Koop to Guy M. Condon, date uncertain but prior to his resignation. NLM Box 86 Cor. For reasons that are unclear, he did not rejoin the board.

47 Michael Horton interview. In 2001, Horton visited Koop at Dartmouth and persuaded him to rejoin the board.

48 There is no title given; it is mainly a reflection on his engagement in AIDS, discussed above in Chapter 11. Wheaton CACE archives.

49 *Chicago Tribune*, February 25, 1990.

50 Not for lack of effort on Koop's part. On October 4, 1993, he sent Johnson detailed fund-raising ideas, including an approach to Richard DeVos, whom he had tried to touch for the museum. "One of the few Christian billionaires in the country . . . has never funded anything I did except minuscule things like lectureships." Koop to Alan Johnson, October 4, 1993, CACE archives. The CACE archives also contain the January 1994, formal proposal.

51 After his retirement as director, Johnson sent Koop birthday greetings in 2000,

396 NOTES TO PAGES 263–266

and Koop replied with much personal news on October 30. Koop to Alan and Rea Johnson, October 30, 2000. CACE Archives.

52 Koop to Alan Johnson, undated (2004?). CACE archives.

53 Koop to Alan Johnson, undated. CACE archives.

54 Koop to Herbert Ratner, June 14, 1993. DA-698 Jan-July 93 KI Cor.

55 Gloria Butland to Koop, January 9, 2003. ACC 2015–011 Box 2.

56 Marcia Martin to Koop, May 14, 2005; Koop to Martin, June 20, 2005. MSC 489 Box 78 Cor.

57 James T. Bennett and Thomas J. DiLorenzo, *Public Health Profiteering* (New York: Routledge, 2001), 138–39.

58 See https://www.lifealert.com and *Forbes*, "The best alternatives to Life Alert," forbes.com, and https://www.bustle.com/articles/37634-that-new-life-alert-basement-ad-its-scarier-than-anything-else-on-tv.

59 Edward J. Marteka to Koop, March 24, 1994. There was evidently a disagreement between Koop and the company that led to the premature ending of the contract. Letter from Marteka to Koop, February 25, 1997. DA-698 Box 1273.

60 See c.v., Ziegler/Koop, 73. Board photo and document at ACC 2014 Box 24.

61 Rick Kogan, *Chicago Tribune*, June 4, 1991. The Time Life Medical video project is discussed in Chapter 15.

62 Neil Romano to Tom Burke, July 21, 1993; to Koop, August 3, 1993. Handwritten note from Burke to Koop, date unclear. DA-698 Box 1273. Burke had been chief of staff to Secretary Bowen. It's unclear whether Burke ever gave up his trademark cigars.

63 Cal Covert to Koop, July 28, 1995. DA-698 Box 1270.

64 Time Life Medical Press Release, November 28, 1994. ACC CEK Papers Box 18. Hyphenation of Time-Life is inconsistent in the name of the parent corporation; there is none in the name of Time Life Medical.

65 *Washington Post*, November 28, 1996.

66 *Washington Post*, November 28, 1996.

67 *Wall Street Journal*, November 28, 1994.

68 "Now, It's C. Everett Koop Inc.," at https://www.bloomberg.com/news/articles /1994-12-18/now-its-c-dot-everett-koop-inc-dot#xj4y7vzkg.

69 It's not clear why Koop agreed to the unfamiliar role of board chair rather than, say, series editor, though the appeal to his ego was palpable.

70 Though he was not an easy person to work with. When he left, *Adweek* reported euphoria among his colleagues. *Wall Street Journal*, November 28, 1994.

71 "Now, It's C. Everett Koop Inc." https://www.bloomberg.com/news/articles/1994 -12-18/now-its-c-dot-everett-koop-inc-dot#xj4y7vzkg.

72 Ellen Joan Pollock, "Health Videos Starring Koop Took Sick, Saw Dismal Sales," *Wall Street Journal*, February 13, 1997.

73 *Wall Street Journal*, February 13, 1997.

74 *Wall Street Journal*, November 28, 1994.

75 *Wall Street Journal*, February 13, 1997.

76 Confidential interview. Time Life is famous for the detailed market research that precedes their products. *Wall Street Journal*, November 28, 1994.

77 Confidential interview.

78 Outside the UK, European systems are not actually "single-payer" but essentially

hybrid. It's notable that the US and the UK are the only developed nations in which healthcare is continually a major political issue.

79 Mullan/Koop, 37. The medical student is identified as "Atua Gwandi;" in fact his name was Gawande. He went on to become a distinguished surgeon and writer, and as of this writing is a senior official with USAID. It's not clear what the content was of all these calls Koop remembers having had with Clinton, or why they did not lead to his being involved in the reform effort at the White House from the start.

80 Clinton appointed Joycelyn Elders to the post in September of 1993, though she stepped down in controversy after just over a year. For the rest of his first term there were only "acting" appointments in the office.

81 Timothy Westmoreland interview.

82 This is surprising, given the reported contacts between Koop and Clinton during the campaign. But as the interposition of the medical student shows, these calls were plainly more significant for Koop than they were for Clinton. The ignored letter in question would seem to be that of March 11, 1993, from Koop and John E. Wennberg, offering their help and that of their respective centers. Clinton Presidential Libraries, https://clinton.presidentiallibraries.us/items/show/42134 at 38. Koop and Wennberg had actually tried earlier to insert themselves into the discussion in a letter dated January 11, 1993, to Judith E. Feder, a political aide who had served as staff director of the bipartisan "Pepper Commission" on healthcare reform and would shortly be appointed principal deputy assistant secretary at HHS. Clinton Presidential Libraries, https://clinton.presidentiallibraries.us/items/show/42134 at 40–41.

83 "C. Everett Koop," unsigned memorandum, Clinton Presidential Libraries, https://clinton.presidentiallibraries.us/items/show/42135 at 30–31.

84 Mullan/Koop, 38.

85 Memorandum from Alexis Herman and Mike Lux, "Remarks to Supportive Doctors . . . ," Clinton Presidential Libraries, https://clinton.presidentiallibraries.us/items/show/46708. One hundred forty-eight invited doctors are listed.

86 Transcript, issued September 20, 1993, Clinton Presidential Libraries, https://clinton.presidentiallibraries.us/items/show/42130 at 30.

87 Address of the President to the Joint Session of Congress, September 22, 1993, Clinton Presidential Libraries https://clinton.presidentiallibraries.us/items/show/42131 at 34.

88 Koop, "A prescription for healthy debate," *Chicago Tribune*, September 29, 1993.

89 Mullan/Koop, 40.

90 Note added to comments on reform document, Koop to Ira Magaziner, August 30, 1993, Clinton Presidential Library, https://clinton.presidentiallibraries.us/files/original/facd5ff518e419768bf25d02e3842577.pdf at 81–88. Separately, Koop wrote on September 7 to Mrs. Clinton to solicit the administration's support for legislation to enable the museum project. https://clinton.presidentiallibraries.us/items/show/42132.

91 Koop to Ira Magaziner, September 8, 1993, Clinton Presidential Libraries https://clinton.presidentiallibraries.us/items/show/46708.

92 Koop file note of April 26, 1993, call; Vice President Gore to Koop, June 8, 1993. DA-698 Box 8298.

93   Clinton, *Living History* (New York: Simon and Schuster, 2003), 216. The Surgeon General, needless to say, has no policy role.

94   Clinton, *Living History*, 234.

95   Koop to Hillary Clinton, January 17, 1993, DA-698 Box 8298.

96   Shape Up America! was formally housed in the non-profit Koop Foundation Incorporated (KFI). KFI would also be the recipient of the substantial research grants Koop obtained for work on bioinformatics. We discuss in Chapter 16.

97   Meeting notes, HRC/Koop Meeting, September 26, 1994, Clinton Presidential Libraries, https://clinton.presidentiallibraries.us/items/show/42130.

98   Mullan/Koop, 17.

99   See https://www.bloomberg.com/news/articles/1994-12-18/now-its-c-dot-everett-koop-inc-dot#xj4y7vzkg. "I always do everything Dr. Koop tells me," Mrs. Clinton declared.

100   Koop to Walter Bortz, September 29, 1994. DA-698 Box 1967.

101   See https://www.bloomberg.com/news/articles/1994-12-18/now-its-c-dot-everett-koop-inc-dot#xj4y7vzkg.

102   Connecticut Marketing Associates (CMA), Preliminary Plan Overview, September 1, 1994. DA-698 Box 1967.

103   *Philanthropy News Digest*, July 26, 2005.

104   *New York Times*, December 1 and 11, 1994; Sally Squires in the *Washington Post*, October 18, 2005. Shape Up was still in business fifteen years later, but as of this writing, the domain shapeup.org is for sale. See "Wearing a Pedometer Can Be a Big Step in the Weight-loss Battle," *Washington Post*, November 12, 2009. Recent research on the causes of obesity and the effectiveness of various kinds of anti-obesity campaign is helpfully reviewed in this article by Helen Lee on *The Breakthrough*: "The Making of the Obesity Epidemic." https://thebreakthrough.org/journal/issue-3/the-making-of-the-obesity-epidemic. It is not possible to discern any statistically significant impact of Shape Up America! on the rising rates of obesity in the United States. See this from the CDC *Morbidity and Mortality Weekly Report*: https://www.cdc.gov/mmwr/preview/mmwrhtml/su6001a15.htm.

105   Bennett and DiLorenzo, *Public Health Profiteering*, 70.

106   Jan Strode interview.

107   Mireya Navarro, "Flight Attendants Reach Settlement in Nonsmoker Suit," *New York Times*, October 11, 1997.

108   Sarah Milov, *The Cigarette: A Political History* (Cambridge, MA: Harvard University Press, 2019), 287.

109   *New York Times*, October 11, 1997.

110   These sums were intended to be placed in a trust fund for healthcare purposes, but—as with similar settlements elsewhere—"state leaders began removing funds from the trust fund to fill budget holes," and the trust was eventually abolished. See Mississippitoday.org for June 26, 2022.

111   *Wall Street Journal*, July 30, 1997. The Koop-Kessler report can be found here: https://pubmed.ncbi.nlm.nih.gov/9396113/. Interviewed years later, Koop reported on another aspect of the settlement talks. "I had two secret meetings with people from the tobacco industry, with great secrecy, in places I didn't usually frequent, go in the back door, go up the backstairs, this sort of stuff. Really seeing if, I would say, I could be bought, but seeing whether in my position of righteousness about

tobacco, I couldn't say things that would be favorable to the settlement, the way they wanted it to go." Mullan/Koop, 50.

112 Milov, *The Cigarette*, 289–90.

113 Milov, *The Cigarette*, 289–90, puts it at $206 billion.

114 David Kessler, *A Question of Intent* (New York: PublicAffairs, revised edition 2002), 361. The states did, however, agree to end their litigation, while individuals and classes continued to be free to sue. Milov, *The Cigarette*, 289–90.

115 "Let's Make a Deal," *Reason Magazine*, October 1, 1997.

116 Quoted in John Schwartz, "The Fox in 'Chick' Koop," *Washington Post*, January 9, 2000.

117 Schwartz, "The Fox in 'Chick' Koop."

118 Koop notes, April 3, 1989. "Dr. C. Everett Koop selects the William Morris Agency for representation. Surgeon General to write book." DA Box 1270.

119 *Tribune* quoted in Schwartz, "The Fox in 'Chick' Koop."

120 Edward Martin interview.

CHAPTER 16: At Dartmouth

1 At a time when little colleges all over the United States have decided to call themselves universities, Dartmouth, founded in 1769 and a member of the Ivy League, has stuck with the name college. This can be confusing, since it refers both to the undergraduate college and also to the wider "university" encompassing several professional schools. Evidently, "Koop got the rumor mill going in 1990, after a brief visit to Dartmouth," when he was "wooed by school officials eager to work with one of the college's most prestigious alums." Stephen C. George, *The New Physician*, December 1993.

2 Dartmouth Hitchcock Medical Center news release, embargoed until 10:00 a.m., May 19, 1992. Koop would be Senior Scholar of the Institute, as well as Elizabeth DeCamp McInerny Professor of Surgery. ACC Box 18. Koop had actually already incorporated a short-lived "C. Everett Koop Institute of Health and Science," with an address in Salisbury, Maryland, and used it to respond to the many letters he received after the NBC specials were broadcast. Its purpose is "exclusively to stimulate and support research, education and knowledge," to improve public health. Copy from family papers. Amusingly, Koop was still using this designation when Johns Hopkins awarded him an honorary degree on May 21, 1992—two days after the Dartmouth affiliation was announced. See https://jscholarship.library.jhu.edu/bitstream/handle/1774.2/36834/commencement1992.pdf?sequence=1&isAllowed=y.

3 Woodie Kessel interview.

4 Bizarrely, shortly before he stood down as Surgeon General Koop had been asked whether he would be interested in becoming dean of the medical school! If so, he was invited to submit his c.v. He sent a polite no thank you. Harold C. Sox to Koop, May 5, 1989; Koop to Sox, May 30. NLM Box 90 Cor.

5 Andrew G. Wallace to Jane Bassick, June 30, 1992. DA-698 Box 8298. Wallace may not have known that Freedman and Koop had history. Twenty years before, Koop had operated on Freedman's son, and Freedman reached out to Koop soon after his appointment as president. "I have the feeling you're up to it," Koop replied.

Freedman to Koop, September 21, 1987; Koop to Freedman, October 26, 1987. Koop also took the opportunity to press the case for his "charming, intelligent, athletic," granddaughter's admission in the fall of 1988! NLM Box 86 Cor.

6 In an obituary in *Dartmouth Medicine*, Spring 2013.

7 Koop to Joan Brundage, July 15, 1992. DA-698 Jan-Dec 1993–94 KI Cor.

8 Stephen C. George, *The New Physician*, December 1993.

9 "Can 'America's family doctor' reshape medical education?" Interview by Berkeley Rice. *Medical Economics*, January 25, 1993.

10 David Serra interview.

11 Duffy also held the rank of Assistant Surgeon General, though as we noted in Chapter 12, there were (and are) many Assistant Surgeons General. *Koop Institute Newsletter* 1:1, Spring 1993.

12 Duffy is quoted in *The Dartmouth* for January 1994. Oddly, he is described here as medical director. Duffy also served as a dean of admissions at Dartmouth, see https://collections.nlm.nih.gov/catalog/nlm:nlmuid-101584930X413-doc. One source told me in confidence that Duffy was forced out, and this is supported by the financials; he received a substantial severance settlement. Confidential interview. Memorandum from Adam Keller to Koop, January 25, 1994. DA-698 Box 8298.

13 Confidential interview.

14 Koop to Paul Brand, January 5, 1994. DA-698 Box 1965.

15 Duffy to James O. Freedman, January 4, 1993; Koop to Freedman, January 12, 1993. DA-698 Jan-Dec 1993–94 KI Cor.

16 Koop to Andrew G. Wallace, November 19, 1992. DA-698 Jan-Dec 1993–94 KI Cor.

17 Koop to James C. Freedman, October 13, 1993. DA-698 KI Cor. 1993.

18 A further set of problems flowing from Freedman's grandiose announcement centered on the decision to establish a single "Board of Overseers" for both the Medical School and the Institute, as if they were co-equal institutions rather than one a tiny component of the other. See Koop to Andrew G. Wallace, May 3, 1993. DA-698 KI Cor. 1993. They were soon separated.

19 David Serra interview.

20 Koop to James C. Freedman, February 11, 1993. DA-698 Jan-Dec 1993–94 KI Cor.

21 Daniel S. Goldin to Koop, April 26, 1994. DA-698 KI Cor. 1/94–6/94.

22 Adam Keller to Koop, January 25, 1994. DA-698 Box 8298. The purpose of the memo would seem to be to give Koop the unwelcome news that Duffy's severance of $90,000 was being charged to the Institute, in line with College accounting policy. "If you feel that this cost should be shared by DMS, let's discuss it next time you are in town." On one occasion, at least, Koop channeled income from his paid lectures into Institute efforts—$25,000 from a lecture in St Louis, put to fund an Institute conference. DA-698 KI Subject Files Box 8298.

23 David Serra interview. He later served as managing director of the Koop Foundation.

24 Koop speech notes, October 7, 1995. DA Box 1272.

25 Details of the personnel of the Institute, particularly after 1995, have been gleaned mainly from the somewhat haphazard records of the Internet Archive "Wayback Machine." The human resources department of the college was unresponsive to a request for information of this kind.

26 Joseph O'Donnell interview. William J. Culp was a long-standing faculty member

at the medical school and an associate dean, who took over as director of the Koop Institute in 1995 and served in this part-time role until 2011.

27 Joseph Walsh interview.

28 Confidential interview.

29 The following chapter picks up on further Institute developments, reviewing Koop's vision for the future of the profession.

30 Confidential interview. Nonetheless, it is a rail journey of approximately eleven hours each way. The Koops soon acquired a small downtown apartment in Hanover, and finally moved house in 1997.

31 Joseph Walsh interview.

32 John Schwartz, "The Fox in 'Chick' Koop," *Washington Post*, January 9, 2000.

33 Stephen C. George, *The New Physician*, December 1993.

34 Woodie Kessel interview.

35 Woodie Kessel interview. Koop's final disillusion with the Dartmouth experience is captured in a 2007 interview in which he reminisces about a banquet in his honor in Washington, DC, hosted by the National Library of Medicine, to which he had donated "970 lectures and 920 videos, all of which I had written or performed in some way." "Nobody at Dartmouth knows what I did in Washington. . . . I think they think the whole thing is a big joke, that it has nothing to do with reality." As he entered the (Capitol Hill) Cannon Building, a car suddenly stopped "and Ted Kennedy hopped out of the back and came ambling over. . . . And if that didn't prove I was in favor, Hillary Clinton came out of her . . . office . . . . So she and Ted Kennedy and I had a little reunion about smoking right there on the corner. It just so happened that the Dartmouth people who had been invited down as guests for this banquet, I think they realized for the first time that yes, he really must have known some people down there." Heininger/Koop, 6–7.

36 One former administrator of the Institute summed up the financial dimension: "$150,000 for the chair, plus $40,000 for a secretary. All the rest needed soft funding." Confidential interview.

37 A not-for-profit 501 (c) 3 organization registered in New Hampshire, #215698, though with a mailing address at 15825 Shady Grove Road, Suite 20, Rockville, MD 20850. Web Archive for April 22, 1999. https://www.nhcompanyregistry.com/companies/the-koop-foundation-incorporated/?__cf_chl_tk=GKu9pbRgnuEyKroLdyzJzibBj8KMiHW4nDhvtIoI1UE-1691933865-0-gaNycGzNC6U.

38 American universities negotiate with federal funding agencies a standing agreed percentage of any awards to be set aside to cover "indirect" as opposed to "direct" costs—a percentage toward general university administration that does not require separate accounting. University authorities then frequently agree to return to the Principal Investigator (the standard term for the chief person to win the grant) a slice of this "indirect" funding to apply to project purposes that are not covered by the terms of the award (such as alcohol at events, certain kinds of travel, and so on). Universities set their own "tax rate" to cover indirect costs for grants and gifts won by faculty and projects such as institutes from other sources.

39 Apparently, these particular awards secured by the Foundation were not available to academic institutions. Michael McDonald interview.

40 The Institute has outlasted him, though after 2013 with a limited level of activity. The failure of Dartmouth's successive leaders to develop any sense of institutional

history for the Institute is striking. Its thirtieth anniversary in 2022 passed unremarked; neither on the website nor elsewhere is there any collation of information about its successive leaders, staff, and projects.

41 Joseph Walsh interview.

42 David Serra interview.

43 Sean David interview.

44 "Smoky Lies," produced by Monica Wilkins. See: https://www.imdb.com/title/tto 936498/.

45 Holcomb B. Noble, "SCIENTIST AT WORK: C. Everett Koop; He's 'Gone Commercial' to Spread Gospel of Health," *New York Times*, February 2, 1999.

46 Virginia Reed and Christopher Jernstedt interview.

47 Virginia Reed and Christopher Jernstedt interview. See also Web Archive, November 17, 2001: https://web.archive.org/web/20011117061351/http://www.dartmouth. edu/dms/koop/programs/outcomes.shtml As of this writing the center continues, accessible here: https://geiselmed.dartmouth.edu/cpde/. The center's website makes no mention of its origins in the Koop Institute.

48 Koop to Naj Wikoff, April 19, 1993. DA-698 KI Cor. 1993.

49 Wikoff is described as "Director of Healing and the Arts" at the Koop Institute, when he writes the lead article for the *Americans for the Arts Monographs* publication for September, 1998.

50 See Joseph M. Rosen, C. Everett Koop, and Eliot B Grigg, "Cybercare: A System for Confronting Bioterrorism," *The Bridge*, Spring 2002. Also, Koop and Rosen to George W. Bush, February 4, 2003; Koop to Fauci, February 5, 2003. ACC 2015–011 Box 2.

51 Confidential interview.

52 Confidential interview.

53 In 1994, for example, a memo mentions plans for the C. Everett Koop Conference and Education Building of ninety-seven thousand square feet, costing an estimated $16.4 million. February 17, 1994, "Health Information Infrastructure Foundation." DA-698 Box 8298.

54 Woodie Kessel interview.

55 Lester Gibbs interview.

56 February 17, 1994, "Health Information Infrastructure Foundation." DA-698 Box 8298.

57 Confidential interview.

58 Joseph Walsh interview. I can add my own report here from a conversation with Koop from the late 1990s. He couldn't understand how the college could have shifted from, initially, promising him a Koop building, to telling him in detail how much money he would have to raise to get one.

59 Joseph O'Donnell interview.

60 "DMS announces new Koop Complex," *The Dartmouth*, November 3, 2006.

61 Joseph O'Donnell interview.

62 Joseph O'Donnell interview.

63 On Lehman, see https://knowledge.wharton.upenn.edu/podcast/knowledge-at -wharton-podcast/the-good-reasons-why-lehman-failed/. Dartmouth immediately instituted a hiring freeze, and on February 12 of 2009 a crisis budget was announced by medical school dean William Green. It included layoffs, no annual raises–and

the postponement of all new building plans. "DMS to cut $25 mil., lay off staff members," *The Dartmouth*, February 12, 2009.

CHAPTER 17: Tomorrow's Medicine

1 *Pennsylvania Medicine*, 1985.
2 *Dartmouth Alumni Magazine*, November, 1993.
3 Joseph Henderson interview.
4 Duffy to William Culp, May 14, 1993. DA-698 KI Cor. 1993.
5 Koop conversation with Goldberg.
6 Koop, "Telemedicine will revolutionize care," *USA Today*, August 23, 1993.
7 Koop conversation with Goldberg.
8 Meeting program. DA-798 KI 1991–94 Box 8298.
9 Koop to Alan Elias, September 27, 1993. DA-698 KI Cor. 1993.
10 ARPA is now known as DARPA. Curiously, the agency's name was originally ARPA, then DARPA, then between 1993 and 1996 ARPA again, then DARPA again. So in 1994 it was ARPA. See Wikipedia, Defense Advanced Research Projects Agency.
11 Meeting between Koop and the First Lady, notes, April 19, 1994. Clinton Presidential Libraries, https://clinton.presidentiallibraries.us/items/show/42130 at 9–10.
12 Letter from Koop to HII Consortium Members, July 20, 1995. Clinton Presidential Libraries https://clinton.presidentiallibraries.us/files/original/53c29e2915671a4faob 3309a848a6faf.pdf
13 Clinton Presidential Libraries https://clinton.presidentiallibraries.us/files/original /53c29e2915671a4faob3309a848a6faf.pdf
14 A not-for-profit 501 (c) 3 organization registered in New Hampshire, though with a mailing address at 15825 Shady Grove Road, Suite 20, Rockville, MD 20850. Web archive for April 22, 1999: https://web.archive.org/web/19990429070359/http:// www.koopfoundation.org/.
15 These figures from James T. Bennett and Thomas J. DiLorenzo, *Public Health Profiteering* (New York: Routledge, 2001), 147–48, 151. Private sector partners included Oracle and A. T. and T. The grant was through the Advanced Technology Program of NIST. Bennett and DiLorenzo suggest that the grant was awarded to the Koop Institute, but this would seem to be in error. On 151 they state that both awards were made to the Foundation. There seems to have been some passing Dartmouth association with the projects, but the awards were not made to the college. Bennett and DiLorenzo submitted Freedom of Information Act (FOIA) requests for paperwork on both, and among the more than five thousand pages of documents they received there was evidence of confusion on the part of NIST administrators as to the relations of the Koop institutions.
16 The total is slightly different—$30,167,952—in a summary of the proposal for the "Health Informatics Initiative" faxed from NIST (unclear to whom) on October 24, 1994. Clinton Presidential Libraries https://clinton.presidentiallibraries.us/files /original/53c29e2915671a4faob3309a848a6faf.pdf at 22.
17 Bennett and DiLorenzo, *Public Health Profiteering*, 150–51.
18 Health Informatics Initiative Consortium, disbanded January 26, 1999, reported *Federal Register* Vol. 64 #159, August 18, 1999, 44958–9. The Koop Foundation was the "convener."

19 *Valley News*, "Published for the Upper Connecticut River Valley," April 20, 1993.

20 See Jeffrey Bauer and Marc Ringel, *Telemedicine and the Reinvention of Healthcare* (New York: McGraw Hill, 1999), 32.

21 Web archive for April 19, 1998: https://web.archive.org/web/19980419230000/http://koop.dartmouth.edu/nnehii_1.html.

22 December 3, 1993, Schedule for the Day. DA-698 Box 8299.

23 Job Description, Project Director, New England Rural Health Information System, undated. DA-698 KI Cor. 1993.

24 Conference brochure. DA Box 1272.

25 Web archive for April 19, 1998: https://web.archive.org/web/19980419214858/http:/koop.dartmouth.edu/contacts/contacts_koopvillage.html.

26 Web archive, see also: https://web.archive.org/web/19980419210916/http://koop.dartmouth.edu/koop_village.html.

27 Sean David interview. See also S. P. David, "The Transatlantic Conference on Tobacco (TACT): A Model for International Tobacco Policy Activism," in *Journal of Cancer Education* 13, no. 4 (1998), 253–54.

28 Michael McDonald interview and see: https://resilientamericancommunities.org/?page_id=10144.

29 Web Archive for April 19, 1998: https://web.archive.org/web/19980419210825/http://koop.dartmouth.edu/projects_dfc.html.

30 Web archive, December 5, 1998: https://web.archive.org/web/19981205135356/http://www.epidemic.org/importantMessage.html.

31 Web archive, February 26, 1999: https://web.archive.org/web/19990224031504/http://koopfoundation.org:80/. In 2020, the reported mortality rates in the United States were 14,863 for Hepatitis C and 18,489 for AIDS. https://www.cdc.gov/hepatitis/statistics/2020surveillance/hepatitis-c/table-3.8.htm https://www.hiv.gov/hiv-basics/overview/data-and-trends/statistics/.

32 Web archive for April 19, 1998: https://web.archive.org/web/19980419210803/http://koop.dartmouth.edu/projects_cbi.html.

33 "Rx for Trouble," *Texas Monthly*, June 2000. A curious statement in light of the evident success of Shape Up America!

34 University of Alabama archives, https://csts.ua.edu/files/2019/09/1993-12-21-John-Zaccaro-to-Eric-Solberg-Internatl-Health-Med-Film-Festival-Award.pdf. The festival would later be acquired by the American Medical Association, which retained Zaccaro as executive director, and in 1998 by Time Inc. Health. http://www.ptca.org/award.html. (Time Inc. Health is a separate Time effort from the ill-fated Time Life Medical company that produced the videos.)

35 "Dr. Koop and the Greed Disease," *Fortune*, May 29, 2000.

36 Per the *Wall Street Journal*, June 9, 1999.

37 Oddly, giving Koop's Bethesda home address at 5924 Maplewood Park Place. By this time the Koops were living in Hanover, New Hampshire.

38 See agreement and related documents at Findlaw. https://corporate.findlaw.com/contracts/operations/agreement-c-everett-koop-m-d-and-empower-health-corp.html.

39 "Rx for Trouble," *Texas Monthly*. It's not clear what this article means by a "relaunch as DrKoop.com." By December 11, 1998, Drkoop.com was already up and running. See: https://web.archive.org/web/19981212013704/http://drkoop.com/.

40 DrKoop.com opened the next morning at $12.25, closing that afternoon at more

than $16—a very healthy premium on its offering price. The company was now valued at almost half a billion dollars. Seven percent of this half billion, or $41 million, was the 2.5 million shares owned by the eponymous Dr. Koop himself. See the *Wall Street Journal*, June 9, 1999.

41 Confidential interview.

42 Edward Martin interview.

43 Per the *Wall Street Journal*, June 9, 1999.

44 "Just call him Doc.Com: Koop's Web IPO Clicks," *Washington Post*, June 9, 1999.

45 By email from Hackett, February 29, 2024.

46 *New York Times*, September 5, 1999. It is striking how long and complex the road has been to enable health records to be accessible online. There is a handy summary with links at www.nethealth.com/blog/the-history-of-electronic-health-records-ehrs.

47 "Charting drkoop.com's rapid decline," April 5, 2000. https://www.zdnet.com/article /charting-drkoop-coms-rapid-decline/ "Marcus Welby M.D." was an immensely popular television series, screened by ABC from 1969–1976. See https://www.imdb.com /title/tt0063927/.

48 Confidential interview.

49 Confidential interview.

50 See "Dr. Koop and the Greed Disease," *Fortune*. AOL: confidential interview.

51 "Irrational exuberance" was a phrase made famous by long-time Federal Reserve chairman Alan Greenspan in a 1996 speech.

52 "Dr. Koop and the Greed Disease," *Fortune*.

53 The 1999 filing with the Securities and Exchange Commission (SEC), full of fasci- nating details, essentially offers an understated obituary for the company. https:// www.sec.gov/Archives/edgar/data/1073794/0000930661-00-000842.txt.

54 For an explanation of the short swing rule, see: https://www.investopedia.com /terms/s/shortswingprofitrule.asp.

55 *Chicago Tribune*, September 4, 1999.

56 "Dr. Koop and the Greed Disease," *Fortune*. Fisher continued: "I just couldn't make sense of it. All the revenues were going to AOL and Disney."

57 Holcomb B. Noble, "E-MEDICINE—A Special report: Hailed as a Surgeon General, Koop Is Faulted on Web Ethics," *New York Times*, September 5, 1999. The actual figures were 2 percent for existing prod- ucts, and up to 4 percent for certain new products. See agreement and related documents at Findlaw: https://corporate.findlaw.com/contracts /operations/agreement-c-everett-koop-m-d-and-empower-health-corp.html. In 1998 and 1999 Koop had accrued a little under $42,000 in these royalties. See Securities and Exchange Commission filing for 1999: https://www.sec.gov/Archives /edgar/data/1073794/0000930661-00-000842.txt. The royalty arrangement was replaced by a further stock option, to buy 214,000 shares of stock at the then traded price of $17.88, at a rate of 8,900 shares per month. (The assumption of stock options is, of course, that the traded price will rise.)

58 *New York Times*, September 5, 1999.

59 Fred Charatan, "DrKoop.com Criticised for Missing Information with Advertising," *British Medical Journal*, September 18, 1999.

60 "Developing Rules for the Web," *American Medical News*, July 31, 2000.

61 *Dartmouth Alumni Magazine*, January/February 2001, cover story.

62 See "Drkoop.com Gets $20 Million Bailout, Appoints a New Executive Team," *Wall Street Journal*, August 23, 2000.
63 *Los Angeles Times*, July 16, 2002.
64 We don't know whether he considered bidding for it himself; at that price it would have been money well spent. Perhaps it did not occur to him that it could go for so little.
65 The internet directory of URL ownership Whois shields the current owner's details from public scrutiny.
66 See "DrKoop.com Sold at Knockdown Price." www.digitalhealth.net/2002/07/drkoop-com-sold-at-knockdown-price/.
67 Nelson D. Schwartz, "Dr. Koop and the Greed Disease," *Fortune*. The late 1990s phenomenon of internet start-ups grabbing investment and turning entrepreneurs into overnight millionaires was thrilling to watch but easy to pillory. It's now common to frame efforts like Koop's effort very differently—as social enterprise, when a profit-seeking business is established to secure worthy ends. See, for example, Paul C. Light, "Social Entrepreneurship Revisited," the *Stanford Social Entrepreneurship Review*, Summer 2009.
68 *Tedium*, January 22, 2021. "Dr. Koop's Digital Korner." https://tedium.co/2021/01/22/c-everett-koop-drkoop-com-history/.
69 October 30, 2000. Wheaton CACE Archives. He did not however walk away empty-handed. The *Boston Globe* reported on April 19, 2000, that he managed to sell stock worth $1 million.
70 *New York Medical Quarterly* 6, no. 2 (1986), 80–82.
71 An apparently lone exception: While the final disposal of the case is unclear, Koop and another physician were sued for malpractice in the Superior Court of New Jersey by one Louise Brinson, on behalf of her infant son Donnell, on April 8, 1983. MSC 489 Box 74.
72 Well, as we saw in Chapter 3, as a young doctor Koop cared a great deal about money, or the lack of it!
73 *New York Medical Quarterly* 6, no. 2.

Part VI: PERSPECTIVE

1 We recount their courtship in the introduction to Part 1.
2 Kenneth Larter interview.
3 Kenneth Larter interview.
4 Confidential interview.
5 Koop to John McClenahan, June 15, 2005. MSC 489 Box 78 Cor.
6 Koop handwritten memo, page 7 alone in the file. MSC 489 Box 78 Cor.
7 Koop to John McClenahan.
8 Anne Koop interview.
9 Howard Filston interview. Koop and Filston shared a special bond. As we noted in Chapter 8, the Filstons too had lost a son (killed by a drunken driver).
10 Larter's first career had been as a nurse. Bailey had been hired as a carer for Betty and stayed on for a period as an aide.
11 Kenneth Larter interview.
12 Kenneth Larter interview.
13 Koop to John McClenahan.

14 Koop to Howard K. Koh, August 4, 2008. ACC 2015–11 Box 2. Sadly, there is no record of what they were!

15 Koop to Hillary Clinton, November 22, 2008. He goes on to propose—to the Secretary of State!—three potential candidates to be Surgeon General. ACC 2015–11 Box 2. Two years later, on his 93rd birthday, he received a call from President Obama, seeking his support for the Affordable Care Act ("Obamacare") then going through Congress. Koop declined. Lester Gibbs interview.

16 Michael DellaVecchia interview.

CHAPTER 18: The Long Diminuendo

1 Gibbs did not feel comfortable calling Koop "Chick" to his face. Though they became close, he could never quite forget that he was dealing with a Vice Admiral. So he called him Dr. Koop, and Koop called Gibbs Captain. His rank had actually been that of Sergeant Major. Lester Gibbs interview.

2 Lester Gibbs interview.

3 Koop organ dedication. Wrfnet.org no longer functioning March 2024. Koop served as lead donor in funding the organ purchase. Confidential interview.

4 Cora Koop interview.

5 The problem was solved by their switching to the same carrier, so they could "talk extensively but not expensively." Michael DellaVecchia interview.

6 *Valley News*, June 5, 2010.

7 Michael DellaVecchia interview. He was also treating Koop for eye ailments

8 Michael DellaVecchia interview.

9 Koop to Gauderer, March 6, 2007.

10 Rhoads in 1990 at the age of around 83, three years after his first wife's death. See https://en.wikipedia.org/wiki/Jonathan_Rhoads#cite_note-:%22a%22-2. Rickham's wife Elizabeth died in 1998. He remarried a year later at approximately 81.

11 Confidential interview.

12 Anne Koop interview. As she implies, it was not only the scheduling issues that kept the sons from the wedding. Moreover, a Koop friend shared with me that one of them actually called him to persuade him to stay away, which he did. Confidential interview.

13 Lester Gibbs interview.

14 Confidential interview.

15 Michael DellaVecchia interview.

16 Linda Boice, email August 4, 2023. The wedding ceremony is available on Vimeo: https://vimeo.com/11177661. Jeff Frazier, a friend of Koop's who was present at the reception, shared a memorable story. Koop rose and said, "I want to thank you all for coming." "There was a deafening silence in the room as at least I thought, and probably like others, that he was done. Then, and with head still bowed forward and into the microphone, which he put a little closer to his mouth, he said in classic C. Everett Koop style, and commandingly: 'Cora has never had something, and I'm gonna give it to her, tonight.' There was COMPLETE silence in the room." Frazier email April 15, 2021.

17 Linda Boice interview.

18 Michael DellaVecchia interview. One long-time Koop friend shared that he could not understand why Cora had agreed to the marriage. "It was basically a nursing job," he reflected. Confidential interview.

19 Confidential interview.

20 Woodie Kessel interview.

21 The dance and Henningfield's speech are on YouTube: https://www.youtube.com /watch?v=QN7LshKzHGw.

22 See Chapter 5.

23 Dotty Brown, "C. Everett Koop and a Choice between Lives," *The Schmooze* February 21, 2012. https://forward.com/schmooze/151687/c-everett-koop-and-a -choice-between-lives/.

24 Koop maintained subscriptions to the various local theater and musical offerings. Lester Gibbs email, March 2, 2024.

25 Joshua Drake interview. A precursor effort was named the David Foundation, "providing scholarships to Christian children," in process of establishment in late 2003, though its details are not clear. Lynn S. Carter to Koop, October 14, 2003; Koop to Allen Koop and Betty Koop, November 4, 2003. MSC 489 Box 78 Cor.

26 Lester Gibbs interview.

27 Michael DellaVecchia interview.

28 Lester Gibbs interview.

29 Kenneth Larter interview.

30 Jack Henningfield interview. Koop had been a keen collector since his teens. At this stage collections included Koop cartoons, walking canes, and orchids. And over one hundred bowties.

31 Christina Koop interview.

32 Memorial Service, April 6, 2013, at 29m: https://www.youtube.com/watch?v=FBm6x ZSmgro&t=9977s.

33 Joshua Drake interview. Drake told me that most of those Koop funded would write him a nice thank-you, whereas he decided to send updates from seminary every couple of months. The relationship deepened, and Koop and Cora were guests at the Drakes' wedding in 2011.

34 Harold O. J. Brown passed just ten days before Betty Koop. As we have noted, Brown was a keen climber; his cancer was first diagnosed a decade earlier, after a fall attributed to problems with his eyesight. Thereafter, he raffishly wore a black eye-patch.

35 Colin Duriez, *Francis Schaeffer: An Authentic Life* (Wheaton, IL: Crossway, 2008), 202, quoting Edith Schaeffer, *L'Abri Newsletter*, July 17, 1984.

36 *Christianity Today*, July 9, 2007: "Theologian Harold O.J. Brown dies at 74."

37 There is a brief Boice bio at: https://www.alliancenet.org/tab/about-dr-boice.

38 He also shares that the *Légion* process is highly political. He had the help of two highly placed friends when he first secured the honor for Koop. The upgrade effort unfortunately failed, since by then they were both dead. Carcassonne to Koop, March 8, 1996; Koop to Carcassonne, July 15, 1996. DA-698 Box 1273.

39 See Jean-Michel Guys, "Michel Carcassonne 1927–2001," *Journal of Pediatric Surgery*, 36, no.12 (December, 2001).

40 Zachary: Obituary, *The Independent*, March 18, 1999. Rickham: Obituary, London *Times*, December 1, 2003. Rhoads: https://almanac.upenn.edu/archive/v48/n17 /Rhoads.html.

41 Rhoads' obituary of Ravdin, *Surgery*, 127, no. 5 (2000), and Royal College of Surgeons, Plarr's Lives of the Fellows: https://livesonline.rcseng.ac.uk/client/en_GB/lives.

42 When we spoke, Johnson said he regretted that the original footage of their encounter was no longer available since he believed their lively discussion crystalized the issue. Timothy Johnson interview. During the interview, they discovered they were slated

to attend the same dinner that evening, and Koop suggested Johnson join him in his official car. Once dinner was over, Koop invited him back to his home on the NIH campus, where Johnson told me they didn't get to bed until "the wee hours." In Koop's later years, Johnson told me, he made a point of visiting him in Hanover around once a quarter, less often after his marriage. Timothy Johnson interview. Later, they wrote a book together: *Let's Talk. An Honest Conversation on Critical Issues: Abortion, Euthanasia, AIDS, Health Care.* (Grand Rapids: Zondervan, 1992).

43 Woodie Kessel interview.

44 Woodie Kessel interview.

45 Koop to Larter, June 17, 1993. DA-698 Box 1965.

46 Kenneth Larter interview.

47 Michael Fiore interview.

48 National Memorial Service, April 6, 2013, at 2h 19m: https://www.youtube.com/watch?v=FBm6xZSmgro&t=9977s.

49 Larter, homily.

50 Larter, homily.

51 Larter, homily. He leaves it open whether Koop was referring to his late father, whom he had often called his best friend, or his God.

52 Linda Boice interview.

53 A private family funeral followed at First Congregational Church of Woodstock, Vermont, of which son Norman was pastor. Koop was interred in Hanover's Pine Knoll cemetery, near the graves of Betty and their son David. Koop's gravestone reads: "C. Everett Koop, 1916–2013. 'For I am not ashamed of the gospel, for it is the power of God for salvation to everyone who believes, to the Jew first and also to the Greek.' Romans 1:16." The text is from the New American Standard Bible. Gibbs was asked to stay on in the house as it was prepared for sale, and departed eventually in May of 2014. Lester Gibbs interview.

CHAPTER 19: A Life

1 Paul Murray Kendall, *The Art of Biography* (New York: Norton, 1965, repr. 1985), xiii. We note the convention, still widely accepted in the 1960s, of using generic "man" to refer to both men and women.

2 Kendall, *The Art of Biography*, 14–15.

3 Michael Gauderer and Moritz Ziegler, "Charles Everett Koop MD, DSc October 16, 1916–February 25, 2013," *Journal of Pediatric Surgery* 48, no. 6 (2013).

4 Arias, "C. Everett Koop."

5 Quoted in "Doctor, Not Chaplain: How a Deeply Religious Surgeon General Taught a Nation About HIV," *Atlantic*, March, 2013.

6 "C. Everett Koop, the Nation's Doctor," *Washington Post*, March 4, 2013.

7 *New York Times*, April 8, 2023.

8 Confidential interview.

9 Michael Horton interview.

10 Philip Yancey, *Sole Survivor* (New York: Penguin Random House, 2003), 179.

11 James T. Bennett and Thomas J. DiLorenzo, *Public Health Profiteering* (New York: Routledge, 2001).

12 Quoted in the *Washington Post*, May 24, 1987.

13 Heininger/Koop, 37.

14 His friend Harold O. J. Brown was critical of his time in office, though the same logic rears its head in Brown's reported statement that he would hand out condoms in Virginia's high schools if doing so would prevent pregnancies and thereby abortions. Robert Case interview, quoted in Chapter 6.

15 Koop to George Anders, November 13, 1996. DA-698 Box 1273.

16 Confidential interview.

17 Confidential interview.

18 Quoted variously, for example: https://www.ft.com/content/2f8ee5f4-e66a-11e7-a685 -5634466a6915.

19 Joshua Nelson interview.

20 Confidential interview.

21 Koop to Waxman, October 5, 1988. MSC 489 Box 87 Cor. And confidential interview.

22 Holcomb B. Noble, "E-MEDICINE—A special report. Hailed as a Surgeon General, Koop Is Faulted on Web Ethics," *New York Times*, September 5, 1999. The biblical quotation is from the King James (Authorized) Version of Proverbs, chapter 15, verse 1. The verse reads in full: "A soft answer turneth away wrath: but grievous words stir up anger."

23 "The Ins and Outs of 1999," *Boston Globe*, December 30, 1999.

24 E.g., John Schwartz, "The Fox in 'Chick' Koop," *Washington Post*, January 9, 2000.

25 Confidential interview.

26 Koop to James E. Eckenhoff, February 8, 1956. ACC 2014–016 Box 24/33.

27 Woodie Kessel interview.

28 Edward Martin interview.

29 Confidential interview.

30 David Serra interview.

31 Schwartz, "The Fox in 'Chick' Koop."

32 Schwartz, "The Fox in 'Chick' Koop."

33 *Newsweek* May 23, 1989.

34 Woodie Kessel interview.

35 *US News and World Report*, May 30, 1988.

36 Quipped fall, 1986; the author was present. Among many favorites, Koop loved omelets, Diet Coke, shrimp cocktails, and Fisherman's Friend (extra strong mints). Conversation with the author. He was also partial to a finnan haddie, an originally Scottish smoked haddock dish made famous in Cole Porter's song, "I belong to daddy." Edward Grant interview.

37 Woodie Kessel interview.

38 Highsmith: from conversation with the author. And: Koop to Waxman, October 5, 1988. MSC 489 Box 87 Cor.

39 Autobiographical sketch, Freshman English, between October 1933 and March 1934. ACC 2017–018 Box 1/3.

40 "The Early Days of AIDS, as I Remember Them," *Annals of the Forum for Collaborative HIV Research*, 13, no. 2 (March 2011), 9.

REFERENCES

Interviews

All interviews with me were conducted between 2020 and 2024. In certain cases, as indicated, an interview, or part of one, was conducted "on background"—that is, on condition that the interviewee's name be withheld. Minor edits have been made for clarity.

Archival resources

Koop's long and industrious life generated a substantial quantity of archival material, and to the inconvenience of the researcher it is distributed around several collections. Thanks are due to various librarians and archivists for aiding me in a research process that was made yet more complex by the vicissitudes of the Covid pandemic. I'm listing below archives and oral materials, beginning in each case with abbreviations or short titles I have employed in relevant footnotes and endnotes. Let me add my special appreciation for "oral history" interviews, both of Koop and various of his collaborators, that have preserved voices and memories otherwise lost.

Archives
Dartmouth, DA, ACC, DB, CE: *Dartmouth College, Rauner Special Collections Library*
HML: *Historical Medical Library, College of Physicians, Philadelphia*
NLM, Box AB Cor., MSC: *National Library of Medicine, Bethesda*

Penn: *University of Pennsylvania Archives*

PHS: *Presbyterian Historical Society, Philadelphia*

Trinity Henry Archive: *Trinity International University, Deerfield, Illinois.*

Wheaton: *Wheaton College Library, Special Collections; Center for Applied Christian Ethics (CACE), Wheaton College, Illinois*

Oral History Interviews and Similar

Ehrhart/Bishop: Mindy Ehrhart interview with Harry Bishop about Louise Schnaufer. https://collections.countway.harvard.edu/onview /items/show/13408.

Ehrhart/Koop: Mindy Ehrhart interview with Koop about Louise Schnaufer. https://collections.countway.harvard.edu/onview/exhibits /show/fhwim-oral-histories/item/13412.

Ehrhart/Melhuish: Mindy Ehrhart interviews Melhuish about Louise Schnaufer. https://www.digitalcommonwealth.org/search/common wealth-oai:fq978r3of.

Ehrhart/O'Neill: Mindy Ehrhart interview with James O'Neill about Louise Schnaufer. https://www.digitalcommonwealth.org/search /commonwealth-oai:fq978r31q.

Ehrhart/Taylor: Mindy Ehrhart interview with Lesli Ann Taylor about Louise Schnaufer. https://collections.countway.harvard.edu/onview /exhibits/show/fhwim-oral-histories/item/13416.

Ehrhart/Ziegler: Mindy Ehrhart interview with Ziegler about Louise Schnaufer. https://collections.countway.harvard.edu/onview/index .php/items/show/13419.

Grosfield/Beardmore: Jay L. Grosfield interview with Harvey Beard-more. https://downloads.aap.org/AAP/Gartner%20Pediatric%20 History/Beardmore.pdf.

Heininger/Koop: Janet Heininger interview with Koop about Edward Kennedy. The Miller Center has not yet opened this interview to the public, but Koop lodged a copy in the public domain. MSC 607 AIDS Cor. 1982–1990 Box 6/10. https://millercenter.org/the -presidency/presidential-oral-histories/c-everett-koop-oral-history.

Heskel/Koop: Children's Hospital History Project, interview by Julia Heskel, November 22, 2002. ACC 2015–011 Koop Papers 1942–2009. Box 2/4

Holcomb/O'Neill: George W. Holcomb III, interview with James O'Neill, Koop's successor at the Children's Hospital. https://downloads .aap.org/AAP/Gartner%20Pediatric%20History/ONeill.pdf.

Knott/Sullivan: Stephen Knott et al. interview with Louis Sullivan.

Emphases original. https://millercenter.org/the-presidency/presiden
tial-oral-histories/dr-louis-sullivan-oral-history.

McComb/Stewart: David G. McComb, interview with Surgeon General
William H. Stewart. https://www.discoverlbj.org/item/oh-stewartw
-19681202-1-74-44.

Mullan/Koop: Fitzhugh Mullan interview with Koop. https://profiles.
nlm.nih.gov/spotlight/qq/catalog/nlm:nlmuid-101584930X1101-doc.

Mullan/Martin: Fitzhugh Mullan interview with Edward Martin. NLM
Box 144 F33 39,40.

Smith/Brandt: David Smith interview with Edward Brandt. https://
www.cms.gov/files/document/cmsoralhistorypdf.

Williams/Fauci: Brien Williams interview with Anthony Fauci. https://
www.aai.org/AAISite/media/About/History/OHP/Transcripts/Trans
-Inv-034_Fauci_Anthony_S-2015_Final.pdf.

Yancey/Koop: Courtesy of Philip Yancey, Yancey interview with Koop.
Copy of Koop/Yancey papers with the author.

Jim Young, et. al: Interview with Otis Bowen. https://millercen
ter.org/the-presidency/presidential-oral-histories/otis-bowen-md
-oral-history.

Ravdin, Reminiscences: Reminiscences of I.S. Ravdin, at Columbia
University. https://oralhistoryportal.library.columbia.edu/document
.php?id=ldpd_4072868.

Ziegler/Koop: Moritz Ziegler interview with Koop. https://downloads
.aap.org/AAP/Gartner%20Pediatric%20History/Koop.pdf.

Books by C. Everett Koop

Visible and Palpable Lesions in Children (Grune & Sratton, 1976).

The Right to Live; the Right to Die (Tyndale House Publishers, Inc.,
1976).

*Whatever Happened to the Human Race?: Exposing our Rapid Yet
Subtle Loss of Human Rights* (Francis A. Schaeffer and C. Everett
Koop, MD, F. H. Revel Co., 1979).

Sometimes Mountains Move (with Elizabeth Koop, Tyndale House
Publishers, Inc. 1979).

Koop: The Memoirs of America's Family Doctor (Random House, 1991).

*Let's Talk: An Honest Conversation on Critical Issues, Abortion,
AIDS, Euthanasia, Health Care* (with Timothy Johnson, MD,
Zondervan, 1992).

INDEX

Orangutan patient, Chickie, 107–8
Organ dedication, David and Elizabeth Koop Memorial organ, 34
Organ Procurement Workshop, 168
Owens, Walter, Baby Doe's obstetrician, 172–75

Panem, Sandra, 203, 383n16
Papadopoulos, Maria, Koop colleague, 99–100
Partners in Health, Koop Institute initiative, 285–86
Parvin, Landon, Reagan speechwriter, 215–19
Pasquariello, Patrick, Koop colleague, 29
Pearl Harbor, 51–52
Pediatric Intensive Care Unit. *See* NICU
Pediatric surgeons, full-time, 356n7
Pediatric surgery, name of the specialty, 72–73, 111, 355n47; specialisms at the Children's Hospital, 364n159
Pediatrics (journal), 69
Penicillin, 43
Penner Lecture (Wheaton College, IL), 262
Pennsylvania Hospital, 50
PEPFAR, President's Emergency Plan for AIDS Relief, 328
Pepper Commission, 397n82
Personal Medical Records Inc., 297
Philadelphia College of Osteopathic Medicine, Koop commencement speech, 128–29
Philadelphia General Hospital, 50
Philadelphia Inquirer, 33
Philadelphia Zoo, 108
Philadelphia's skid row, 22, 338
Philip Morris, 144, 194; on Koop's impact, 195
PICU (Pediatric Intensive Care Unit) 102. *See also* NICU
Picuris, Indian tribe, 161
Pipes, Ralph, Koop trainee, 51
Planned Parenthood, 129
Plath, Sylvia, poet, 351n22
Pneumocystis pneumonia, 198
Pollack, Shepard, president, Philip Morris, and Koop patient father, 144
Pornography and Public Health Workshop, 168
Potomac Restaurant, 217

Potts, Willis J. (1895–1968), Koop friend, 66–67, 76; vascular clamp, 67; antisemitism, 67
Presidential Commission on HIV, Watkins Commission, 206, 213–15
Presidential Medal of Freedom, 365n168
PriceWaterhouseCoopers, accountants to DrKoop.com, 299
Prisons, Koop concern for AIDS spread, 198–99
Professionalization of pediatric surgery, 109–11
Prohibition, 15
Pro-life movement, evangelical, launched by Koop, 118. *See also*, Koop, C. Everett, support and criticism of the pro-life movement

Quinn, Father Luis, 104–5

racism, at the Children's Hospital, 56, 338
Randolph, Judson, 59, 71
Rappaport, Milton, 87–88
Ravdin, I.S. (1894–1972), surgeon and Koop's chairman at the University of Pennsylvania, 35–36, 43, 52–62, 68, 70, 74, 76–77, 111; Brigadier General, 53; Columbia memoir, 81–82; concern about Koop fees, 79; death, 317; and Goulding, 95; importance as a surgeon, 353n7; importance of grand rounds, 79, 80; irascibility, 78; I.S. Ravdin Institute, 79, 80; and Koop, 78–82; Koop effort to get him a Dartmouth degree, 250, 392n43; Koop recruitment, 49–50; and married staff, 353n9; opening editorial, *Journal of Pediatric Surgery*, 82; Ravdin/Koop relationship, 95, 358n21, 369n1; spelling of first name, 70, 353n12; use of nickname Rav, 355n51; and women trainees, 88
Ravitch, Mark. M., 68; and pediatric surgery as a hobby, 72
Ray family with hemophiliac kids, firebombed in Florida, 201
Reader's Digest, 25, and "What I Tell the Parents of a Dying Child," 100; early cancer report, 190
Reagan, First Lady Nancy, 202, 215–19; role in AIDS speech, 215

NIGEL CAMERON is a graduate of Cambridge and Edinburgh universities. His most recent academic appointments have been as Research Professor of Bioethics at the Illinois Institute of Technology, and Fulbright Visiting Research Chair in Science and Society at the University of Ottawa. For a decade, he directed a Washington, DC think tank on technology policy. He has published on ethics, religion, and history, including as lead editor for a collection of essays on the societal impact of nanotechnology, and for a million-word encyclopedia of the history of religion in his native Scotland.

Cameron has served on US diplomatic delegations to the United Nations and UNESCO, and was a US Government nominee for UN Special Rapporteur for the Right to Health. He served four terms on the US National Commission for UNESCO, and was chair of its Committee on Social and Human Sciences.

He and his wife Anna divide their time between homes in Belgium and France.

Printed and bound by CPI Group (UK) Ltd, Croydon, CR0 4YY

28/04/2025

14662974-0003